TEACHING THE PRACTICE OF NURSING

Teaching the practice of nursing

Second edition

J M Mellish
DN BA MCur(Ed) MCur(Admin) DCur RGN RM RCN RNA RNE
Emeritus Professor of Nursing Science
University of Port Elizabeth

In consultation with and with contributions from
Hilla Brink
DN DNA BAHon(Psych) MACur DLitt et Phil RGN RM RCN
Professor of Nursing Science
University of South Africa

BUTTERWORTHS
Durban

© 1982
Butterworth Publishers (Pty) Ltd
Reg No 70/02642/07

First edition 1982
Reprint 1985
Second edition 1986

ISBN: 0 409 11146 5

The Butterworth Group

South Africa
Butterworth Publishers (Pty) Ltd
8 Walter Place, Waterval Park, Mayville, Durban 4091

England
Butterworth & Co (Publishers) Ltd
88 Kingsway, London WC2B 6AB

Australia
Butterworths (Pty) Ltd
271 – 273 Lane Cove Road, North Ryde NSW 2113

Canada
Butterworths – A Division of Reed Inc
2265 Midland Avenue, Scarborough, Ontario MIP 4S1

New Zealand
Butterworths of New Zealand Ltd
205 – 207 Victoria Street, Wellington

USA
Butterworths (Publishers) Inc
80 Montvale Avenue, Stoneham MA 02180

Asia
Butterworth & Co (Asia) (Pte) Ltd
30 Robinson Road, Unit 12-01 Tuan Sing Towers,
Singapore 0104

Printed and bound by Interpak Natal

This second edition brings the text in line with changes in the pattern of training and education of nurses in the Republic of South Africa. It also presents additional material on andragogy and discusses several additional teaching techniques.

The South African Nursing Council also lays down that study for the student nurse means involvement at the cognitive, psychomotor and affective levels, and that these skills should be developed within the clinical situation while the student is being trained.

The participation of the student as a member of the nursing team, as well as of the multidisciplinary team in the clinical situation, is indispensable for the development of the student into a mature, professional practitioner.

Policy of SANA regarding basic training of nurses and midwives for registration (1986)

The policy of the South African Nursing Association is that –

- The basic training of nurses and midwives for registration with the South African Nursing Council forms part of the post-secondary education system in the Republic of South Africa.
- The financing of nursing education should be done on a national basis in order that available funds can best be utilised and that a separate budget is available that will not be influenced by changes in the health services.
- The student corps should not be seen as work force, but student status should be accentuated and bursaries be awarded that are adequate to stimulate the training of sufficient nursing manpower for the Republic of South Africa.
- The student is expected to contribute financially towards her training.
- Simulation can never replace learning experiences in the practical situation, although it can be used to develop skills in the teaching situation.
- Clinical instruction is an integral part of the total curriculum and is aimed at achieving specific goals. It is therefore essential that the teaching staff be involved in both the presentation of theory and clinical practica. It is further essential that registered nurses and midwives in training hospitals should be active members of the teaching team and that the staff establishments should provide for the optimal guidance and support of the student.
- Learning situations should be purposefully used in clinical practice in order to attain specific teaching goals, and these goals and the accompanying evaluation criteria should be explained to the student at the outset.
- An atmosphere conducive to training should be deliberately created in the practical situation. Professional nurses and midwives should be encouraged to develop a positive attitude towards training and towards the students themselves.

ADDENDUM

to

Teaching the Practice of Nursing 2nd ed.

J M Mellish   H Brink

Butterworth Publishers (Pty) Ltd 1986. ISBN 0 409 111465

See pages 72 – 74:

Statements on pages 72 – 74 regarding the training of nurses and midwives for registration have been superseded by:

POLICY STATEMENT OF THE CENTRAL BOARD OF THE SOUTH AFRICAN NURSING ASSOCIATION 1986

BASIC TRAINING OF NURSES AND MIDWIVES FOR REGISTRATION

Introduction

The principles of a comprehensive health service, and its availability to the entire population, underlie the whole health care system and health legislation in the Republic of South Africa.

The nurse, by virtue of her availability and her comprehensive training that prepares her for providing a comprehensive service, is recognised as an indispensable part of the health care manpower in the Republic of South Africa.

As a statutory body, the South African Nursing Council is empowered in terms of the Nursing Act, 1978 (Act 50 of 1978), *inter alia* to prescribe minimum standards for the training of nurses and midwives and to approve training schools.

The South African Nursing Council has determined that, in future, nurses and midwives at diploma level will only be trained at nursing colleges in co-operation with universities, and those at degree level only at universities that have a department of nursing.

The aim of training nurses and midwives is to produce informed, critically thinking, skilled and creative professional persons, who can act and take decisions independently within their nursing frame of reference. It therefore aims to promote the personal as well as the professional development of the individual.

Contents

1 Nursing, nursing education and the philosophy of nursing

In a book dealing with teaching the practice of nursing, the concept of nursing must surely be defined before the didactics relating to it can be discussed.

1.1 NURSING

This has been defined in many ways, by many people, depending on their orientation, personal philosophy and experience. The word has also gained many connotations throughout the long history of the English language, so that 'nursing' can be used to denote the action of one who suckles a baby, as a 'nursing' mother; for 'tending' animals or plants; in the sense of 'protecting or cherishing', as in 'nursing' a plant to maturity until it reaches a state of blooming. It can even be used in speaking of business matters where statements such as 'nursing' an ailing economy are not unusual, and in general terms – expressions such as 'nursing' a grievance are common.

The origin of the word is from the Old French *norrice* (French *nourrice*), Latin *nutrix, nutricius, nutrire,* to nourish, while a list of the meanings of the verb 'to nurse' include:

- to suckle
- to tend, as an infant or sick person
- to bring up
- to cherish
- to manage with skill and economy
- to play skilfully, manipulate carefully, keep watchfully in touch with, in order to obtain or preserve the desired condition
- to hold or carry *(Chambers Twentieth Century Dictionary)*.

To these *The Concise Oxford Dictionary* adds the following:

- to foster, tend or promote the development of
- to try to cure
- to wait upon a sick person
- to manage with solicitude
- to hold or clasp (baby, one's knee or foot) caressingly.

How many of these meanings can be applied to the profession, that is to the art and science of modern nursing?

- *To suckle* in the form of direct 'breast'-feeding or *giving suck to*, hardly applies. Perhaps artificial feeding by means of a bottle which the baby sucks in order to obtain nourishment is an extension of *suckling*, but this is a somewhat remote connection that can only be applied if one stretches one's imagination to the full.

- *To tend, as an infant or sick person,* certainly applies, for *to tend* means *to take care of, or look after,* and nursing definitely involves tending.

- *To bring up* relates more to the field of the parent and the teacher. Nursing is only involved inasmuch as health education is given to mothers so that they may bring up their children more effectively. Nurses, as part of their nursing activities, also give health education to pre-school and school children. When children are entrusted to nursing care for long periods of time, the bringing-up element enters the field of nursing.

- *To cherish* means to tend with affection, to promote the growth of. This is certainly a function of nursing. Thus nursing involves cherishing.

- *To manage with skill and economy:* At first sight this phrase may appear irrelevant, but the nurse, in tending the patient or the client, has to manage both human and material resources, that is personnel and equipment, medications, etc, with *skill and economy* in order to personally give or ensure that the best possible treatment and care are given to those persons entrusted to her care. The unit (or ward) professional nurse and many others engaged in nursing manage patient care, equipment, personnel and other resources with skill and economy.

- *To play skilfully, manipulate carefully, keep watchfully in touch with, in order to obtain or preserve the desired condition:* The *desired condition* in nursing is the optimum state of health for the patient or client. To *obtain* or *preserve* this health requires skilled and careful *manipulation* of the environment, the persons available and the other resources to promote good health and prevent ill-health. In order to do this the nurse *keeps watchfully in touch with* the patient's condition, needs and treatment plan, as well as with all the new developments in the medical and nursing fields. Thus nursing also fulfils this definition.

- *To hold or carry:* In supporting those whose state of health makes it impossible for them to manage on their own, nursing holds and helps to carry where necessary. In the care of the young this is self-evident, but it also applies at various times and to different degrees. Thus nursing involves holding or carrying.

- *To foster, tend or promote the development of:* The first two concepts have already been discussed, while the last one, *promote the development of,* can be readily understood. A midwife aims at promoting the development of a healthy baby and a healthy mother; child health care is directed at the same *promotion of development* as are the *school health* services. The examples are endless. Thus nursing is involved in promoting the development of healthy people.

- *To try to cure* needs no explanation. Nursing is involved in trying to cure. It actually goes further, for if cure is impossible, nursing sustains and supports people to make the most of what is still left to them.
- *To wait upon a sick person* is so obviously part of nursing that it needs little discussion. It is, however, 'waiting upon' with a definite purpose, that is to help the person who is sick to regain health, or where possible, to regain his ability to cater for his own needs.
- *To manage with solicitude* adds a dimension of caring to the previous *management with skill and economy*. Such solicitude is a vital part of nursing.
- *To hold or clasp* has really been dealt with under *to hold or carry*.

What has emerged so far? Nursing involves:

- *Tending* infants and sick people
- *Cherishing* those in need of it
- *Managing* with skill, economy and solicitude, the nursing care of patients and clients
- *Playing skilfully* and *manipulating carefully* the environment and all available resources in order to provide nursing treatment and care both preventive and promotive, curative, rehabilitative and terminal, as well as keeping *watchfully in touch* with the patient's condition and needs as well as with new developments in the nursing and medical fields
- *Holding, carrying or clasping* in the literal as well as the figurative sense by giving psychological and physical support to patients, clients and their families or friends
- *Fostering, tending* or *promoting the development* of health and healthy people
- *Trying* or assisting to cure
- *Waiting upon sick people* in order to ultimately place them in a position to provide for their own needs where at all possible. Where this is not possible, nurses wait upon sick people as long as is necessary, that is until life itself ceases.

It will be seen that beyond the tending, cherishing, fostering and waiting upon sick people some other points have emerged – the first is *skill,* that is to manage with *skill*; the next is *management;* the third is the *solicitude* or *caring* underlying the nursing act, while *knowledge* is needed in *trying to cure*, in *keeping watchfully* in touch with, and *promoting the development of* as well as being essential to the development of skill.

3

(a) Let us first consider *knowledge*. The art and science of nursing is based on knowledge derived from the *natural and biological sciences* as well as the *human sciences*. Therefore nursing has a scientific foundation. Skills which are purely automatic or technical, and not based on scientific knowledge, do not form part of the art and science of modern professional nursing. They are only accessory to it.

(b) *Management* is perhaps one of the least thought about, talked about and understood facets of nursing, but one that occurs all the time. To *manage* means to *control, take charge of* or *conduct*. If we apply this to the provision of health care, it is the nurse, by virtue of the availability of nursing service on a 24–hour basis 365 days of the year for those who need it, who ensures that health care is given, *health care,* and not only *nursing* care. The nurse is *the* co-ordinator of the whole gamut of health services which the patient may need. The unit or ward 'sister' (professional nurse) co-ordinates cleaning services, the provision of a safe environment, the physical care of the patient in respect of his hygiene, feeding requirements, and even recreation. She co-ordinates the care given by paramedical personnel and social workers, the patient's rest periods and his visitors, such as relatives, the pastor, minister or priest, lawyers, insurance agents, etc. Whenever necessary, she calls in medical help over and above routine visits.

One could continue endlessly in this vein. The nurse caring for one patient in a private home also has a management function and though it is more limited than that of a unit 'sister', it is nonetheless important.

(c) *Solicitude* is based on respect for the person who needs nursing care, be it preventive or promotive, curative, rehabilitative or terminal, as a person, a human being with human needs, and with emotional needs as well as purely physical ones. In order to care for people, knowledge of the human sciences is essential. Nursing thus has a very *human* component.

From all this it will be clear that arriving at an easy definition of nursing is difficult if not impossible, because nursing has so many facets. Perhaps the following would encompass most of these.

Nursing is an art and science directed at providing a human health-care service which is based on *scientific principles*. It requires *knowledge* derived from the *biological* and *natural* as well as the *human sciences* in order to apply *personalised treatment and care, of a highly skilled nature, to people and their families* who are exposed to, or may be suffering from *physical or mental ill-health*. This treatment must be given with *care and concern*. It covers *personalised care from before birth until death* at, hopefully, *a ripe old age*. It is concerned with solicitous care, with the *quality of life* and the *human dignity* of those needing care.

Nursing co-ordinates and manages health care. It applies the nursing process of assessment, planning, implementation, evaluation and record-keeping to the promotive, preventive, curative and rehabilitative, long-term and terminal aspects of the total health care of people, so that they may, whenever possible, attain and maintain good health. Where this is impossible, nursing provides and co-ordinates the care given by others so as to enable the person receiving that care to make the maximum use of his remaining potential and, in the terminal stages of life, to die in peace and with dignity.

This definition combines the practicalities of nursing with an underlying philosophy, namely that it is people, as individuals, who count and that all the knowledge and skill (based on science) that are required to give nursing care are directed at one goal – the care of people, to prevent illness, to promote health and to treat ill-health where necessary. The care of people is the fundamental aspect on which everything else is based to form a picture of the whole that is nursing.

In reading literature on the subject, students will come across many points of view. People have said that nursing is an art and a science, with some believing that the art takes precedence over the science and vice versa. The growth of interest in the application of the nursing process with its facets of *assessment, planning, implementation, evaluation* and *recording* to the practice of nursing has, perhaps, served to highlight the *scientific* aspect of nursing, for the nursing process as such is based on the methods of science. It is important that everyone engaged in teaching the practice of nursing should not lose sight of the basic concern of all nursing, that is the person needing nursing care. Without this person, be he patient or client, no nursing would be necessary. A salutary thought when one is confronted with an inflated ego situation where the convenience of doctors, nurses, paramedics and even domestic personnel is paramount, and that of the patient receives scant attention.

A method is not an *end* in itself, it is only a means to that end. Nursing is practised for the benefit of human beings in need of the care of nurses. The art must not be lost in the science, the science must complement the art; the two need to be wed into a working, understanding partnership.

The South African Nursing Council has recently defined nursing as follows:

> Nursing Science is a human clinical science that constitutes the body of knowledge for practice of persons registered or enrolled under the Nursing Act, as nurses or midwives. Within the parameters of nursing philosophy and ethics it is concerned with the development of knowledge for the nursing diagnosis, treatment and personalised health care of persons exposed to or suffering or recovering from physical or mental ill-health.

5

Professional nursing is practised by independent practitioners whose field of work is health care. Nursing is aimed at total health and not only the care of the sick. Nurses give care to people, well or ill, to promote as complete a state of health as is possible for each individual.

Nursing, in its pride in its own profession, must not be afraid of making use of other disciplines. Today a multidisciplinary approach to health care is essential.

The biological, psychological, sociological and spiritual dimensions of the human being must all be part of the study of nursing care and nursing courses must be structured so as to comprise these dimensions in the correct relationship to one another.

The science of nursing, like all sciences, must take from others that which has relevance, and synthesise what it needs into a meaningful, organised, stable whole, which is applied with skill to the art of nursing, so that an art and a science can truly be said to exist. It must be focused on the *human being* for whom the profession of nursing exists. The form and content of what is taught must be ordered and related to all the dimensions of the human being. If this is clearly understood, then the design of nursing curricula and the planning of nursing education programmes will be so broadly based that the student will be able to function, at the end of her basic period of education, as a competent, understanding, self-organising practitioner of nursing. She will have a firm knowledge of the needs of her patients, both physical, psychological, spiritual and social, an ability to assess priorities and act upon her assessments, and a dedication to keeping her professional knowledge and skills at optimum level so that excellent health care can result.

1.2 NURSING EDUCATION

Nursing education is designed to prepare students to give nursing care of a high standard which meets all the above criteria.

Education, from the Latin *e* (= from) and *ducere* (= to lead), may be considered to be the leading of someone from the known to the unknown. It implies giving guidance, providing opportunities and facilities for learning, and giving assistance to those studying. *Learning* as such can only be done by the *learner*. *Nursing education* is the method by which students are guided, assisted and provided with means which enable them to learn the art and science of nursing so that they can apply it to the nursing care of people in need of such care.

When students join the profession as neophytes, one may assume that they know nothing, or at most very little about nursing. They must therefore be guided along the path of knowledge to the stage where they can assume responsibility for their nursing actions; thus until they attain professional adulthood. After attaining this stage they must be ready to accept responsibility for the continuous learning which is part of their professional practice.

The meaning of nursing, education and nursing education has now been examined. Nursing education has only one aim – the production of a skilled practitioner of nursing. In teaching the practice of nursing the level of the practitioner to be prepared will, of course, play a part.

The practice of nursing makes provision for various categories of nurses to provide the necessary care of the patient, and each of these will be dealt with. However, it must be borne in mind that there are many areas of practice where the different categories perform similar functions and that similar education is thus necessary.

The ultimate goal in nursing education is the production of a highly skilled *professional* practitioner at the first level, which is that of *registered nurses*.

Professionalism has been adequately discussed in other works, and it suffices to recapitulate the characteristics of a professional person; in this case, a professional nurse. She has been prepared over a long period of time, by a specialised form of education at a recognised education institution and her licensure to practise follows on examination before being registered with the approved registered body. In the case of the Republic of South Africa, this body is the South African Nursing Council. She is a member of a professional organisation, the South African Nursing Association.

The specialised theory which is part of her education is based on the natural and biological sciences and other learning disciplines which are relevant to her field of study. The well-developed technical skills which she must acquire are founded on this theory.

The South African Nursing Council, which licenses her to practise, determines professional standards and the ethical control of professional conduct rests with this body.

The work of the professional nurse is based on the motive of service, the welfare of the patient or client being the overriding consideration. There is a high degree of accountability inherent in her work.

The profession of nursing involves a feeling of exclusiveness, and has a recognised status in law. It also enjoys a high social status and has considerable social power.

The profession itself determines the subjects to be studied in order to prepare a competent practitioner, and the activities of the profession are subject to constant critical analysis by its members. The aims set are in accordance with what can be realistically attained by members of the profession.

The individual professional nurse has independent functions for which she is accountable. She has the power of exercising not only discretion, but also initiative. She is expected, at all times, to use all her abilities and endeavours for the benefit of clients and she must continually strive for excellence; competence is not enough.

It is thus obvious that those entrusted with the preparation of the professional nurse must be fully cognisant of what aims to strive for, what the set criteria are, and what the end product of the education must be.

The professional nurse in embryo is being prepared to function in many areas, for instance in the general hospital ward, the specialised unit, the outpatient department or detached clinic, the community, the work situation, and private homes, to name but a few.

The preparation of such a professional person entails a great deal of responsibility, and needs constant thought and endeavour to make a success of a dynamic work situation.

The next category of nurse who has to be prepared is the *semi-professional or enrolled nurse*. Here the guide-lines laid down by the South African Nursing Council are of value. A further category is that of the *enrolled nursing assistant*. By considering the regulations regarding the practice of all three categories as laid down by the South African Nursing Council, clarification of their roles, and thus of the preparation needed to fill these roles, is obtained.

1.2.1 The scope of practice of registered nurses

The scope of practice of a registered nurse shall entail the following acts or procedures, which may be performed by scientifically based physical, chemical, psychological, social, educational and technological means applicable to health-care practice:

- diagnosing a health need and prescribing, providing and executing a nursing regimen to meet the needs of a patient or group of patients or, where necessary, referring the patient to a registered person
- executing a programme of treatment or medication prescribed for a patient by a registered person
- the treatment and care of and the administration of medicine to a patient, including the monitering of the patient's vital signs and of his reaction to disease conditions, trauma, stress, anxiety, medication and treatment
- preventing disease and promoting health and family planning by teaching and counselling individuals and groups
- prescribing, promoting or maintaining hygiene, physical comfort and reassurance of the patient
- promoting exercise, rest and sleep with a view to the healing and rehabilitation of a patient

- facilitating body mechanics and preventing bodily deformities in a patient in the execution of the nursing regimen
- supervising and maintaining a supply of oxygen to a patient
- supervising and maintaining the fluid, electrolyte and acid base balance of a patient
- facilitating the healing of wounds and fractures, protecting the skin and maintaining sensory functions in a patient
- facilitating the maintenance of bodily regulatory mechanisms and functions in a patient
- facilitating the maintenance of nutrition of a patient
- supervising and maintaining elimination by a patient
- facilitating communication by and with a patient in the execution of the nursing regimen
- facilitating the attainment of optimum health for the individual, the family, groups and the community in the execution of the nursing regimen
- establishing and maintaining, in the execution of the nursing regimen, an environment in which the physical and mental health of a patient is promoted
- preparing for and assisting with operative, diagnostic and therapeutic acts for the patient
- co-ordinating the health-care regimens provided for the patient by other categories of health personnel
- providing effective patient advocacy to enable the patient to obtain the health care he needs
- caring for a dying patient and a recently deceased patient within the execution of the nursing regimen. (SANC Reg no R2598 30 November 1984.)

1.2.2 The scope of practice of the enrolled nurse

This should state that the scope of practice of an enrolled nurse encompasses certain acts and procedures which have been planned and initiated by a registered nurse or registered midwife, and which are carried out under her direct or indirect supervision as part of the nursing regimen.

- carrying out nursing care to fulfil the needs of a patient or a group of patients
- caring for a patient and *executing* a programme of treatment for a patient, including the monitoring of vital signs and the observation of reactions to medication and treatment. The enrolled nurse executes (carries out), but does not plan or initiate the patient's programme of treatment and care

- preventing disease and promoting health and family planning by means of providing information to individuals and groups.
- maintaining hygiene and physical comfort and reassuring the patient
- promoting exercise, rest and sleep with a view to healing and rehabilitating a patient
- preventing physical deformity to a patient in the execution of nursing care
- maintaining a supply of oxygen to the body cells of a patient. The enrolled nurse is not expected to know the actions and treatment necessary to promote the physiological and anatomical basis for effective oxygenation of the body systems. However, such essentially practical aspects as maintaining clear airways, positioning patients to improve breathing, resuscitation in the event of drowning or cardiac arrest, exercise to improve oxygen intake and the administration of oxygen by mechanical means fall within her scope of practice, and she must be adept at identifying the need for carrying out such life-saving activities
- maintaining the fluid balance of a patient
- promoting the healing of wounds and fractures, protecting the skin and maintaining sensory functions in a patient
- maintaining body regulatory mechanisms and functions in a patient
- feeding a patient
- maintaining elimination in a patient
- promoting communication by and with a patient in the execution of nursing care
- promoting the attainment of optimal health by the individual, the family, groups and the community
- maintaining an environment in which the physical and mental health of a patient are promoted
- preparing for and assisting with diagnostic and therapeutic intervention for a patient
- preparing for and assisting with surgical procedures under anaesthetic
- caring for a dying patient and a deceased patient.

1.2.3 The scope of practice of an enrolled nursing assistant

The scope of practice of an enrolled nursing assistant will be published shortly as an amendment to R2598 of 30 November 1984. The scope of practice of an enrolled nursing assistant is extemely limited and will be restricted to:

(a) assisting the registered nurse, registered midwife and enrolled nurse with those acts and procedures which are part of the nursing regimen planned and initiated by a registered nurse or registered midwife for a patient or a group of patients

(b) performing those procedures concerned with maintaining the hygiene and comfort of the patient under the direct or indirect supervision of a registered nurse or registered midwife.

This scope of practice makes the enrolled nursing assistant responsible to a registered nurse or registered midwife at all times, but she is nevertheless accountable to the South African Nursing Council for her acts and omissions. She is legally responsible for any criminal act she may commit.

A detailed discussion of the scope and functions of various categories of nurse will be found in Searle (1985: 188–192).

The *student nurse* who is being prepared for *registration* must be made ready for the exercise of independent professional judgement in the exercise of these independent functions. She must be prepared for the supervision and direction of other categories of nurses. The enrolled categories of nurses are prepared to work under the direct or indirect supervision of a registered nurse. True, this 'indirect' supervision or direction may be long distance, but it is nevertheless supervision or direction.

The following are translated exerpts from Searle's Credo (1980a: 3,4).

Nursing can only fulfil its allotted task if it has an intellectual, philosophical and disciplined approach to man's health needs.

She saw the philosophical landmarks of nursing as follows:

- The *belief* in the essential *meaning* and *worth* of every human life
- The *recognition* of the *uniqueness* of every human life
- The *responsibility* that the Creator has placed in the hands of man for the welfare of his fellow-man
- *Trust* that there will always be an inner strength that will enable one to cope and will help one to make the right decisions
- A *yearning* to be a worthy servant of mankind and of medical science
- *Acceptance* of the fact that nursing has instrumental and expressive dimensions and that it is not disease that matters, but patients who are ill and threatened
- *Overcoming* a tendency toward a nurse/patient relationship in favour of the relationship between one human being and another and an overcoming of all obstacles in the provision of health care
- *Change* and *conservation* – conservation of a precious human life and assistance to those who are vulnerable through change. All nursing is aimed at prevention, promotion, change, balance and conservation
- *Help and support*, not only to those in need of health care but also to fellow-workers
- The development of a nursing *technology* in the application of scientific principles, knowledge and skills
- The therapeutic use of self.

1.3 THE INDEPENDENT, INTERDEPENDENT AND DEPENDENT FUNCTIONS OF A NURSE

In 1982 Professor C Searle, with her usual insight, clarified thought on these functions of the nurse. In the past it has been customary to talk of the independent and dependent functions of the nurse, without examining the subject in-depth. Today health care is given in the team context. Each member has a specific role and function, with a legal right to practise. The medical man has specific levels of expertise which lead him to make major diagnostic and therapeutic decisions, which will be implemented largely by other members of the health team who are then accountable for their own actions. One of these persons is the nurse whose functions will now be examined.

1.3.1 The independent functions of a nurse

These may be listed as follows:

(a) *Supervision of the patient or client so as to ensure his safety and security:* This includes aspects such as asepsis and cleanliness which are part of the safe environment, and security from physical as well as emotional hazards. The patient must be unable to injure himself or others. Safety includes ensuring that the patient is identified clearly.

(b) *Observation of the patient or client:* This includes signs and symptoms of disease, any change in the patient's condition during the course of the illness or treatment and any reactions, untoward or otherwise, which may occur.

(c) *Recording and reporting* observations made, instructions received and given, care and treatment carried out, including the patient's reactions to treatment or other events. Recording and reporting must be accurate, precise and easily comprehensible by those who have to continue the treatment.

(d) *Assessment of the patient's response to treatment:* Decisions involving changes in the planned therapeutic programme may have to be taken because of this assessment.

(e) *Nursing diagnosis,* for nursing care, for referral to a medical practitioner or for emergency action which the nurse may have to carry out before a medical man can arrive on the scene.

(f) *Performing nursing procedures* as required by the prescribed treatment, the patient or client's conditions, the reason for the procedure, the availability of equipment and other factors. Nursing procedures must be carried out accurately, competently and with due regard for the patient's physical and mental comfort and his safety. Record-keeping is also necessary.

(g) *Supervision of personnel,* so that duties are delegated to those with the knowledge and ability to carry them out. Teaching staff members is an important part of their supervision.

(h) *Education of the patient or client,* and relatives or friends where necessary, so that where possible, self-care is undertaken, therapy is continued for as long as is necessary and community resources are made known to the person being treated or to those caring for him in the home, and are used when and as the need arises. Preventive aspects of health care must be emphasised.

Thus eight independent functions of the nurse have been identified. Many interrelate as interaction takes place between members of the health team. The nurse does not need a prescription to know that she must observe the patient's condition carefully after surgery. It is part of her independent professional responsibility to do so.

1.3.2 The interdependent functions of a nurse

These relate to the interrelationships of the nurse with the patient and with other members of the health team, particularly the interdependence of nursing and medicine.

Neither the nurse nor the doctor can provide all the health-care needs of a patient. Co-ordination of activities and acknowledgement of each other's field of expertise is essential. These are perhaps the most important functions of all in the light of today's nursing practice.

1.3.3 The dependent functions of a nurse

The dependent function of a nurse is based on the law which authorises her practice, as well as on common law and relevant statutory laws. The Nursing Act, as amended from time to time is the law which empowers the nurse to practise, and the regulations promulgated in terms of the Act govern this practice. It is the law, and only the *law* that authorises the professional practice of the nurse.

There are other Acts which have to be taken into consideration, such as those governing the control and handling of medicines, and it is the duty of the nurse to be aware of her responsibilities under common law and specific laws which affect health care. Ultimately, the nurse, practising within legal boundaries, is responsible for her own acts. The nurse, whether she practises within an institution or as a private contractor, remains personally responsible and accountable to the registration authority which, in the RSA, is the South African Nursing Council. She is also answerable, in the broader sense, to the courts of law.

Only the nurse herself can be held personally responsible for her actions. Inefficient work on her part may be the concern of the doctor and of the employing authority if reported. She is accountable for the standard of care she gives in carrying out a prescription. The acceptance by the nurse of a doctor's prescription for patient care is an unwritten agreement between professional colleagues. She accepts the order and must then see that it is carried out. No other person, be he or she senior to the nurse in question, may interfere with the order or attempt to change it.

It is imperative that nurses in South Africa understand that:

(a)   The registered nurse and the registered midwife both have diagnostic, therapeutic and care responsibilities that can be carried out without a patient's having a doctor in attendance or being even remotely responsible for him.

Both these categories of nurses can book patients independently of a relationship with a medical practitioner and both can prescribe certain medications and treatments without having a doctor in attendance. In the case of the registered nurse, she can prescribe all medications that can be sold directly to the public without a doctor's prescription (unscheduled medicines) and carry out all nursing treatments and care where a patient does not have a doctor or is not in obvious need of one.

Regulations relating to the keeping, supply or prescription of medicines by registered nurses are set out in Regulation R2418 dated 2 November 1984. Readers should be aware that regulations may change and should keep themselves informed regarding any such changes.

A registered nurse can (according to R2418) supply, administer or prescribe any medicine or substance listed in Schedules One, Two, Three or Four of the Medicines and Related Substances Control Act, 1965 (Act 101 of 1965).

An extract from these regulations is included for the sake of completeness.

Conditions under which an authorised nurse may supply, administer or prescribe a prescribed medicine

An authorised nurse who supplies, administers or prescribes a prescribed medicine to a patient in terms of these regulations shall –

(a)   directly after supply, administering or prescribing, enter –
(i)   the diagnosis made by the nurse in respect of the health condition of the patient;
(ii)   the name, quantity, strength and dosage of the medicine supplied, administered or prescribed, as the case may be;
(iii) the number of the Schedule to the Medicines Control Act in which such medicine is listed (if any);

(iv) the date and time of supply, administering or prescribing on the patient's file or treatment record, as the case may be, and against that entry the date and time of the entry, his name and category of registration in block letters as well as his signature.
(b) ensure, that in the case where such medicine is supplied to a patient, the medicine is an original or in a replaced form and the container in which the medicine is supplied is labelled with –
(i) the approved name, quantity and strength of the medicine;
(ii) the number of the Schedule to the Medicines Control Act (if any) in which such medicine is listed;
(iii) the name of the patient and his file or treatment record number, as the case may be;
(iv) the dosage of the medicine; and
(v) the address of the body which supplies the medicine.

Note (i) – Attention is drawn to the fact that, in terms of section 38A, the Director-General, the relevant director of hospital services, the relevant medical officer of health or the medical officer in charge of a relevant organisation which renders a health service and who is designated by the Director-General in consultation with the South African Pharmacy Board, must authorise the registered nurse and must determine, after consultation with the South African Nursing Council, the acts which such a nurse may perform.

Her duty is to exercise judgement about referring the patient to a doctor should the need arise. She acts unprofessionally if she does not do so when the patient obviously needs medical attention.

In the case of the registered midwife, she is entitled by law to carry and prescribe scheduled drugs in addition to having the same rights as the registered nurse in respect of mother and baby.

(b) Where a doctor is in attendance on a patient he in reality shares the patient with the nurse. It is her patient as much as it is his patient. Doctors tend to forget this. Legally as the person in charge of the patient, either as a ward professional nurse (or her deputy) or as a private duty nurse, she has co-responsibility for and to the patient, and is totally accountable for her acts and omissions in respect of such responsibility. The doctor is not held responsible for her acts and omissions, for she is an independent registered practitioner accountable for her own acts.

The doctor diagnoses the disease or condition and prescribes the necessary therapeutic modalities, whilst the nurse diagnoses the needs of the patient for nursing care, carries out such therapeutic modalities as the doctor prescribes and which require her assistance or total responsibility, provides care and the therapeutic climate, provides the continuous observation, support and recording facilities on which so much of the further action by the doctor rests, and by the quality of the nursing process contributes to the total therapeutic regimen of the patient.

(c) When nursing action moves up and down the health-care continuum where, depending on the circumstances, she may be performing acts that are normally performed by doctors, she is not practising medicine, she is practising nursing. It is illegal in terms of the Medical, Dental and Supplementary Health Professions Act for anyone other than a registered medical practitioner to practise as a medical practitioner, but this provision cannot detract from the responsibility of the nurse, as a nurse, to do whatever she can for her patient depending on the situation. Similarly, when a doctor performs an act that is normally performed more frequently by nurses, he is acting as a doctor and not as a nurse.

The whole issue depends on the situation in which the care is required, the nature of the intervention required, the urgency thereof, and the ready availability of a more knowledgeable health-care professional, that is the doctor.

When you act, you always act as a nurse and never, never as a medical practitioner or dentist or as a supplementary health professional, irrespective of the task that you do. It is nursing when a nurse does it.

Nurses employed in the primary health-care situation may well perform a variety of professional acts that are normally performed more frequently by doctors, but that does not mean that they are engaged in medical practice. They are nurses, doing what they can to alleviate a position where doctors (for a variety of reasons) are not readily available.

1.4 THE PHILOSOPHY OF NURSING

In the preparation of a skilled practitioner of nursing, the educator will develop her own philosophy of nursing. If some of what has been said here inspires the tutor to further reading and thought, then the writer will have achieved her objective.

Nursing is concerned with people, and the nurse must be *with* the people who need her. The patient needs to *see* the nurse, to know that she is available when needed. When a large amount of clerical work keeps the 'sister' or any nurse out of the ward, and in a duty-room or professional nurse's office, the matter needs to be investigated.

Professor Searle emphasises that:

> The most important role of the registered nurse or sister is the *actual nursing of the sick* and her *management* and teaching functions are intertwined with this for the patient is the focus of all her activities. She is an administrator only so far as to safeguard the well-being of the patients and/or to co-ordinate all the services he needs. She is an educator so that he may receive safe care at the hands of co-workers and junior personnel. She has

to function independently, dependently and interdependently in the total health team (Searle 1980a: 5).

If the nurse–educator prepares her students with this in view, the product of her education will be a credit to her, the institution where she receives her education, and the profession as a whole.

Nurse–educators need to look at the philosophies of education as a whole, for nursing education is part of general education. It is not the aim of this book to expound upon any educational philosophies. Nevertheless, a brief look will be taken at a few ideas from the field of general education which have special meaning for nurse–educators.

Education, in order to take place, needs one who *educates*. In the case of nursing education, this is the lecturer, the tutor, clinical instructor and/or unit 'sister' (professional nurse) with all the means at their disposal to facilitate the education of the student. The education is structured according to a deliberately planned pattern. It requires a person *to be educated*, that is the *student nurse* (or, in the case of other categories, the pupil nurse) and it also requires a *purpose* or *aim*. In the case of nursing education, this aim is the production of a person who is able to nurse efficiently, humanely and safely, someone who not only provides excellent nursing care herself, but is able to supervise its provision by others and to pass her knowledge and skills on to neophytes in the profession. In other words, to produce someone who is capable of exercising educated judgement in her nursing care, and who acts calmly and efficiently in an emergency situation and who is in all senses of the word a professional person.

Education is a social phenomenon which is characteristic of human society. The educator and the educand(s) are placed in a special situation where one expects to guide and lead the others to the discovery of what, to them, is as yet unknown, while those others expect to receive the necessary guidance and assistance. There must be communication between the educator(s) and those receiving education, as well as mutual acceptance of the situation, directed towards a specific goal.

The tutor and others in the nursing education situation expect to guide and lead the student nurse towards her aim of becoming a professional adult, and they accept this role as well as the necessary authority that goes with it. The student expects to be led to professional maturity, and accepts the authority of the guiders or leaders. There must be mutual respect and trust for the goal to be reached. A student who loses respect for, or trust in her teachers, will not progress well. The teachers, on the other hand, must respect and trust the student's integrity and willingness to learn.

Both the teacher(s) and those being educated are actively engaged in the learning event. True, only the learner can learn, no one can do it for her, but the educator(s) must be actively engaged in the whole occurrence; must prepare herself, keep up to date and provide a good role model. The educator must provide meaningful material and make the best use of the facilities available and spur the student to greater efforts on her path towards professional adulthood, where she can become an independent practitioner who is able to assume complete responsibility for her actions in her professional life.

The subculture of nursing must be passed on to the one striving to master its intricacies, with its values, norms and ethical standards, as well as the scientific knowledge and technical skills necessary for good practice.

The educators are educating the person who will practise nursing. They are, or should be producing educated persons who are experts in a specialised field of endeavour. An educated person must not only know, but must know 'why', and must be able to assess the different dimensions of a situation. As training tends to imply skills only, it would be more correct to talk of the educated *and* trained nurse.

Before closing this chapter, a word about existentialism in nursing philosophy. It is a form of thought that has gained a great deal of popularity with many modern nurse-thinkers.

Existentialism is concerned with the individual person as he experiences the actuality of his existence. He exists in an individual world of his own. Existentialism is also concerned with a belief in the worth of the individual and with this unique being's responsibility for shaping his own life. He must help those for whom he is responsible to accept responsibility for themselves. In the final analysis, man alone is responsible for what he makes of his life. Man is forever 'becoming' – he is never complete. He must make his own choice about the direction he will follow or what he will become. He faces adversity with courage and participates in his personal growth and development.

In accepting responsibility for her own life, the nurse-educator also accepts that she must guide and help those for whom she is responsible so that they can ultimately accept responsibility for themselves. The nurse-educator must understand that each student is a unique being with her own potential, her own life to shape and her own professional way to make. The nurse-educator must help and guide the student in developing her own abilities, so that she can participate in her own professional development.

The student must come to the realisation that, in the final analysis, it is she and only she, who can learn or not learn – that she is responsible for her own growth and development in her chosen field of work. Only then will there be meaningful participation in the learning event.

2 The history of nursing education: An outline

2.1 INTRODUCTION

Nursing, in some or other form, is as old as man's history. Nursing education, or the formal preparation towards becoming a competent practitioner of nursing, is of comparatively recent origin. The development of nursing probably began in response to the primitive man's need for nurture, for care when his health broke down as a result of disease or injury. The history of the evolution of nursing runs parallel to that of medicine.

Palaeontologists have found signs of pathological conditions in ancient human remains, and there is evidence of surgical intervention in ancient skulls that were dug up in various parts of the world. How and when medical practice originated is shrouded in the mists of antiquity, but it seems likely that it originated in magic. All frightening and inexplicable things were thought to be the work of devils, evil spirits and such agents. The medicine man, sorcerer, priest or doctor, call him what you will, sought to propitiate these evil spirits, or to drive them out of the affected person's body by diverse methods, including making holes in the skull.

There is little doubt that the women of the tribe, as in all primitive societies, cared for the sick and injured. They probably carried out the 'treatments' prescribed by the witchdoctor. In primitive cultures too, it has been found that the 'wise women' very often have a store of remedies derived from herbs, which they use to treat disease conditions. In the early cultures treatment was purely empirical, based on observation of the effects of the administration of herbal remedies or on the effects of surgery.

The history of medicine has always been closely allied with religion, for both seek to protect man from the effects of evil. As civilisation developed, medical practice, such as it was, became established in temples and sanctuaries. Any form of training that took place, both in medicine and in nursing, would have been learned in the course of service to the sick.

Throughout history, medicine has been concerned with the diagnosis of ailments and the prescription of certain treatments. Some of these such as surgical intervention, have been carried out personally by the doctor, but there has always been the need for the existence of a colleague in health care who carries out the doctor's prescription and provides the constant care required by the sick. This colleague is the nurse. As medical knowledge progressed from the empirical and magical towards the scientific with its accompanying technology, the education for medical practice also underwent great changes. Nursing has kept pace and the education of the professional nurse of today differs greatly from that of her predecessors, as does that of the medical man.

The level of performance expected from the semi-professional group of today is higher than that required from the professional nurse at the beginning of the century. Added to this, it is now recognised that the professional nurse has many functions in her care of the patient, which she must carry out without medical prescription. These functions include attending to the physical comfort of the patient, ensuring the safety of his person, property and name, looking after his nutritional needs, organising the environment and resources to promote recovery, providing emotional support, rendering promotive and preventive services for those who are well and teaching patients, relatives and friends, as well as neophytes in the profession.

Modern nursing services form the biggest component of any health-care facility. They interrelate with and co-ordinate the other health services into a meaningful whole. Round-the-clock care must be provided. Health services are only as good as the nursing services that they provide. This sophisticated approach to health care is a development of social change, the explosion of knowledge and the growing awareness of the public of their own health needs. The ratio of nurses to medical personnel has probably always been the same.

As training or education of other health professionals developed, so did that of the nurse.

Specialised education for the nursing profession probably began towards the end of the 18th century, although St Vincent de Paul, as early as 1630, expressed a wish that the religious sisters be taught nursing. What teaching there was, was probably in-service training, passed on by one to the other.

In 1781 Professor Franz May of Mannheim, Germany, persuaded some of the authorities who were responsible for the running of hospitals to provide a series of lectures to successive groups of nursing attendants. This was, in effect, the beginning of the training of secular nurses in hospitals. Many of his colleagues opposed this step, for they were afraid that trained nursing attendants would compete with medical practitioners (Searle 1965: 135).

That attitude is still found today among some doctors, and in countries where there is an apparent oversupply of medical practitioners the quality of nurses' training has not kept pace with world standards.

Figures exist which show this discrepancy in the number of doctors per 1 000 of the population in the EEC countries. According to these figures, Britain in 1971/72 was at the bottom of the list with 1 doctor per 1 000 while

Italy had almost twice as many doctors, that is 1,97/1 000, West Germany had 1,79/1 000 and Belgium 1,55/1 000.

The so-called threat to medical practice would seem relative for even when there is an overproduction in some countries, there is a gross underproduction in others where the professionally trained nurse then forms the backbone of the health services.

In countries where there is still a backlog in the preparation of both doctors and trained nurses it is very difficult to provide adequate health services.

Professor May gave a series of lectures to medical men at the University of Heidelberg in 1797, during the course of which he convinced the medical practitioners of the day of the need for training their hospital attendants. The result was that he was asked to establish a university course for the education of nurses in 1797 (Searle 1965: 135).

Professor May was convinced that poor nursing, engendered by ignorance and lack of a scientific background, was the major cause of the high mortality rate in hospitals. In the interests of his patients he began lecturing to his nursing attendants. The fact that he was asked to start a university course at all, and at a university of the high standing of Heidelberg University, was proof of his ability to persuade others of the validity of his views. This was 50 years before the Nightingale School was established in London. It was thus in Germany that the first course of formal theoretical and practical instruction was organised. On satisfactory completion of the course a certificate was issued to candidates. This event, which is so often overlooked in considering the history of nursing education, was a major landmark, for at that time no other country in the world provided any formal training for nurses, even of an elementary nature.

In 1793 an Italian, Professor Sannazaro, published an article in which he pointed out to doctors and hospital authorities that the role of the nurse was of great importance in the care of the sick, and he pleaded for more understanding of this fact (Searle 1965: 135).

A Dr Valentine Seaman gave a series of lectures to nurses at a New York hospital in 1798.

Several other schools of nursing were started in Germany between 1782 and 1815 as part of the general interest in public health. The deaconess training centre of the Fliedners at Kaiserwerth was started in 1833 by Pastor Fleidner. At this centre formal courses were organised for nurses, teachers and social workers.

In France too, the medical profession started to show interest in the education of nurses in medical subjects as opposed to their purely religious instruction up to that time. In 1819 Bishop Grégoire appealed for a system of teaching nurses in France, and the improved education in the science of nursing of the nuns in the religious orders was instituted.

It is also significant that a doctor, writing in *Blackwoods Magazine* in 1825 advocated the teaching of nurses and the examination of their proficiency.

The realisation that nurses need a formal, systematised form of education to fulfil a meaningful role in the care of the sick was thus recognised in the 18th century, although it took some time for this to gain general acceptance.

Florence Nightingale, who is considered by many to be the pioneer of modern nursing education, visited Kaiserwerth for two weeks in 1850, and in 1851 spent three months there. She also spent some time with the Sisters of Mercy of the Catholic Hospital, the 'Hôtel-Dieu', in Paris.

The interest in the scientific preparation of nurses stimulated the re-employment of Protestant deaconesses in the care of the sick, as well as the establishment of training schools, especially in Germany, and the improvement of the medical education of nurses in religious orders.

After the Crimean War a fund was established to honour Miss Nightingale in some permanent way and £45 000 was raised by public subscription. This was a very large sum of money, considering the time in which it was collected and the then value of money. She used it to establish a training school for nurses, The Nightingale School, at St Thomas Hospital in London in 1860.

Florence Nightingale met with considerable opposition to the establishment of this formal training school for nurses. A Mr South, a surgeon, led the group who stated that he and his colleagues were 'not at all disposed to allow that the nursing establishments of our hospitals were inefficient, or that they were likely to be improved by any special institution of training'. 'Nurses,' said the doctors 'were in the position of housemaids and needed only the simplest instruction' (Baly 1973: 72).

The training course at the Nightingale School was subject to strict discipline. However, this was not discipline for discipline's sake, but was intended to avoid all causes of disapproval of the training programme. The first 'probationers' had to be above suspicion. Character training was emphasised. The connotation of the nurse being a sleazy servant of the type described by Charles Dickens in *Martin Chuzzlewit* in the person of Sairey Gamp had to be avoided at all costs. Carefully selected students with a good background of general education and impeccable moral standards were selected. These students lived in a nurses' home under the strict supervision of a home sister. This, in Victorian times, was very important, as it ensured that no breath of scandal was allowed to taint Miss Nightingale's ladies. It must also be remembered that work outside the home was not, at that time, considered proper for 'ladies'. This training scheme, considered by Miss Nightingale to be suitable for any intelligent girl with some education and an aptitude for caring for the sick, actually found favour with the upper class. The middle class, in whose minds the idea of gentility was bound up with a life of busy idleness, did not at first take to the idea of nurse training readily.

The training of nurses, according to Florence Nightingale, should take place in a hospital, the bulk of the curriculum being concerned with practical experience gained at the bedside. Nurses were at that time the only personnel in a hospital who provided service to the sick. They therefore had to be taught how to prepare food and what types of food were considered suitable for various disease conditions. They had to learn to give toilet care as well as the specific nursing care which the patient required.

The patient was in bed and nursing was at the side of that bed, a very different concept from today's ambulant patients, preventive and promotive care and rehabilitation. The education of the nurse was tailored to meet the needs of the time. As times change, the pattern of nursing education must necessarily also change.

The idea of training women for professions, due to the initiative of Florence Nightingale, actually spread to other spheres of life as well. In the second half of the reign of Queen Victoria (1837 – 1901) the idea that upper class and middle class women, more particularly those who were unmarried, should be trained to support themselves and to be of some use to the world, gained considerable ground. With it was realised the need for secondary education for women.

The one-year nursing course included daily lectures by medical men, sisters and also by chaplains. Mrs Wardroper, the matron of St Thomas hospital, drew up a monthly report on the progress of the students. The form used for this report was designed by Miss Nightingale and was subdivided into detailed headings (Baly 1973: 73). Students were also required to keep a personal diary of their work and observations. After seven years of this training system, a method of admitting students for training was developed. Two groups of women were considered eligible for training: the first was 'lady' probationers who paid for their training themselves, which was of one year's duration, while the second group consisted of ordinary probationers who received free board, a uniform and a £10 training allowance. Eventually all training was done over a two-year period. The fact that some groups paid for their training while others did not, had an adverse effect on the development of nursing education. Paying for 'service' led to the exploitation of students. It was never Miss Nightingale's intention that the student nurses should become the labour force of the hospital or conversely that all the sick should be nursed by 'trained' nurses (Baly 1973: 73). The Nightingale School aimed at training hospital nurses to supervise non-trained nurses and to train others as well as training district nurses to nurse the sick poor. Despite the problems mentioned earlier, the Nightingale system began a proud tradition of nursing education in England, which was later to spread to many parts of the world. With it unfortunately, spread the idea that the nurse was not an independent practitioner in her own right, but subservient to doctor's 'orders', a point of view that has taken a long time to be discarded.

When considering nursing education it must be kept in mind that it is a specialised part of the field of general education and is closely allied to medical education. Medical practice had to break away from the routine treatments of bleeding and purging, a throwback to the era when these methods were used to rid the body of evil spirits. As medical knowledge became more complex and extensive, medical education followed suit. Lord Lister, father of antiseptic surgery, stated that the greatest discovery medical science made during the 19th century was 'the discovery of the professional trained nurse who has helped the medical practitioner to revolutionize the care of the sick, to extend his own sphere of usefulness, to increase his personal income and to apply his scientific discoveries to patient treatment' (Searle 1965: 283).

The pattern of nursing education in the USA followed similar trends, developing from the assistance given to the sick by relatives and neighbours to the present organised pattern aimed at the production of a highly skilled professional nurse, serving the society in which she lives and works in an ever evolving role.

The role and status of the nurse in the USA were low in the 18th century. Care of the sick was primitive, conditions in big city hospitals were poor and those giving care were often inmates of a penitentiary.

A few progressive physicians appealed, during the latter half of the 18th century, for better nursing care of the sick, and leading personalities such as Benjamin Franklin, urged that kindness and consideration for those unfortunate enough to be sick, should be shown in the name of humanity. The education or training of the people who must give this care was not even considered.

Mother Elizabeth Seton, who founded the order of the American Sisters of Charity, was responsible for some attention being focussed on nursing needs, and a Nurse Society established in Philadelphia, organised a short course in 1839 to train respectable young women in maternity nursing.

An attempt was made in 1859 to establish a training course for nurses, but when the Civil War broke out in 1861 this came to nothing, and there were no trained nurses available for the care of the sick and wounded soldiers. The real beginning of nursing education in America was the founding of schools of nursing in New York, New Haven and Boston in 1873 (13 years after the founding of the Nightingale School). The training was at first based on the Nightingale pattern, though it later developed its own individual style.

Florence Nightingale was not the first to establish a school of nurse training. Religious nursing orders had already started some training of their members and even the training of deaconesses for nursing had a religious connotation. She was not even the first to found a school for the training of 'lay' nurses (those not attached in some way to a religious congregation), for the first such school was established in Lausanne in Switzerland in 1859. Nevertheless, her influence on nurse training was so great that she is generally regarded as the pioneer of modern secular nursing. Florence Nightingale had to tailor her training system to the existing system of 'voluntary' hospitals in England where the matron was an established hospital official, and, as such, could also be placed in charge of training. The Nightingale School, because of the fact that it received financial endowment from the Nightingale fund, was in a unique position. This financial independence was not as easily attained in other schools, and led to the service aspects becoming more important than the educational needs of students.

The Nightingale pattern did not always fit the established patterns of hospitals in other countries, nor did it always conform to their customs. The position of matron, as head of the training school, could not always be accommodated in the nursing systems which had developed in other countries, as was the case in England. Nevertheless, the pattern Miss Nightingale established could be adapted to meet different needs – and this is what happened.

The field of general education has undergone many changes; in fact, all formal education was, until comparatively recently, limited to the wealthy. It was not until the latter part of the 19th century that the luxury of education was available to anyone outside the moneyed social classes apart from the few with special intellectual gifts who were fortunate enough to have these recognised.

Teaching was confined to lectures, demonstrations and private study. The supply of books was limited, the variety was small and textbooks as we know them were almost non-existent. Technical skills were passed on from master to apprentice in specific trades or occupations. It was only in the early 1900s that a proper study of learning and methods of teaching was undertaken. This brought about drastic changes in the ideas of what education entailed and of the methods which could be used to educate.

General education of the public at large only became possible in the latter part of the 19th century, and even today there are large numbers of people who have never received any formal education at all. The general education of women was even slower to become established. The idea that it was sufficient for a woman to read, write, do some simple arithmetic, sew and do household tasks was prevalent. It was considered unnecessary for her to study anything in depth. In fact, a woman was considered incapable of real intellectual feats. The few exceptions that did emerge were regarded as freaks. The fact that secondary education for girls was a late starter is significant for nursing education, for it limited the number available for training in a predominantly female profession. In certain countries today many women still find it difficult to gain admission on equal terms with men, to education institutions. This also limits the development of nursing service based on professional training in these countries.

Added to all this is the tremendous, almost daily increase of knowledge. The term 'knowledge explosion' of the 20th century has become commonplace in our language. The addition to present knowledge is being made by those who themselves have had the education which has enabled them to search for what is as yet undiscovered in our universe and beyond. Education is groping through this massive accumulation of new knowledge in a search for new and better methods of imparting knowledge to those seeking to acquire it, and of facilitating learning. Minds have to be trained to think, and to probe into the future, as has been man's wont since he first inhabited the earth. Nursing education is no different, it dare not stand still; it must also be shaped to meet the demands of the future. It must not only prepare its practitioners for today and tomorrow, but also its own scientists, researchers and educators.

2.2 THE NIGHTINGALE SYSTEM

This system, as designed by Florence Nightingale, had the following basic pattern:

(a) The matron of the hospital was to have supreme responsibility for:
  - the *nursing care* of the patients
  - the nursing personnel
  - the *training* of nurses
  - the hospital kitchen, linen room and laundry
  - the domestic staff.

She was answerable only to the Hospital Board and *not* to the medical superintendent.

(b) The student nurses (or probationers as they were then known) had to live in a nurses' home, supervised by a 'home sister'.

(c) The theoretical education of the nurse had to include basic sciences.

(d) The *ward sister*, under the matron's direction, had a two–fold responsibility, namely patient care and *teaching of student nurses*. The professional nurse in charge of a ward was actually paid an extra allowance in recognition of her *essential teaching function*.

The two groups of students who attended the Nightingale School, as mentioned earlier, were:

(a) The *ordinary* probationers who at first underwent one year's training (which was later extended to two years) followed by three year's supervised practice. These students were paid a stipend.

(b) The *educated* probationer, who followed a formal curriculum which, per week, included:
- 12 hours of anatomy and surgical nursing
- 12 hours of physiology and medical nursing
- 12 hours of chemistry, foods and sanitation
- talks on ethical and professional subjects, lectures, quizzes, notes, case studies, library work and the keeping of diaries.

This group underwent one year of formal training (also later extended to two years) and two years of supervised practice. They paid fees for their training.

The latter group of nurses were 'trained to train' as their main function. It is because of this that many St Thomas nurses were sent out by Miss Nightingale to give advice and help in the founding of training schools. This became the pattern throughout the British Isles, and in many of the then British Colonies, including South Africa.

Miss Nightingale's principles of nursing education included the following:

(a) A school of nursing should be attached to a medical school and a teaching hospital.

(b) The nurses' home should be a place where a disciplined way of life prevailed and character could be formed. (It must be remembered that the reputation of lay nurses of that time was not good and the Nightingale probationers had to be kept free from any chance of gaining such a reputation. This strict discipline was necessary at that time.)

(c) The matron should have the responsibility for the entire education programme for the nurses, including theoretical and practical teaching and experience and should control the nurses' home, its rules and regulations.

This pattern is easily discernible in our early education of nurses. South Africa still uses the term matron, although it is falling into disuse even in Britain.

The new terminology in South Africa for 'matron' is 'nursing service manager' which is officially being used, and is gradually coming into general use.

2.3 THE AMERICAN SYSTEM

This is an adaptation of the Nightingale system, and is found in Canada, the USA and other countries. The main features include:

(a) Training schools attached to hospitals: The Superintendent of nurses is responsible for patient care, the term 'matron' not being used, except for a housekeeper grade.

(b) A dietician to control the catering department and its personnel (This is another area where changes are occurring throughout the world.)
(c) A housekeeper or 'matron' controlling the domestic department
(d) The Superintendent of Nurses being responsible to the Board, or the superintendent of the hospital who could be a doctor, nurse or layman
(e) Students living in a nurses' home or outside
(f) A very broadly based theoretical instruction programme
(g) A head nurse is the person in charge of a ward, while a supervisor is in charge of a department consisting of several wards. She is responsible for the teaching and disciplining of students, and the management of the wards in her department.

2.4 THE MOTHERHOUSE SYSTEM

This is a modern adaptation of that developed by the old religious orders. It is found where a school is maintained by a religious sisterhood, Catholic or Protestant, as well as in the Red Cross Schools of Switzerland and Germany. The theoretical instruction may be quite elementary, the ward professional nurse has an important teaching function, and professional nurses are supported for life, living in a nurses' home.

2.5 THE CONTINENTAL SYSTEM

Found all over the European continent and in Latin America, this system exists side by side with the Motherhouse system and has adopted certain features from both the Nightingale and the American systems. There is, however, no equivalent of the matron or the superintendent of nurses. Each 'service' block (eg medical nursing) has its own head nurse who is directly responsible to a doctor in charge of the block and also to the director of the hospital who may be a layman or a doctor.

The training school may form an integral part of the hospital, or it may be an independent educational institution. Theoretical instruction is given and students are given practical instruction by various means. They are supernumerary in the wards. The teaching role of the ward professional nurse also varies. In the early days training was hampered by the illiteracy of the masses, but this improved with the increased availability of general education.

In most countries today there are at least three systems of basic education of the nurse, namely:

(a) The preparation for professional practice with registration of qualifications. This may be offered at baccalaureate, associate degree or diploma (or in some countries at certificate) level.

(b) Preparation of nurses on a sub-professional level, who are usually prepared for enrolment or licensure at hospital training schools.
(c) Preparation of a group of qualified assistants to the first two categories. These are nurses' assistants, or assistant nurses who assist registered and/or enrolled nurses.

The programmes offered vary throughout the world and changes and adaptations are constantly being made. Courses vary in duration and in admission requirements and in many countries students pay for their training. Basic university education for nurses is provided in the USA, Belgium, Great Britain, New Zealand, Canada and the RSA. Other countries are working towards this. In some countries where degrees cannot be obtained in nursing, nurse leaders often study the arts, social science, philosophy or economics at degree level.

The history of nursing education is no different to that of other professional education. Medical men teach medical students; sociologists teach sociology students; pharmacists teach pharmacy students and nurses teach nurses. When nursing education programmes were first introduced there were no 'trained nurses' to teach students. There were certainly no nurse-educators, that is people with a background in education as well as in nursing. Empirical skills learned in practice, were taught by those who had taught themselves and nursing education became very technique or procedure oriented. The need to know the reason for a technique and the inherent dangers, so as to safeguard the patient, was not at first recognised.

2.6 THE DEVELOPMENT OF NURSING EDUCATION IN SOUTH AFRICA

Sister Henrietta Stockdale introduced nurse training into South Africa when she instituted a training programme at the Carnarvon Hospital in Kimberley in 1877. Lectures for the first group commenced in February 1877. A ward for Black patients at the Digger's Central Hospital was used for practical training purposes as well as the wards of the Carnarvon Hospital. Later these two hospitals were united to form the Kimberley Hospital.

The first training course lasted for one year, and the knowledge obtained was tested by written examinations. The students had to serve another year as staff nurses before they gained recognition as trained nurses. Sister Henrietta was greatly assisted in her training programme by eminent medical men. She was a great advocate of nursing education being part of the general education system of the country, but unfortunately for the progress of nursing education in this country, she did not succeed and the struggle continues to this day. In the 1980s at last, significant progress is being made to reach this goal.

The part of the training programme which is interesting in the light of later developments, is that the lectures were concentrated in the winter months. A 'block' system in embryo? Subjects included anatomy, physiology, practical nursing, surgery and cookery for the sick. Instruction in ethics was also given. A second course of lectures was included in the second year while nurses were serving as staff nurses and a second examination was conducted towards the end of the second year. Thus theoretical and clinical instruction was combined with practical experience. The Kimberley-trained nurses (much as the Nightingale nurses in Britain) spread their influence far and wide and, among others, started training nurses at Barberton in 1877, at the Volkshospitaal in Pretoria in 1890 and at the Frontier Hospital, Queenstown in 1890. Sister Henrietta also helped Sister Mary Agatha to start training at the Somerset Hospital, Cape Town, in 1886 when three ladies of 'education and refinement' were admitted as probationers.

By the end of the 19th century there were 18 hospitals in South Africa where the training of nurses was undertaken and a Kimberley-trained nurse was associated with each of these training schools. This was no mean achievement! The examination of nurses became the responsibility of the Colonial Medical Council in 1892. Prior to that examinations were conducted by the hospitals themselves. The first Afrikaans woman to train as a nurse was Alice Eveline de Beer in 1886.

The educational requirements laid down by Sister Henrietta for admission to training were that prospective students should be 'cultured young women' who had a thorough command of the three Rs, who had read widely, knew Latin, and played some musical instrument. So highly was the training at Kimberley valued that educated women had their names entered on a waiting list, and some had to wait as long as five years to obtain admission to training. At the same time, it must be remembered that the number admitted to training at any one time was limited. Nurses at Kimberley Hospital who were in training were supernumerary and paid a fee for tuition.

From small beginnings come great developments. The examination and certification of nurses were taken over by the various Medical Councils as they became established, until the passing of the Medical, Dental and Pharmacy Act, 1928 (Act 13 of 1928), when the South African Medical Council came into being. This provided for recognition of the certificates issued and registration of nurses, granted by the various Medical Councils. The South African Medical Council then became the registering body for midwives and nurses, with disciplinary powers and powers to approve of training schools, conduct examinations and grant certificates. It also provided for recognition of additional qualifications.

By the time the South African Medical Council assumed responsibility for nurse training, the training period was three years in Class I training schools, and four years in Class II training schools. Unfortunately for the education of the nurse, Sister Henrietta's plan for nursing education as part of general education was not implemented and an apprenticeship system of training was introduced which greatly exploited the students and from which we have not yet entirely escaped. Lectures were only given near examination time and in the off-duty time of the student. Nurses were taught how to do something, but seldom told why. This was against both the Nightingale and the Stockdale principles of how nursing education should take place.

In 1937 the South African Medical Council increased the training period to three and a half years and four and a half years for Class I and Class II training schools respectively. A preliminary training school system was introduced at the Johannesburg Hospital in 1921 where the first qualified sister-tutor in South Africa, Miss MEG Milne, was appointed in October of that year. In June 1943 Miss EM Pike established a full block system at Groote Schuur Hospital. After a period of struggle for professional control of nurses by nurses, the Nursing Act was passed in 1944.

When the South African Nursing Council took over these responsibilities in 1944, the apprenticeship system of training was still in force, with the exception of Groote Schuur Hospital, where the block system was used. Gradually changes were brought about. Hours of practice were reduced, lectures were given in 'duty' time and students were less exploited. In 1945 there were only 29 trained nurse-tutors in the Union of South Africa, of whom six were able to teach in Afrikaans. In 1985, 40 years later, there was a registered total of 1 883 of whom 1 102 were White, 135 Coloured, 34 Indian and 612 Black. It is realised that not all of those are actively engaged in teaching. Nevertheless an improvement is obvious, although the numbers are still too small, and there is a great maldistribution among the races to meet their own needs. It must be remembered that in those groups basic nursing education on a large scale is of recent origin, and a great deal of teaching in Black training schools is done by White tutors.

More and more teachers of all race groups are being prepared for nursing education and in 1975 an increase of 40 in Black tutors registered out of a total of 52 new registrations was encouraging. The increase in Black registered tutors was 45 out of a total increase of 74 in 1977. In 1945 the educational standard required of those who could be admitted to training for registration was only Standard VII. Today it is Standard X (12 years of schooling). The number of practical training hours required in Class I training schools by the South African Medical Council was 8 664 and the minimum number of hours of lectures prescribed was 100 plus 100 demonstrations. It must be pointed out that the minimum was seldom exceeded. A minimum of 3 000 hours of clinical practica and a minimum of 960 lecture periods or 640 hours of theoretical instruction was laid down for the educa-

31

tion of a registered general nurse.

The new comprehensive course, which prepares the student for registration as a nurse (general, psychiatric and community) and as a midwife has altered this considerably. In terms of the regulations published on 22 February 1985 (R425) the requirements are:

Subjects

(a) The curriculum shall consist of at least the following subjects and the approach shall be the integration of the various fields of study, particularly in their clinical application:
  • Fundamental nursing science, ethos and professional practice – at least one (1) academic year
  • General nursing science – at least three (3) academic years
  • Psychiatric nursing science – at least two (2) academic years
  • Midwifery – at least two (2) academic years
  • Community nursing science – at least (2) academic years
  • Biological and natural sciences – at least two and a half (2½) academic years
  • Pharmacology – at least half (½) an academic year
  • Social sciences – at least two (2) academic years.

(b) Systematic professional practice instruction, which includes laboratory and clinical training, shall extend over the full period of the course of study.

(c) Such education and training shall include at least the following aspects:
  • General nursing science – at least 2 700 hours
  • Psychiatric nursing science – at least 800 hours
  • Midwifery – at least 800 hours
  • Community nursing science – at least 320 hours.

(d) The total period of clinical training at night shall not exceed 960 hours and shall not be continuous: Provided that no clinical training shall be done at night in the first semester of the first year of study.

Examinations

(a) Subject to the provisions of paragraph (b), examinations shall be conducted in all subjects prescribed and an examination mark of at least 50% shall be obtained in each subject.

(b) In the case of nursing science subjects with practica components, the theory and the practica shall be examined and passed separately in terms of the requirements of the nursing school concerned.

More details are given in Directives, as are specific practica requirements.

The entire system of providing these courses has been altered. All students who commenced preparation as a nurse for the first time, from 1 January 1986, are required to take this comprehensive course.

It will also be clear that the course is offered by approved nursing schools which consist of:

(a) a university with a department or sub-department of nursing, or a nursing college which has entered into an agreement of co-operation with a university which has a department or sub-department of nursing
(b) the course of study has been approved by the Council
(c) the head of the department or sub-department of nursing or the head of the nursing college where education and training is offered, is a registered nurse who holds at least a baccalaureate degree and against whose name additional qualifications in nursing education and in nursing are registered.

These regulations require that the curriculum be submitted by the university or nursing college in terms of section 15 of the Nursing Act, 1978 (Act 50 of 1978 as amended by Act 71 of 1981). This includes the subjects to be offered and the minimum duration of each, the examinations to be conducted by the university or nursing college and the nursing science subjects to be conducted by the university or nursing college as well as the nursing science subjects with practical components, where the theory and practica must be examined and passed separately.

This means, in effect, that the responsibility in many cases for conducting examinations (for the 'new' comprehensive course) has passed from the Nursing Council to the universities and nursing colleges as stated in the regulations.

The Nursing Council still conducts examinations for students completing courses under the old regulations, and for post-registration courses, although it is envisaged that these too will eventually be conducted by universities in co-operation with nursing colleges. Universities with their own departments or sub-departments of nursing have in any case conducted their own examinations, their students being registered by the Nursing Council on completion of the various post-registration courses offered. This also applies to those qualifying for basic registration. University departments or sub-departments of nursing are subject to inspection by the Nursing Council, as are colleges of nursing, including the areas where practica (clinical education and training) is undertaken by the students.

The examination of nurses for qualification as enrolled nurses is still the responsibility of the Nursing Council.

The period of training required for registration in the disciplines is now four years. Midwifery training programmes have also been drastically altered and today a registered general nurse completes the course in one year, while an enrolled nurse takes two years. The training of singly qualified midwives has been stopped. The period of midwifery training for the registered nurse has been increased first from six months to nine months and then to one year, except where the comprehensive approach is used.

The South African Nursing Council constantly reviews training programmes. New regulations are made after careful consideration and consultation with experts in the different fields. Many factors have to be taken into consideration when framing regulations. These include

(a) the needs of the public for well-trained persons in all categories to supply nursing care of a high standard;

(b) the educational needs of students and pupils;

(c) admission requirements which will ensure that the educational programme objectives will be met, while at the same time being realistic; and

(d) the necessity for tailoring training regulations flexibly enough for them to be adapted to meet constantly changing needs created by new techniques employed in nursing and medical practice.

The South African Nursing Council issues directives to training schools which are constantly under review. These set out the purpose of the courses, the course content and the minimum qualification of lecturers as well as the minimum number of teaching periods required. Because they are not embodied in regulations where amendments take a considerable period of time, they are easily altered. Regulations are framed in very broad terms whereas directives include more details.

The South African Nursing Council registers general nurses, midwives and psychiatric nurses after completion of a prescribed period of training and the passing of examinations. Similarly it enrols nurses after a shorter, less intensive training period as well as nursing assistants who have a still shorter period of training which is mostly practical in nature. It also registers additional qualifications after the student has either followed a course prescribed by the South African Nursing Council, and is examined by it, or after a student has followed a course of study and examination conducted by another institution which has been approved by the Council for that purpose. Postbasic registration can be obtained after having specialised in the following:

- Nursing education
- Nursing administration
- Community nursing science
- Paediatric nursing science
- Orthopaedic nursing science
- Operating theatre technique
- Intensive nursing science
- Ophthalmic nursing science
- Advanced psychiatric nursing science

34

- Advanced midwifery and neonatal nursing
- Geriatric nursing science
- Oncology nursing science
- Advanced paediatric and neonatal nursing science.

As needs change, courses are changed, new ones are introduced and others are withdrawn.

The first Nursing College was established at the Johannesburg General Hospital. Today there are many throughout the country. University education for nurses commenced with the establishment of courses leading to the Diploma in Nursing (Tutor) at the Universities of the Witwatersrand and Cape Town which admitted the first students in 1937. The first six students obtained their diplomas at the University of the Witwatersrand on 11 March 1939. In 1949 the University of Pretoria instituted a one-year diploma course for tutors. This was the first one offered in the Afrikaans medium.

Other universities have followed suit. In 1956 the University of Natal instituted the first course specifically for Black nurse-tutors. The University of the North offers a similar course. Some Black students have, of course, obtained diplomas in nursing education at other universities and the Transvaal Provincial Administration ran a tutor's course based at Baragwanath Hospital for a short time. The Diploma in Hospital Administration was pioneered by Professor C Searle, when she was directress of Nursing Services of the Provincial Administration at the Pretoria College of Nursing. This course can now also be followed at universities where in some cases it is offered in combination with community nursing science.

The need for the inclusion of community nursing science in post-registration courses, and for its continuation as a 'single' course will disappear eventually as more basic students complete the comprehensive course. The need may be felt to replace it in time by an advanced community nursing component.

3 Purposes and objectives of nursing education

3.1 INTRODUCTION

In chapter 2 it was stated that the purpose of nursing education was to prepare the student to nurse efficiently, humanely and safely, which is the main objective of any programme of nursing education.

The student is educated to become a nurse in the fullest sense of the word, to become someone who could not only provide nursing care of the highest quality, but could also supervise its provision by others and who could pass her knowledge and skills on to the neophytes in the profession. She should be capable of exercising educated judgement in her nursing care and should act calmly and efficiently in an emergency situation. Someone who is, in all senses of the word, a professional person . . .

In any programme where objectives are stated there is always one *main objective* and a number of *subsidiary objectives*, all of which are planned to ultimately fulfil the principal objective. The subsidiary objectives can be subdivided further into *intermdiate* objectives and *specific* objectives. Objectives can be seen as markers along the way which must be followed and are milestones on the road to the achievement of some definite goal.

The word objective comes from the Latin *objectus* and in Roman times it referred to a post used to denote the turning point in a chariot race. It was not the final goal but a mark along the way. If objectives are used to mark out the nursing education pattern, a large number will be needed along the path to the achievement of the main goal.

In setting objectives, care must be taken not to adopt a purely behaviouristic approach, for we are dealing with human beings, being prepared to care for other human beings, and the stimulus-response reaction can cause pitfalls for the unwary.

Bloom defined a taxonomy of educational objectives, namely the cognitive domain, the affective domain and the psychomotor domain, which have had an influence on educational thought.

The *cognitive domain* deals with knowledge and understanding. Bloom defined six levels of cognitive behaviour, which were arranged in hierarchical sequence:

Knowledge → comprehension → application → analysis → synthesis → evaluation.

Too much of nurse teaching has been, and unfortunately still is, simply to present students with facts, to expect them to memorise these facts and then recall them when necessary. *Learning* was then said to have taken place. The guiding of students to the acquisition of facts, their comprehension of what lay behind this knowledge and the application of knowledge to the practice of clinical nursing and to the administration of patient care, in other words the correlation of theory and practice, was forgotten. Analysis of the nursing situation, of the type of care most suitable for the person in need of that care, the synthesis of knowledge from different fields of learning into a meaningful nursing theory and critical evaluation of what was good or bad, necessary or unnecessary and what the results of nursing intervention would be, were disregarded. Nevertheless it is possible to set relevant objectives in the cognitive domain, provided the persons behind the actions are always kept in mind.

Bloom's second domain, *the affective domain*, had a hierarchical structure similar to that of the first one and concerns *feelings*, beliefs and values. The hierarchical structure consists of five main categories:

- Receiving or attending
- Responding
- Valuing
- Organising
- Characterisation by a value or value complex (internalisation).

There is less unanimity about the possibility of setting objectives in this domain. Indeed, it is quite difficult to do so. In nursing education one is concerned with guiding the student towards acquiring the values and norms of the profession and with the cultivation of attitudes and feelings towards patients and clients and their emotional as well as their physical needs, which would be consistent with good nursing care. It is an aspect of learning which must not be forgotten. But setting clearly defined objectives to be obtained according to a behavioural stimulus-response pattern would be very difficult indeed.

The third domain, the *psychomotor domain,* can be defined as behaviour which includes muscular action and which requires neuromuscular co-ordination. Five categories are distinguished:

- Imitation: copying
- Manipulation: performing acts on instruction
- Precision: producing a high level of proficiency
- Articulation: co-ordination of a series of activities
- Naturalisation: an act is performed with maximum proficiency and minimum expenditure of energy.

The nurse–educator might be inclined to seize on this as an area where pure behavioural objectives can be set. Yet the administration of an injection or the dressing of a wound entails far more than a technical skill; it involves knowledge and all aspects of the *cognitive domain* for it deals with persons and their feelings, with the nurse and her attitudes, the emotional support given to the patient. It thus also encompasses all aspects of the *affective domain* as well as the purely technical skills inherent in the *psychomotor domain*. All are interrelated. In setting objectives, cognisance must be taken of the *persons* concerned and not just of the techniques. Nursing education or training has been obsessed far too long with *procedures* and *technical skills*.

This does not mean, however, that objectives cannot be usefully employed in nursing education. All that is asked is that they be designed with thought given to the main objective of *preparing a human being* – the nursing student – *to nurse another human being* – the patient or client – *with competence, knowledge, understanding and humanity*.

An educational programme has a greater chance of success if its objectives have been clearly stated. If you have not defined the purpose of your course, you cannot have any criteria against which to measure your product; in this case the registered nurse. You will have no yardstick against which to judge your success. So often we are called upon to produce 'good examination results', without giving any thought to the use to which this knowledge, tested by examination, is to be put. True, one of the criteria of a profession is that admission to its ranks is obtained after some form of testing. But do we set our objectives clearly so that we are testing competence for practice in the role of a registered nurse, or do we only expect regurgitation of *book knowledge*, without judging its relevance to the job in hand?

Properly stated objectives will mark the way to this attainment of competence as a registered nurse. This role requires the synthesis of knowledge, skills, technical know-how, observation, judgement, human understanding, vision and decision making.

A professional nurse does not follow prescribed activities blindly. She uses the process or system of nursing, with all its facets, in order to provide good nursing care.

A framework of values is also built up during nursing education which is generally shared by all members of the profession. The educated professional nurse must act with judgement based on knowledge, with skill and with clinical competence. The clinical component may never be neglected in teaching the practice of nursing.

Students must be guided theoretically *and* in practice, so that they can ultimately:

● care for individual patients or clients according to their diverse needs

38

- manage and co-ordinate the nursing and health care of groups of patients or clients
- apply theoretical knowledge to practical situations
- devise nursing care plans based on observation, knowledge and critical judgement according to observed and perceived needs
- become full members of the health care team with a vital contribution to make to any therapeutic action
- develop their own unique approach to nursing care, and initiate action where necessary
- be competent in nursing skills
- be able to pass these skills on to others
- use their intellectual and motor abilities and continue to practise and develop these throughout their professional lives.

This somewhat detailed preamble leads to the next section.

3.2 THE SELECTION OF EDUCATIONAL OBJECTIVES IN NURSING EDUCATION

3.2.1 Decide what students need to know

This does not mean that 'experts' should sit down and decide, in an arbitary fashion, what they think the student of a basic nursing programme needs to know. The whole exercise would be too subjective, and the curriculum, thus devised, would be overloaded. A more impersonal assessment in the actual practice situation of what is to be expected of the registered nurse in that situation would produce data of more value. What does the average, competent registered nurse actually do in a general nursing situation?

This would include an analysis of tasks, of dealing with people, of skills and planning.

A research project along these lines would probably revolutionise our curricula. The objectives then determined could be realistically designed to meet proven needs.

In deciding what the student needs to know, the following should be borne in mind:

3.2.1.1 Main objective

The main objective will be broadly stated and will combine the overall objective of the institution at which the student receives her clinical experience, with the need to produce a registered nurse who can meet these needs.

The overall aim of a health-care institution would perhaps be *to provide preventive, promotive, curative and rehabilitative as well as long-term and terminal health care to the community it serves.* Thus the educational objective, broadly stated, could be to *'produce registered nurses* capable of providing the *nursing art and science component* of preventive, promotive, curative, rehabilitative, long-term and terminal health care to people of all ages in the community she serves, and in varied states of health, with *competence* based on knowledge and skill, with *understanding, judgement,* and *humanity'.*

3.2.1.2 Intermediate objectives

In order to achieve the main objective, intermediate objectives can be defined, such as acquiring

- knowledge of the ethos of nursing and of professional practice;
- knowledge of the structure and functioning of the human body based on the natural and biological sciences, and including the developmental aspects;
- knowledge of the changes in the human body as a result of disease and deformity;
- knowledge of man in his interaction with other men;
- knowledge of man's psychological functioning;
- knowledge of the causes and preventive aspects of all ills which may befall man;
- knowledge of and practice in the technical skills in nursing with due regard to the needs of patients – physical, sociological and psychological – and the scientific principles on which these technical skills are based;
- knowledge of teaching and management skills required – for professional competence;
- the ability to think, synthesise, plan, implement and evaluate;
- the ability to maintain personal mental and physical good health; and
- the ability to initiate change so as to improve the quality of nursing care given.

This would lead to the laying down of a broadly structured syllabus, which would include the following aspects:

- The ethos of nursing
- Professional practice
- Applied natural sciences
  - Physics
  - Chemistry
  - Medical biophysics
  - Medical biochemistry
  - Pharmacology

- Biological sciences
  - Anatomy
  - Physiology $\Big\}$ including all phases of development
  - Microbiology
- Pathology
- Nutrition
- Basic medicine and surgery
- The humanities, especially sociology and psychology
- Disease causation
- Community health nursing science, including epidemiology
- The art and science of nursing, including clinical practice
- Unit teaching and administration
- Health education, etc.

3.2.1.3 Specific objectives

Having established a syllabus for the course, it is then the task of the educator to take each intermediate objective and break it down into specific objectives which can be very detailed indeed.

A *specific objective* can again be stated in terms of a main objective, subsidiary or intermediate objectives and specific objectives. An example of this might be:

(a) *Specific objective:* The administration of an intramuscular injection. This is also the *main sub-objective*.

(b) *Intermediate sub-objectives:* These include knowledge of sites, purpose, material to be injected (including side-effects), disease to be prevented or treated, asepsis, instruments to be used (syringe and needle), patient/ client fears and attitudes, legal requirements (such as checking, recording, etc), and positioning of patient.

(c) *Specific objective:* The clinical skill required to draw up under aseptic conditions the required dose of the prescribed drug and to administer it to the right person at the right time in the correct manner at the most suitable site, causing as little discomfort as possible, with due regard to the patient/client's physical and psychological needs, and his safety; to leave the patient/client comfortable, to record the dose, to watch for side-effects and to be able to deal with them if they occur; to dispose of the discarded apparatus and materials safely and efficiently; to be able to pass this skill and knowledge on to others.

3.2.1.4 Overall considerations

The above has indicated in broad outline how use can be made of objectives in nursing education. There are some general points which should be borne

41

in mind by those planning to set up objectives as markers along the pathway to the achievement of nursing efficiency. The following general points must be remembered:

(a) *Prerequisites* must be determined, such as admission requirements for a course level reached in training, for example previous knowledge, skills and attitudes before commencing study of the next section.

(b) *The objective* must state what the student should be able to do, with the basic knowledge required for the safe care of humans, at the end of a specific learning period.

(c) *Intermediate objectives* must point the way to the ultimate objective in broad but definite stages.

(d) *Specific objectives* must be
- relevant to the needs of the learner and the recipient of care;
- reasonable – consistent with what has gone before;
- unambiguous – incapable of misinterpretation;
- realistic – they can be done;
- observable – they can be seen to be done;
- measurable – their achievement can be measured.

(e) *Words used in writing should cause no confusion:* They should be open to only one interpretation where this is at all possible. Such words are *active* and good examples include:

administer	avoid	collect
analyse	care for	compare
apply	categorise	control
arrange	change	decrease
ask	chart	define
assemble	check	demonstrate
assist	clean	detect
determine	operate	select
draw	order	send
estimate	organise	set
explain	outline	simplify
formulate	pick	solve
get	place	sort
give	plan	specify
guide	point	state
identify	position	supply
increase	practise	support
indicate	prepare	synthesise
inform	present	tabulate
insert	prevent	take responsibility
isolate	promote	teach

label	protect	time
list	provide	trace
locate	raise	use
maintain	read	utilise
make	rearrange	verify
measure	relate	wash
move	reload	weigh
name	remove	work
obtain	replace	write

(f) It may be necessary to *explain* the meaning of an objective.
(g) An educational objective consists of the following aspects:
- *Activity* which must be identified in writing the objective
- *Content* of the section
- The *conditions* under which the activity must occur
- *Criteria,* such as the minimum level of performance.

A simple *example* to illustrate the point is as follows:

Objective: The student must identify the name from memory, on a diagram of the heart, the chambers of, and the valves and blood vessels entering and leaving the heart and the flow of blood through the heart.
- Activity: Identify and name
- Content: Anatomy of the heart
- Condition: From memory
- Criterion: *All* the chambers, valves and blood vessels entering and leaving the heart, and the flow of blood through the heart must be identified.

3.2.2 Plan

Having decided upon and written objectives for the course, plan how these are to be offered: at what stage, and at what level? Test your objectives: are they clear, can they be followed?

3.2.3 Implement the plan

Using your tested markers or objectives, implement the educational programme, always bearing in mind the main or co-ordinating objective.

3.2.4 Evaluate

Evaluate the results by using your markers as criteria. This will lead to re-writing, replanning, re-implementation and re-evaluation in the education cycle. A dynamic system of leading students to the discovery of what, to them, is as yet unknown, leads to the ultimate production of the professional person defined in the main objective.

Finally, it is important to realise that all goals and learning objectives determined for the nursing profession must take into account the health needs of the community, the means of meeting these needs, the authorities which provide the health-care facilities and the interaction with the medical and paramedical professions. The learning needs of the student will be geared to preparing her to meet these health-care needs as a well-prepared colleague. The health of the nation depends on this.

The objectives stated must fall within the matrix of nursing care of the person who is the recipient of that care so that the societal, psychological and personal needs as well as the technological skills backed by knowledge and educated judgement are given due consideration.

4 Authorities responsible for providing nursing education in the RSA

It has already been mentioned that Florence Nightingale, in designing her nursing education programmes, did not see a nurse's 'service' as more than only a part of her education. It was never intended that the care of patients should rest mainly in the hands of the students, without whose 'service' the care of patients would suffer. She did not intend that those learning to nurse should provide the labour force of the hospital. It was also pointed out that paying for service had a detrimental effect on nursing education, and this is still valid. Sister Henrietta Stockdale was also an advocate of nursing education being made part of the general education system of the country, and not a 'service' situation, a change she unfortunately could not bring about. Sister Henrietta advocated that nursing education should be paid for and governed by the authorities responsible for general education, in much the same way as the training of teachers for primary and secondary education is financed. This system, she felt, should meet national needs and not only the needs of local services, and in this way the student of nursing would have been accorded the student status enjoyed by others training for professions. Unfortunately this did not take place. In order that trainee nurses be available to nurse the sick, the education of nurses was assumed by hospital authorites who had no knowledge of education as such. They were thus able to meet their staff needs at relatively low costs, the student nurse becoming the work force in hospitals rather than a student professional.

The situation in the RSA today is that there is no direct legislation which authorises any national body to spend any money obtained from the public on nursing education.

A great deal of such money is made available for the provision of nursing education facilities, based on the concept 'that persons in the service of health authorities should receive adequate preparation to enable them to render effective service' (Searle, 1980: 53).

The money used to finance education for service comes from the various health and hospital service provisions in the budget. Money for nursing education comes chiefly from the taxpayer, and is channelled via the various authorities charged with the provision of health services. The allocation of money depends on the types of services which the Department of National Health, Welfare and Population Development, provincial administrations and other health-care bodies are entitled by law to render.

The Cape Provincial Administration promulgated Ordinance No 12 of 1948 in September 1948 which provided for the establishment and control of the training of nurses, midwives and other hospital personnel.

The Ordinance came into operation on 1 April 1948.

This important piece of legislation was the first of its kind in the country. It led to the present-day establishment of nursing colleges, which, in accordance with articles of agreement with the various universities in the Cape Province (namely the Universities of Cape Town, Stellenbosch and the Western Cape, and Unisa which serves the whole of South Africa and is used by nursing colleges situated away from resident universities) provide for the education and training of their students. The original Ordinance was replaced by the Cape Training of Nurses and Midwives Ordinance 4 of 15 June 1984.

This Ordinance entitles the administration of the Cape of Good Hope to establish and maintain nursing colleges, and to enter into agreements with educational institutions in association with these nursing colleges.

Further, it makes provision for

(a) the presentation of training courses and the examination of students, with the approval of the South African Nursing Council
(b) the admission of students to nursing colleges and their release from service to attend such colleges
(c) the establishment of a College Senate, under the authority of the College Council and
(d) the making of regulations which do not conflict with the Ordinance.

Section 4(2)(e) of the Transvaal Hospitals Ordinance (No 14 of 1958) stated that the Administrator could establish and maintain in connection with one or more hospitals 'colleges of nursing or other institutions for the training of persons for service in the Department'. Similar provisions exist in other provinces.

No special provision was necessary for expenditure by the Department of National Education, for once a course is approved at a university or a technikon it automatically qualifies for subsidy (Searle 1980b).

The Health Act, 1977 (Act 63 of 1977) spelt out the functions of the then Department of Health, provincial administrations and local authorities in this regard, so that, broadly speaking, the current *Department of Health, Welfare and Population Development* is responsible for the co-ordination and provision of additional health services necessary for a comprehensive health service for the RSA; the establishment of a national health laboratory service; the promotion of a safe and healthy environment; the promotion of family planning; research in connection with any matter falling within the department's functions; and the provision of services related to the procurement or evaluation of evidence of a medical nature with regard to legal proceedings. Any of these functions, except the first, may be delegated to a provincial administration.

Provincial administrations are charged with the provision of hospital facilities and services, ambulance services, facilities for the treatment of persons suffering from acute mental illness, maternity homes, personal health services, either alone or by delegation to a local authority, and the provision of out-patient facilities.

The whole structure of provincial administrations, their place in the complex pattern of government and their place in the health-care system, which includes the education and training of nurses, is under review. Regional councils may replace these administrations in the future. Under the present constitutional dispensation, health care has been designated as an 'own affair', but details of functions have not yet been worked out, and it is essential that readers watch the development of the supply of care to the population as this occurs.

Local authorities are in accordance with the Act, charged with the maintenance of hygiene and clean conditions in its district. Furthermore, they must prevent the occurrence of a nuisance or any other condition harmful or dangerous to the health of any person, or if a nuisance has occurred, take steps to remove it; prevent the pollution of water and/or purify water; and render approved services in its district for the prevention of communicable diseases, the promotion of health of the inhabitants, and the rehabilitation of any person cured of a medical condition.

Functions of the Department of National Health, Welfare and Population Development or a provincial administration may be delegated to a local authority.

Finance to carry out the above functions of all three health bodies is provided by the taxpayer.

Comprehensive education of the nurse to meet national needs was not possible under the system which developed. Nursing education was a by-product of hospitalisation of the sick who needed treatment of a medical or surgical nature, the mentally ill or mentally defective persons, and those needing the services of midwifery and obstetrical care. Because the education of the nurse was fragmented according to the type of service in which she was 'trained', it was unavoidable that her education was limited and did not meet the total needs of the community for nurses to work in preventive, promotive, curative, rehabilitative, maintenance and terminal-care institutions, non-institutional services, in state health services as well as in the private sector.

Many of the authorities, leading medical men and nurses were very conscious of the deficiencies of the existing system of nursing education but they were unable to change the system.

The fact that nursing education has progressed as far as it has, and that it is broadly based as possible to meet the needs of all citizens of the country, is due in large measure to the foresight of the leading nurse educationalists, and because the South African Nursing Council has been able to tailor nursing education programmes to meet the total health needs of the country. Nursing education must never be seen as the preparation of practitioners to meet local needs only. Taxpayers are not limited to one area or one race and the needs of all of them are the concern of nursing education. Legal barriers to comprehensive nursing education must be circumvented until they are removed.

At present nursing education is financed in the following ways:

(a) Degree and diploma courses at universities are financed from the appropriation of funds of the Department of National Education, by fees from students and in some cases by subsidies or joint appointments for lecturers' posts from provincial appropriations.

(b) Diploma courses at technikons are financed from the appropriation of funds of the Department of National Education, and its counterparts for Black, Coloured and Indian Education.

(c) Nursing schools run by the Department of Health and Welfare from the financial appropriation of funds of that department.

(d) Nursing schools in the self-governing national states from the health budgets of those states.

(e) Nursing schools and colleges run by the provincial administrations from the appropriation of funds by the provincial authorities, and by fees paid by students (nominal).

(f) Nursing schools conducted for the mining industry are financed by the industry itself.

(g) Private (proprietary) hospitals finance nursing education from patient fees, although these hospitals may also receive a provincial subsidy.

It is felt that, because the provision of adequate nursing education facilities is a national rather than a provincial or local matter, the matter of financing nursing education should be put on a different basis and greater use could be made of larger private hospitals which could provide valuable clinical experience for students. These institutions are major consumers of trained nurse labour, but make no contribution towards that training although this is changing. A national policy which could plan and co-ordinate nursing education where the education of the nurse in its totality could be seem as a national priority, would facilitate matters. Autonomous colleges linked with universities now form part of the reform in the financing and implementation of nursing education which is seen as 'education for service'-oriented instead of being a haphazard service with incidental education. The new comprehensive course makes provision for this.

This does not mean that practical aspects of training must be neglected. They are indispensable but they must be properly planned and co-ordinated. The number of hours spent in a unit, however, is not necessarily correlated to experience gained. The student nurse must be primarily a student, with her practical experience related to her educational needs. Such experience should not be tied to a monetary 'payment for service'. The incorporation of various types of clinical experience, from private hospitals, other health services and various types of general hospitals, if it were made financially possible, would produce a far better all-round practitioner of nursing.

The method by which nursing education in this country is financed is under review. As long as nursing service needs predominate, with nursing education as the stepchild of such service, there will never be progress. The education will not be of the standard which it should and can attain, service will suffer, and in the long run the *patient*, who should be the centre of all this activity, will suffer because of this.

The whole matter of the provision of nursing education is so variable at the moment of writing, that only in-depth study of the various educational and training facilities presently available will give a clear indication of the actual state of affairs.

The privatisation of many services is advocated, and independent nursing colleges are coming into being. Again, investigation *in situ* is necessary for the student to understand the education and training facilities presently available in the area in which she works.

5 Regulations affecting nursing education

This chapter will not deal with specific regulations in any detail, but will only highlight the part played by such regulations in determining the planning and organisation of nursing education programmes in the RSA.

Regulations regarding training are drawn up by the South African Nursing Council in terms of the powers invested in it by the Nursing Act. They are then sent to the Minister of Health, Welfare and Population Development and eventually published in the *Government Gazette*.

Changes in regulations are not made lightly. They are carefully considered by specially appointed committees who have the power to co-opt experts in any particular field, and are framed and altered to meet the changing needs of health services. It is the duty of everybody concerned with nursing education to keep an up-to-date file of all regulations relating to the courses offered by the institution in which she works and of changes made to them.

The South African Nursing Council draws up training regulations in broad outline, and supplements them with directives which are more flexible and can be changed as the needs change.

Apart from the regulations of the South African Nursing Council, which must be adhered to by all schools where nurses of all categories are following pre-registration, pre-enrolment or post-registration courses, there are those drawn up by various training institutions such as universities and technikons. These regulations must incorporate *at least* the minimum requirements of the South African Nursing Council, but they may, and often do, require more. Bodies which conduct their own examinations (ie, where the students do not write the South African Nursing Council examinations) make their own regulations regarding internal examinations. The South African Nursing Council, before registering students who receive their nursing education at such institutions, have to approve the programmes followed, and it also has the right to carry out inspections of training programmes. This right is exercised regularly. University and technikon programmes are inspected in the same way as are those of nursing colleges, hospital schools and others.

5.1 REGULATIONS OF THE SOUTH AFRICAN NURSING COUNCIL

Regulations drawn up by the South African Nursing Council follow a broadly based common format under the following headings:

- Definitions
- Conditions for registration
- Conditions for the approval of a nursing school
- Admission to the course of study
- Duration of the course of study
- Curriculum
  - Programme objectives
  - Subjects
- Examinations

The details under each heading will, of course, vary with each course. It would be advisable for nurse-educators, as well as nurse-administrators, to pay attention to these differences, particularly where integrated as well as separate courses are offered.

5.2 SOUTH AFRICAN NURSING COUNCIL DIRECTIVES

The South African Nursing Council directives, which are much more easily changed than are the regulations, supply a great deal more detail. The headings under which directives are framed include at present:

- Philosophy of the Council
- Policy concerning the educational task of the South African Nursing Council
- Subject and subject content
- Annexures to serve as examples for the planning of the curriculum

Changes in syllabi do not necessarily mean that *more* lectures must be given, but that the subject-matter be rearranged according to a new format. For example, when the subject of preventive and promotive health was included in the nursing syllabus and specified as such, many nurse-educators did not stop to think, but metaphorically threw up their hands in horror at all the 'extra' material to be presented. What had really happened was that material which had previously been taught as hygiene, the preventive aspects of infectious diseases, nutrition for health, and many more, were lifted from the theory and practice of medical and surgical nursing, and given a composite name. There was, in reality, very little extra material, simply a rearrangement of what was already there.

There also seems to be a reluctance on the part of nurse-educators to discard outdated subject-matter and techniques, so that a great deal of irrelevant material may still be taught, 'in case it is asked in examinations'. Not a very intelligent approach to nursing education which is aimed at preparing the present and future practitioner, and not some mythical body from the past. With universities and colleges now setting their own examinations this practice should disappear.

5.3 THE SOUTH AFRICAN NURSING COUNCIL: ASPECTS OF ITS EDUCATION, TRAINING, REGISTRATION AND ENROLMENT

The Nursing Act makes provision for the control of nursing education and training in the following ways:

(a) Approval of persons or institutions who offer education or training which is intended to qualify any person to practise the profession of nursing or midwifery. Such courses must be specified and approved
(b) Appointment of examiners and moderators and the examination of persons preparing for registration or enrolment at specified intervals, or approval of the education and examination of other institutions
(c) Registration or enrolment of students or pupils who are undergoing periods of training
(d) Registration or enrolment of persons who have complied with regulations regarding training, or whose qualifications meet the Council requirements for registration. Limited registration, for a period not exceeding two years, is also available under certain conditions, for persons who have trained in other countries and are registered in those countries
(e) Approval of nursing schools in accordance with the prescribed conditions
(f) Inspection of training schools
(g) Approval of training schools for and registration of additional qualifications according to prescribed conditions.

The regulations and directives of the South African Nursing Council provide a basis according to which the discerning nurse-educator could organise her programme in order to educate and train the student to function with technical expertise, so that the patient/client and the attending physician may have confidence in her ability. The patient must be safe and emotionally supported. The patient must be seen in his social setting which the nurse is educated to recognise.

The regulations make it possible for the nurse-educator to concentrate on fundamentals, on principles and meaningful experience correlated with the theory necessary to prepare the nursing professional.

Properly handled and interpreted, such regulations do not restrict, but provide guide-lines and markers along the road to the achievement of professional adulthood by the student of nursing.

5.4 TYPES OF COURSES AVAILABLE

5.4.1 Registration

For the basic training of nurses for registration in General Nursing, Midwifery and Psychiatric Nursing, the following courses have been approved by the South African Nursing Council and regulations have been promulgated:

(a) Diploma in General Nursing for registration as a general nurse. Duration: Three years (except when already registered as a psychiatric nurse, when the training is 18 months). The South African Nursing Council will not conduct further examinations after 31 December 1990.

(b) Diploma in Midwifery for registration as a midwife. Duration: If already registered as a nurse, one year; all other categories, two years.

(c) Diploma in Psychiatric Nursing for registration as a psychiatric nurse. Duration: The registered general nurse, one year. The old three-year course has been discontinued.

Other exemptions can be made at the discretion of the Council.

(d) Integrated courses: It is possible, according to regulations issued by the South African Nursing Council, for basic courses to be combined or *integrated*, when the period taken for the course or the duration of the course is shortened. At present these include:

- A Diploma in General Nursing and Midwifery for registration as a general nurse and midwife. Duration: Three and a half years.
- A Diploma in General and Psychiatric Nursing for registration as a general nurse and psychiatric nurse. Duration: Three and a half years.

In both these diplomas it is possible to add an additional *optional* course in psychiatric nursing or midwifery to give registration in all three *basic* disciplines. This extends the course by a further six months.

The aim of the integrated courses is to present subject-matter on an integrated basis throughout, and to avoid unnecessary repetition.

These courses are not offered at every training school, but many larger centres do train nurses according to this formula.

Examinations conducted by the South African Nursing Council in these courses will also cease on 31 December 1990.

These courses will exist until those presently enrolled in them complete their courses, and those presently registered as general nurses have had the opportunity to be registered as midwives, psychiatric nurses and community nurses (at present a post-registration course, offered mainly at technikons).

53

(e) Comprehensive course: This is a four-year course leading to registration as a general nurse, psychiatric nurse, community nurse or midwife.

This course, which became compulsory from 1 April 1986 for all students registering for the first time to train for registration as a nurse, combines the above disciplines.

The course is run by universities as well as by nursing colleges in conjunction with universities which have a department or sub-department of nursing.

The objective is to produce a nurse capable of analytical, evaluative and creative thinking and able to exercise independent judgement of scientific data. The nurse must be able to supply the nursing component of a continuous, comprehensive health service, that is be able to provide for all the nursing care needs of the community in institutional and non-institutional services.

Subject-matter and practica are integrated throughout the course, so that maximum use is made of the nurse, without unnecessary repetition. The nurse must be seen as a student, whose participation in patient care is part of her learning experience, and not simply part of 'getting the work done'.

5.4.2 Enrolment

The following certificates for *enrolment* as a *nurse* or a nursing assistant are available. Regulations have been promulgated by the South African Nursing Council:

(a) Certificate for enrolment as a nurse. Duration: Two years. A common core with electives in various branches.
(b) Certificate for enrolment as a nursing assistant. Duration: 100 days, to be completed within a period of two years.

It is impossible to give details of these courses in a work of this nature, as changes occur frequently. It is incumbent on the student and the teacher of nursing to keep up to date with what is currently in force.

6 *The student of nursing*

Anyone who is preparing to teach nursing, or is already engaged in this exercise, should pause and consider very carefully the characteristics of the student entrusted to her care. This should lead to an understanding of student needs.

6.1 CHARACTERISTICS OF STUDENT NURSES

6.1.1 Age

Seeing that at least a Standard 10-certificate is required for admission to a course leading to registration, the person concerned will have had a minimum of 12 years successful schooling. This will make the student of nursing approximately 18 years old. There will of course be exceptions, such as those who decide on a nursing career later, but they are very much in the minority. A young person, only 18 years old, coming from the sheltered school environment with its discipline, regular hours, and study and leisure patterns, now finds herself (or himself) in a completely different world with many strange experiences, and the necessity of adapting to clinical practica as well as to human suffering.

At this age, the student is not really out of the adolescent stage, is still seeking a complete self-image, and needs to exert self-discipline in a way never required before. She is subject to changes in mood, with heightened emotionality, which can be compounded by coming into contact with ill persons. No matter how high the service motive may be, there are bound to be times of emotional tension. Understanding on the part of the nurse-educator as well as other members of the registered nurse corps, can do much to reduce this tension and channel it into productive patient care.

The older adolescent, which is what the young student nurse is, may have fewer actual fears than when she was younger, but tends to worry more about more things. In a changed environment such as the nursing laboratory or ward, worry about doing the wrong things, about actually doing harm to a patient, or not being able to measure up to requirements, is ever present. Feelings of inadequacy are not infrequent. She may even withdraw from a situation which is fraught with too many anxiety-producing conditions. Again, understanding based on knowledge of this phase in the development of the human being who is the student of nursing, can do much to reduce tension and prevent unnecessary dropouts.

Social adjustments to the new world of nursing are necessary. The older adolescent has a great need for recognition, affection and understanding. As she grows towards emotional maturity, the student nurse also treads along the path to professional maturity.

As the student it guided in the theory and practice of the art and science of nursing towards independent decision making and the achievement of the ability to plan, implement and evaluate nursing care, the adolescent world is gradually left behind, physical as well as emotional strength is attained and a well-rounded, competent, mature practitioner of nursing is produced.

As long as those in the class-room as well as in the clinical area guide, assist, understand and deal with the problems which may arise without prejudice, from a basis of discernment of what the student really is, the progress towards that professional adulthood should be smooth and give satisfaction to both student and teacher, in whatever situation teaching occurs.

6.1.2 Sex

It has already been pointed out that the majority of students of nursing in the RSA are females. Only 3% of the registered nursing population (1980) are male. This is true of many, if not most of the Western nations. The proportion of males to females is far too low, but it is a fact of life. Male students may find this predominance of the female sex in nursing disconcerting, and may have to make special adjustments to the situation. At present we are dealing with a predominantly female student as well as registered nurse population.

The largest number of males in the nursing profession is to be found in the semi-skilled category, although even here females predominate.

Investigation into the reasons for the lack of males where they are greatly needed, especially in the psychiatric field, is an urgent necessity.

6.1.3 Education

Although the South African Nursing Council has laid down Standard 10 (or 12 years of satisfactorily completed schooling) as a minimum educational requirement for admission to training for *registration as a nurse,* and Standard 8 (or ten years of satisfactorily completed schooling) for admission to training for *enrolment* as a nurse, the subjects which students take for these examinations vary greatly and students recruited into the nursing profession often have a very inadequate background in the scientific subjects. There are various reasons for this, such as:

(a) Insufficient teachers to teach mathematics, physics, chemistry or biology. This applies to all population groups, and is one of the problems of education in the RSA. The limited number of school leavers with a scientific background in turn restricts the number who can be trained as teachers. Science teachers themselves require more than a basic knowledge of science before they can undertake to study science in preparation for teaching. Science graduates are also snapped up on completion of their studies by commerce and industry. Degree study, particularly in the science subjects, is a long and difficult course and the financial rewards in teaching are far lower than those in the private sector. This further limits the teachers, and thus a vicious circle develops.

(b) The selection of 'soft options' as subjects at school. This problem is often compounded by poor advice given to those who indicate that they wish to follow nursing as a career. The lack of knowledge regarding the requirements of a modern nursing course in the way of scientific background by many so-called 'career guidance' officers, is deplorable.

(c) Competition for school leavers with the 'right' (that is the science) subjects, so that many are attracted by commerce and industry, where excellent bursaries are also available for university education.

Because of these factors, large numbers of students are recruited into the nursing profession without the basic scientific preparation necessary for them to cope adequately with the course of preparation for modern professional nursing. It is from those who do pass the course that the teachers of future nurses are drawn. Their shaky scientific backgrounds then have to be made more secure before they can face their usually inadequately schooled students. This adds a great burden to the course for preparation of nurse-educators. Nurse-educators have to teach professional applied science courses of three to four years' duration in a tertiary education course. Many of the older nurse-teachers in the profession and, of course, large numbers of older 'ward sisters' did not themselves receive a good scientific background in their own nursing education. Some have remedied the deficiency in one way or another, but those who have not are left with feelings of inadequacy, which does not make good teachers of nursing practice in the 1980s.

With this lack of educational background, the numbers who can be recruited for degree study at universities where the minimum requirement is matriculation or matriculation exemption, are not sufficient to meet the needs of the country. As a result, students without science subjects have to be accepted by some universities for degree study provided they have the required educational admission standard. These students have a disadvantage from the start.

6.1.4 Population group

The population of the RSA is made up of a multiplicity of population groups, including Asians, Blacks, Coloureds and Whites. Because of this, the students of nursing come from a variety of cultural backgrounds with different home languages. The medium of instruction in nursing education is one of the two official languages of the RSA, that is either Afrikaans or English. The fact that neither of these languages is the home language of the Black population which consists of nine main ethnic groups using different languages such as Xhosa, Zulu, South and North Sotho and Tswana, only compounds the problem. English or Afrikaans is taught at all the schools catering for the different Black national groups, but they remain the second language of the people. It is not the colour of the skin that causes problems, but the difficulty students have in coping with scientific study in a second language, that needs to be fully understood by those teaching nursing students of different population groups.

Language is only one of the problems. Different cultural norms and customs pose another. Various food taboos cause difficulties in teaching nutrition, child care and even hygiene practices.

Normlessness or anomy amongst urbanised groups, who are caught between the traditional cultures from which they have become isolated and Western cultural patterns which they have not yet made their own, is another factor with which the nurse-educator is often confronted.

The fact that there is a backlog which will take time to remedy, is very strongly felt in the lack of teachers for the science subjects. This is an even more acute problem amongst the Asian, Coloured and Black population groups than amongst the White, where it is serious enough. The lack of true competition amongst school leavers, which makes nursing a status profession amongst the Black groups, will also change with time as more career opportunities become available, and nursing will have to compete with other professions to attract the students of the future.

The care of the sick knows no boundaries of colour, race or creed, but the nurse-educator who does not take the problems caused by these difficulties into account, is inviting failure.

6.2 RECRUITING STUDENT NURSES

Nursing cannot hope to gain its proper and necessary share of school leavers without a realistic and co-ordinated recruitment policy. The majority of health-care workers in the RSA are nurses, and as such are vital to the health services.

The RSA covers a vast area, with a multinational population. As various national states become independent, the actual size and constitution of the total population of the RSA changes. The density of the population also varies a great deal, being high in urban areas and low in large rural areas.

Health services have to be provided in areas varying from desolate desert regions to lush subtropical regions, from vast plateaus to very mountainous terrain, from coastal areas to high mountains. There are densely populated, highly industrialised areas, and small, isolated rural communities. There are fishing communities, farming communities and mining communities. Student nurses have to be recruited and trained for all these communities, from remote clinics where there is, at most, a visiting doctor, to the highly sophisticated modern research hospitals.

The disease pattern of the community is as varied as the geographic, social and health-care service depicted. The nurse, when trained, is confronted with a great variety of health-care problems, ranging as they do from elementary community health problems to highly complicated medical treatments, such as transplants. There are old and young people, and all have to be served by nurses.

If the health needs of the nation are to be met, potential students must be recruited for training in the profession. Numbers, however, are not enough – quality is also important. Because, as has already been pointed out, there is great competition for school leavers from the commercial and industrial world, and because of the great ignorance which still exists among school-girls (and boys) regarding nursing as a career, it is necessary for a realistic recruitment programme to be undertaken by all schools where nurse training is offered. The attrition rate which occurs as a result of students not completing their courses can in many instances be attributed to the misconceptions which many potential students have about nursing.

Before embarking on a recruitment campaign, those who will be involved in recruiting should themselves have a clear picture of the characteristics required from student nurses.

6.2.1 A profile of the requirements for nursing students

(a) *Educational requirements* laid down by the South African Nursing Council are the minimum requirements. Every school has the right to raise its own educational requirements, or make them more stringent, by determining which subjects and/or symbols are acceptable to it. By eliminating students with unsuitable subjects and/or poor symbols, the school can reduce the attrition rate, avoid frustration among students, and eventually gain the reputation of being a 'good', that is, a successful training school.

Nursing as a career requires intelligence, academic potential, and the ability to combine study with practical work. During recruitment, the potential student must be made aware of the 'learning' component of the course, for this component forms a major portion of her education.

Often one finds that pupils who are academically weak at school are advised to make a career of nursing, with consequent frustration all round. The situation also arises far more frequently than it should, where nursing students resign when confronted with their first 'block', because they do not wish to follow any career involving study and have thought, or worse, been informed that nursing did not involve study. When confronted with the reality of the situation, with compulsory study and annual examinations, they realise that this is not what they want, and leave.

(b) *Good health,* physical as well as mental: Nursing is not only a physically taxing profession, but involves a great deal of emotional strain, especially for the adolescent student who has not previously been in contact with sickness and suffering. Strict medical examinations before acceptance are essential. A history of emotional instability should not be disregarded.

(c) *Motivation:* The student with a slightly weaker academic record who is truly motivated towards nursing as a career, will usually do as well as, if not better than, one with a very good academic record who is not really interested in nursing.

(d) *A desire to help others:* A sick person is seldom attractive and needs another person's help and care. A young person who seeks to make of her chosen career something worthwhile, someone who seeks a service motive in her life's work can fulfil this need.

(e) Good *interpersonal relationships* with loyalty, reliability, a high moral code, high ideals, patience and tolerance for other people and their failings, are important attributes.

(f) *A strong sense of realism* and the ability to combine practical work with understanding based on learning. An 'all-round' ability is needed.

The recruiter is now armed with a picture of the qualities she is seeking in would-be students. Now comes the most difficult task, that of recruiting enough of such people she has identified as most likely to succeed.

6.2.2 Methods which can be used in nursing recruitment

6.2.2.1 Literature

Many excellent brochures, pamphlets and recruiting literature have been prepared for distribution. Others tend to present an unrealistic, overglamourised idea of nursing.

Brochures are expensive to produce and can be misleading, as information in them may need constant updating. In designing a brochure the comparatively static information, that is that which does not change much, as well as supplementary sheets or leaflets to supply constantly changing information such as training allowances and differences in service conditions should be incorporated. Some form of information leaflet that can be sent to anyone who enquires about courses should be readily available. Brochures could be sent on a regular basis to schools, career guidance officers, parent-teacher associations and women's organisations, where the mothers of possible recruits could be given up-to-date information.

When preparing recruitment literature, the following points could well be borne in mind:

- Use plenty of space.
- Headings must be clear.
- Personalise words and phrases.
- Include illustrations which, although adding to the cost, can be very effective, and attention catching.
- Compile all relevant information such as the educational standard required, subjects which should be taken, the theoretical as well as the practical aspects of the course, training allowances, examinations, working conditions, uniforms, etc.

6.2.2.2 Films, slide-shows, TV presentations and the use of radio interviews

The cost of using media can be quite high, but also very effective. Slide-shows are, perhaps, least expensive to prepare, and outdated slides can easily be replaced. An imaginative slide-show, presented at a 'careers day' or 'careers evening', can be of great interest. If the presenter watches audience reaction and invites questions throughout the presentation, a very lively, informative session can result.

In the making of films or any form of presentation using media, care must be taken that information, both visual and given by the spoken word, is absolutely accurate.

6.2.2.3 Career days

These are popular at schools and universities and can do much, if properly used, to improve recruitment. A static display of photographs is not sufficient. A display of hospital equipment, a mock theatre scene, or some other form of simulated presentation will arouse a greater deal of interest. If well-informed people are available to answer questions, quite a fair amount of recruiting can take place.

It is often a good idea to have student nurses in uniform available, so that prospective students can talk freely to young people who have entered the profession. Questions are much more likely to be asked and answered in this sort of situation, which would never be voiced in the presence of adults, particularly those regarded as 'sisters' or 'matrons' by the schoolgirls, and consequently far removed from themselves.

6.2.2.4 Visits to schools

If nursing is to gain its fair share of recruits among school leavers, a concentrated effort must be made to have access to all the high schools from which possible recruits may be drawn. These schools should be visited regularly, and pupils given information and guidance regarding the career of nursing. Again it is advisable to include student nurses in the recruitment team. The career-guidance teachers should also be contacted and kept up to date with new developments. It is important that the persons chosen to visit these schools be well-informed, have excellent interpersonal relationships, especially with young people, and believe in the necessity for recruitment.

People who do not have a very positive approach can do more harm than good. A person who could do a great deal towards recruiting, but who is often forgotten, is the school nurse. Are these nurses ever approached in a positive way to help with recruiting, and supplied with up-to-date recruiting material? Perhaps an excellent recruitment source is being neglected. A great deal could be achieved not only by the positive image of the practitioner of nursing which the school nurse can present, but also by talking to scholars in the course of her work, and handing out informative literature.

6.2.2.5 The appointment of nursing recruitment officers at provincial headquarters

These people, who should be young, enthusiastic and knowledgeable, with a great deal of initiative, could do a great deal to initiate, co-ordinate and implement recruitment campaigns. Again, those appointed to such posts should want to do this type of work. After a few years they could move on to other posts, or they could be seconded to such posts for three to five years.

6.2.2.6 Visits to hospitals and open days

Arranged visits to hospitals, where interested scholars are given talks by various people, shown slides or films, taken on visits to wards and various departments, shown the college and library where possible, and given the opportunity to talk freely to nurses in training, can prove very valuable in presenting a realistic picture of what nursing entails.

Besides such visits, individuals can be given the opportunity to spend a day or two during school vacations in uniform with a student nurse to gain some idea of ward activities. Scholar nursing where schoolgirls were appointed to the staff for a week or two, and actually worked in the ward, seems to have run into difficulties. Provided the ward and the type of work she was expected to do were carefully selected, this was a valuable means of introducing realism into recruitment.

6.2.2.7 Future nurse-clubs

This is a means of recruitment which has been tried with success in some countries. These clubs form a part of extra-mural activities, and those who show an interest in nursing can become members. They are taught first aid and elementary home nursing, and are taken on organised visits to hospitals, given talks, films or slide-shows on nursing, and interest is generally stimulated. It may be that scholars have too many extra-mural activities already, but it is an idea worth considering.

6.3 THE SELECTION OF STUDENT NURSES

It goes without saying that where public monies are expended on nursing education, the public has a right to expect responsible use to be made of that money. The attrition rate among student nurses is a cause for concern. Careful selection is essential if this wastage is not to continue. Yet the determination of valid criteria against which to predict success in a nursing career, has so far eluded researchers. Perhaps this is why selection is still so haphazard, depending as it does more on the vacant posts and the number of school leavers presenting for training rather than on well-devised predetermined criteria.

Some criteria obviously exist, such as a Standard 10 school-leaving certificate, and good health. Others have been added by some schools where the subjects taken for the senior school-leaving examination, and even the percentages gained in these subjects, evidence of interest in community work and satisfactory performance and behaviour at school, are taken into account.

Aviva Rothenburg, a lecturer in the Department of Nursing at Tel Aviv University, remarked as follows (1978):

> Psychological tests as one of the influential and, in some instances, crucial criteria in selecting candidates to schools of nursing, have long been used, and during the last 25 years have been discussed in literature. Time limitations do not permit a wide review of the literature here. In general it can be concluded that psychological tests –
> * do not predict success in nursing
> * do not predict success in practice
> * may predict success in theory,
>
> and this is true not only for nursing itself.

63

Searle (1980d: 32) states:

> There seems to be no satisfactory way of determining who will measure up to the demands of nursing, and who will be able to cope with the contents. In some instances a battery of tests was used to screen out those who would not have the academic ability, or the personal characteristics to stay the course. It is very disappointing to state that this method was no more successful than the other hit-and-miss methods. Indeed in many instances the results were far less satisfactory . . . Perhaps the battery of tests was outdated in respect of the requirements of modern nursing, or perhaps the advisers to the test constructors were nurses who did not, themselves, understand the nurses' expanding role, their measure of accountability and their level of scientific expertise.

Other criteria that have been suggested, include:

- Entrance examinations
- Letters of recommendation
- Parents or siblings in a health profession
- Previous interest, and participation in the activities of organisations such as the Red Cross Society, St John's Ambulance Brigade, or the Noodhulpliga
- Participation in team activities at school
- Demonstrations of leadership abilities at school
- Impressions of self-confidence, pleasant personality, etc, on personal interview.

It must be remembered that poor selection is not the only reason for student wastage. Unsympathetic handling of the late adolescent and lack of understanding by members of the teaching staff as well as by registered nurses in the practical or clinical sphere can do untold harm. The 'old dragons' of the past may not be as prevalent as they were, but there are still too many students who leave for 'personal reasons' where the fault in fact lies with more senior nursing personnel. A poor role model can put off young, idealistic nurses, while lack of proper orientation to expected duties and behaviour can also play a part.

6.4 COUNSELLING STUDENT NURSES

The student (or pupil, as the case may be) is the centre around which all nursing education activities take place.

In this chapter, the following aspects of student nurses have been examined:

- Characteristics

- Recruitment
- Selection.

Having thus obtained a picture of the student nurse, having recruited applicants to follow a career in nursing, and selected from those applicants persons who are suitable and likely to make a success of their chosen career, the exercise must be followed through to its logical conclusion, that is, the retention of students and the production at the end of the period of nursing education of a well-rounded, competent registered nurse, who will give excellent patient care, will at the same time obtain work satisfaction, and be a credit to the institution that prepared her and the profession as a whole.

The pressures that beset young students of nursing are many and diverse. They often encounter severe illness and death for the first time. They can be beset by doubts as to their handling of patients with serious illnesses. They are themselves experiencing the problems of late adolescence. They are often away from home for the first time in their lives. Small wonder that there is need in their lives for someone to whom they can turn for help, guidance and counselling.

Counselling is a person-to-person form of communication. It is centred around a problem which is very real to the person seeking counsel. It aims at helping or enabling the person in need of counselling to come to his own decision, to make up his own mind, and therefore the choices open to him must be clarified. This may only consist of verbal discussion, or it may involve other forms of active help in the work situation.

The nurse counsellor has to play a supportive role. She is there to act as a sounding board and to provide additional assistance to those caring for the sick, so that difficulties which may well arise from the stress situations inherent in nursing may be recognised and dealt with to the benefit of all.

Counselling is based on a respect for the individual, for his innate worth as a person, for his humanness and weaknesses, as well as his strengths. It is non-judgemental and all matters dealt with are highly confidential.

6.4.1 The characteristics of a nurse counsellor

In order to select suitable people for nurse counselling, the following should be considered:

(a) Should the counsellor be a *trained nurse* or not? A trained nurse may be better able to understand the problems of the nursing situation, but she may bring built-in prejudices and expectations with this knowledge which a non-nurse may not have. One thing is certain, the nurse counsellor should not be part of the authoritarian hierarchy of the health-care institution. A knowledge of the hospital environment and its particular problems and stresses is, however, essential.

(b) A *stable personality* with integrity, a sense of humour, self-control, sensitivity to the feelings of others, tolerance, tact and adaptability is needed.

(c) The ability to *listen* attentively, to engender confidence, and to see the situation through the eyes of the person in need of counselling.

(d) The counsellor should be *available* to people when needed and not be bound too rigidly to office hours. Thus in the selection of a counsellor, account must be taken of the willingness of the would-be counsellor to accept that inroads may at times be made on her 'free time'.

(e) The counsellor must have the ability to build up excellent *liaison* with the authorities without ever being regarded as one of the authoritarian hierarchy by the students. She must know where to find assistance of a practical nature for students when it is needed. This includes medical advice, social assistance and even legal guidance if necessary.

Counselling, therefore, is a service given to individuals in need of assistance which will help them to clarify in their own minds the problem, identify the cause of the problem and arrive at a decision as to the best way, for themselves as individuals, to solve the problem or cope with the situation.

A counsellor must ensure that the atmosphere is conducive to conversation with the student in need of assistance. She must provide a relaxed, informal environment which encourages communication.

The 'office' used for counselling should be comfortable. An atmosphere of formality and authority, caused by the counsellor being distanced from the student, by for example being seated behind a desk, should be avoided. Cosy easy-chairs should be arranged so that the counsellor and her client, in this case the student, can sit face-to-face in a restful, friendly setting. There should be no physical barrier between them.

The counsellor's 'office' or suite should be situated well away from the nursing administration complex, in a quiet area which is not commonly used by large numbers of nursing personnel. The nurses' residence may be too far away to provide a practical 'office' for the nurse counsellor. The chosen site must be easily accessible yet away from general hospital activities and from curious eyes. If the counselling service is to succeed, a great deal of thought must be given to this aspect. People in need of the counselling service may also be hesitant to use it if the whole world passing by sees them waiting to go in. A discreet 'waiting room' away from questioning eyes is essential.

The actual room used by the counsellor should have two doors so that a client may leave by the second door, thus not walking through the waiting room, if she prefers not to do so.

Comfortable seating arrangements should be supplemented by facilities for making tea and coffee. A chance to visit the counsellor unobtrusively and relax with a cup of tea or coffee may help to break the ice and enable the client to talk freely. This could be hampered by a formal setting. An appointment system can be used, but must never be so rigid that it cannot be broken in times of crises. The counsellor will be away from her office on many occasions as part of her activities. There must be a means of ascertaining, by the use of a notice board in her office, or a message to the telephone exchange, where she may be found at a moment's notice.

Having created a physical environment conducive to counselling, the counsellor must also create the right psychological climate. This will be facilitated if she possesses the characteristics already mentioned, including:

- A relaxed, but attentive attitude
- A non-judgemental approach
- The ability to create an atmosphere which encourages frank discussions
- The ability to respond to the client's expression of fears, doubts and conflicts with sympathetic understanding
- Building up a trust relationship, with an absolute guarantee of confidentiality. The counsellor does not pry into private affairs unnecessarily, nor does she divulge information gained during a visit by a student, unless this is absolutely unavoidable for the safety of the student or others, such as patients. Discretion is essential
- The use of a confidential secretary during office hours should also be considered. The secretary would be part of the counselling team, and would have to be very carefully selected. A pleasant, cheerful, discreet person, with a non-judgemental attitude and the ability to recognise and deal with crisis situations in those needing the assistance of the counsellor is essential
- The ability to refer clients to other persons and agencies where this is necessary, without losing the trusting relationship that has been established
- Displaying interest and a desire to help
- Impartiality – when a problem is brought up for discussion with the counsellor, she should not take sides until the subject has been thoroughly investigated. If the student then appears to have been in the wrong, the counsellor only points out mistakes, and presents the other side of the picture. Causes for the situation which is creating unhappiness must be sought, and the student should be given the opportunity to make her own decision. The student's strengths and abilities must be determined and her limitations recognised. The final decision regarding further action must be left to the student. Open-ended questions can be used, and phrases like 'have you ever thought of this possibility . . .?' or 'what would you have done in a similar situation?' or 'let us consider why this has happened; perhaps . . .' are useful ways of introducing alternatives.

Counselling should always be followed up by showing interest in how the student has coped with the situation, either in the area where the problem arose if it was the working area, or by a follow-up appointment. Further guidance can be given if necessary. Visits to a 'problem' working area should be engineered as part of the routine activities, so that a student who has come for counselling on a work problem is never identified, and is not labelled as someone who has lodged a complaint, which might lead to victimisation if it became known. This would negate the value of the counselling service.

A list of some of the problems which students need counselling on, or seek guidance about, include the following:

- Guilt feelings at having failed a patient
- Difficulties with accepting that all patients will not get well or that some will be permanently disabled
- Difficulties with professional nurses in charge of wards or fellow students
- Feelings of inadequacy
- Learning difficulties
- Social activities and problems relating to off-duty
- Health problems and fears
- The special problems of adolescence
- Difficulties with socialisation into the nursing role
- Problems occurring in sexual relationships – boyfriend difficulties
- Doubts about future plans as training nears completion, etc.

The section on counselling has been dealt with from the point of view of a person who acts as a full-time counsellor. Larger hospitals may even appoint more than one counsellor.

It must never be forgotten that many people can and do act in a counselling capacity. This includes the ward sisters, (professional nurses), matrons (nursing service managers), clinical teachers, and tutors or lecturers. The tutors may be concerned with specific problems, such as difficulties with study, examination panic, and other aspects of the formal teaching situation. Condemning a student for poor performance without trying to find the cause for failure is to be deplored. All tutors must realise that they have an important counselling function.

What has been said of the general aspects of counselling applies to counselling in the teaching situation, just as much as anywhere else. The student of nursing is the person around whom all nursing education is centred to prepare her for the professional care of patients and clients. No one teaching the practice of nursing will succeed if the characteristics and needs of the students, who are her concern, are not considered and understood.

6.5 STUDENT STATUS

This is a very difficult concept for many people to grasp. It is well to pause and examine the meaning so that nurse-educators themselves have clarity on the matter. A few definitions of the word 'student' will bring some perspective on this subject: According to *The Concise Oxford Dictionary* (1961), a student is a 'Person studying in order to qualify himself for some occupation – person devoting himself to some branch of learning – person under higher instruction at university or other place of higher education'. *Chambers Twentieth Century Dictionary* (1901) defines a student as 'One who studies; one devoted to books or to any study; one who is enrolled for a course of instruction in a college or university; the holder of a studentship', while *The Shorter Oxford Dictionary* (1965) defines him as 'A person who receives emoluments during a fixed period to enable him to pursue his studies and as an award of merit'.

Thus a student is one who studies, usually at some institution of tertiary education, probably to prepare himself for an occupation or for further study. He may receive emoluments during a fixed period (studentship). *Status* is defined as a 'person's relation to others' *(The Concise Oxford Dictionary)*, and 'state, condition, standing' *(Chambers Twentieth Century Dictionary)*.

Thus 'student status' is the condition, *state* or *relation to others* of someone who is engaged in a course of study, usually at some institution of tertiary education.

The student of nursing is learning to nurse. Her course includes theory and practica. The service element is contained in the prescribed practica as laid down by the registering body, the South African Nursing Council. This body has laid down the minimum time for obtaining learning experience in the various branches of nursing in the new comprehensive course, such as in *general nursing*, where out of a total of 2 700 hours, 800 hours are laid down for midwifery practica, a minimum of 800 hours must be devoted to the practica of psychiatric nursing science and at least 300 hours for community nursing science.

The confusion that exists in the minds of many regarding the 'service' component of the programme of nursing education, is perhaps compounded by the fact that nurses are paid a 'salary' by the employing authority, which is also the authority responsible for providing the nursing education programme. This 'salary' is, in fact, a training allowance or bursary, and should be seen as such. It is *not*, and *cannot be* a payment for services, for the student does not give continuous 'service'. In the first year the student nurse, under a 'block' system for instance, is engaged in the service areas for seven of the 12 months. Four months will be spent in college in 'block' and one month on leave.

If it is realised that she is only in the practical situation for seven of the 12 months of the year and that, except for students attending university to obtain their basic education, there are no tuition fees to be paid, then the amount paid to students would not be so easily criticised. 'Training allowances' or 'bursaries' are now paid, which should remove many anomalies. If they were accorded true 'student status' student nurses would perhaps be more inclined to apply themselves diligently to study. They are now required to pay fees towards their education, their responsibilities in this regard should thus be brought home to them. While they were regarded as part of the labour force and nothing more, the situation did not improve.

Various organisations have expressed views on this matter of student status. As long ago as 1956, the World Health Organisation (WHO), expressed its views as follows:

> The nursing service assignments of students should be based on the *educational needs of the students* rather than on the needs of the hospital. Therefore . . . schools of nursing should be administered as separate entities . . . The budget should be adequate to provide . . . *scholarships, bursaries or stipends* for students who need financial assistance.

In 1966 the Expert Committee on Nursing of the WHO stated, *inter alia,* that –

> while most nursing schools are maintained in relation to hospitals, both classroom and clinical instruction should be under the control of qualified nurse-teachers, thus avoiding the distortion, dilution, or diffusion of student learning that can arise from institutional service demands. Through co-operative planning with the hospital staff (and other health service staff, instructors) nursing schools should plan, provide and supervise *meaningful learning experiences properly related to* the students' needs and theoretical instruction.

In 1952 the International Council of Nurses made the following statement in a published paper, 'The basic education of the Professional Nurse':

> Sometimes student nurses are referred to as hospital workers or employees. There is no objection to the title of worker but employee status and student status are fundamentally different and the chances for sound educational work are better where distinctive titles are used for the two groups and where no wage element or contract enters in to confuse the issue . . . the chief purpose of education is to help individuals live better and serve better. It is not a case of education or service but of education for service.
>
> Principles of learning and teaching must be applied at all times when the student is engaged on practica. Everything she does should be a

learning experience, and should be based on sound theory (summary by Searle 1980b).

And in 1964, the Royal College of Nursing and the National Council of Nurses of the UK stated:

> The students should not form part of the basic staff of the hospital; and The student must be a student in fact and not in name only; the service which she gives must be governed by her educational needs. The student must be financially independent of the hospital service for the first two years of training.

A degree of consensus is evident in all these statements. The accepted interpretation of student status could be the following:

(a) The student nurse does not form part of the basic nursing force essential to keep the hospital functioning.
(b) The student should be subject to educational control and should be assigned to hospital 'service' units for the sole purpose of undertaking that type of clinical work necessary to complement her theoretical instruction, and forge the clinical and theoretical components into an entity.

The Board of the South African Nursing Association has expressed the opinion that the growing emphasis on student status and the effects which the implementation of an undesirable interpretation thereof would have on the profession as a whole, demand immediate attention. South African nurses, having given the matter careful and thorough consideration, must come to a definite decision with regard to the interpretation and implementation of the term 'student status'.

The issue at stake is whether or not the profession is going to insist that supernumerary status be granted to student nurses. The accepted interpretation of student status is as follows:

(a) That student nurses do not form part of the basic nursing force necessary to keep the hospital functioning; and
(b) That students under the control of their training school should be brought into hospital purely to do that type of clinical work necessary to round off their theoretical training.

We must determine how to provide an adequate training for the student without exploiting her in the service situation. Is it possible to reconcile service and education? Does a service situation make of her an apprentice? Is it in conflict with her student status?

These questions demand an answer and the profession will have to come to an agreement on this issue, because divergence of opinion can totally undermine the ultimate aim of nursing education.

The Board is of the opinion that the crux of the matter is this:

> *who* controls nurse training; and
>
> is the amount of practical work which is expected of the student in the service situation in *accordance* with what she needs to become a competent nurse practitioner? Is it possible that because the student has to make such a substantial contribution to the service needs that the aims of nursing education are sacrificed in the process?

It is necessary to investigate the desirability of the situation in which the control of nursing education and the control of the service situation are in the hands of the same person. It is important to remember that the educational aspect is of *first* importance in the professional preparation of *any* student. This principle applies also to the nursing profession. The primary responsibility of the person in control of the service situation is, however, to fulfil the *service needs*. If an administrator has such dual responsibilities as indeed is the case in the majority of the training centres in our country, we are faced with a paradox.

If we are to see this matter in its true perspective it will be necessary to arrive at an interpretation of the term 'student status'.

The Board feels that student status and supernumerary status are not synonymous. Student status in the strict sense of the word embraces the *development of the person* from the stage of being a young recruit to that of being a true student. It also concerns the opportunities in the training system offered the newcomer in this developmental process. In other words, how do we make it possible for her to become a student – a thinking person who asks questions, investigates and in the process learns how to make use of all available learning sources; teaches her to make her contribution, no matter what her role, in all the many service situations she encounters.

The Board regards the development of the student to be possible only if the training authorities realise that the following requirements form the real basis of the development of the student as an efficient member of the health team, *viz*:

(a) a broad professional training
(b) the application of those teaching methods which will help the student to see the opportunities for acquiring knowledge for the independent development of professional potential and for the insight to analyse problems.

It has also become essential to bring home the idea that the student must be taught and helped to arrive at independent judgements; taught how to weigh up and give opinions; taught how to form her own ideas and use her own initiative. She must also develop the ability and the will to work in a team, to adjust easily to new working conditions and above all to cherish her selfrespect and to show regard for others.

The Board maintains that should the student nurse be granted supernumerary status such development would be impossible. The *professional development of the nurse demands much more than the limited opportunities inherent in supernumerary status*. It is imperative that the student nurse be a *member* of the clinical team for, *inter alia*, the following reasons:

(a) In order to enable the student to cope with the clinical situation in all its multiple problem aspects, it is necessary for her administrative ability to be developed.
(b) As a member of the ward team she is taught the extent and nature of her professional responsibility within the clinical situation as a *whole*.
(c) She becomes aware of her role in the team, of her relationship with other categories of personnel in the team, of the possibilities and limitations of their practice, and the maximum contribution of each member towards the activities and co-operation of the team.
(d) She is taught how to become a group leader, how to organise members of the team and how to give detailed assistance. The latter will enable her to be a skilled practitioner at every level and will prevent a functional breakdown of the team in the absence of any one member. Only thus can she develop into the leader of a multidisciplinary team.
(e) Right from the beginning the student nurse is taught professional accountability because within the team responsibilities are allocated to her. These are gradually increased until complete control of the clinical situation can be entrusted to her.

The only way in which the student nurse can develop such independent and responsible nursing practices is by making her a member of the team in the clinical situation from the commencement of her course.

In order to prevent exploitation of the students' service in the hospital it is necessary to emphasise that the hospital should not depend entirely on student nurses for its *unregistered* nursing service requirements. Other categories of workers must be employed to ensure continuity of service in the absence of the student.

The student nurse is entitled either to a salary, an allowance or a scholarship for whatever service she renders.

The problem as to who should have control of the training of student nurses is not insurmountable. The Board believes that the person in charge of the educational programme should have this control in preference to the person in charge of the hospital where the student obtains her clinical experience. However, this does not exempt the nursing service manager and her clinical staff from their educational responsibilities. The Board regards it as essential for the nursing service manager, in addition to her administrative function in the service situation, to occupy a key position in the education staff structure. In this way she maintains a direct concern in nursing education. Both the person in charge of nursing education and the nursing service manager will of necessity have to *co-operate* very closely and *plan together* to ensure a balance between the service and educational needs. Only thus can both groups benefit and nurse training come into its own in respect of service as well as education.

The clinical staff under control of the nursing service manager should also contribute to the teaching. The ultimate responsibility, however, rests with the person in charge of nursing education. It is of the utmost importance that both the clinical and teaching personnel should have uniform objectives in respect of the student. If in addition to awareness and acceptance of interdependence within these two groups, there is also adaptability, leniency and candour, the balance between service and educational needs can be maintained at a high level. This in itself could be a source of learning which the student would be able to use to great advantage.

Student status is not merely a dignity which can be conferred on a person preparing herself for professional nursing practice. It is the *end-result* of a multidimensional process of growth, and it implies much more than the granting of *supernumerary* status. *The concept of supernumerary status will remain foreign to the vocabulary of the South African nursing profession.*

From this it will be seen that the Board feels that the *control* of nursing education should rest with the person in charge of the educational programme rather than the person in charge of service, but that the student nurse be part of the nursing team. Furthermore it is necessary to prevent exploitation of the student's service in hospital – her educational needs come first. Although the student nurse is entitled to a training allowance, scholarship or 'salary' commensurate with the service she renders, the hospital should not depend entirely on the student nurses for the nursing service requirements provided by unregistered nurses.

It can be seen that the financing of nursing education is not at present satisfactorily spelt out, and that re-thinking and re-allocation of funds from the taxpayer's pocket, should be specifically directed towards providing nursing education facilities as such. It should not be necessary for that money to be allocated, as at present, on an *ad hoc* and indirect basis.

Another aspect which should receive consideration is whether the student of nursing should not pay something from her training allowance towards her own education. When nurses receive adequate training allowances they should, as consumers of nursing education, be prepared to pay towards this education. Nursing must not be a stepchild of education, but take its full and proper place in the main stream of tertiary education where it belongs. (From a statement of the view of the Board of the South African Nursing Association regarding the supernumerary status of student nurses, quoted in Searle 1980b.)

Searle comments as follows:

Student status cannot mean supernumerary status no matter what is said in other parts of the world. If the student strength is over and above the personnel requirements of the clinical departments what will there be for them to do? If they are observers they cannot be true participants. They will also be in the way!

This question must be seen in a different light. The educational authority responsible for organizing nursing education should determine what type of practical experience is required to meet the minimum requirements for registration. It should then plan for something in addition to that. Thereafter the educational authority and the hospital and other health service authorities should plan together for the number of student places.

The number of places allocated should be in accordance with some of the service needs of the participating hospital and health service agencies. Under no circumstances should these services rely too extensively on students to meet the needs of the service.

The student force should form part of a pre-determined staffing ratio. The ward personnel structure should consist of registered nurses (and midwives if necessary), enrolled nurses, enrolled nursing assistants, clerical and domestic personnel, and a proportion of student nurses (or pupil nurses as the case may be).

Students should not be paid a salary, but should receive generous scholarships. Such scholarships should be equal to the value of care the student provides. Each service agency should also agree to accept the student as a full member of the team for the period during which the student is assigned to it. It should also help to provide the student with the necessary clinical teaching. For this purpose joint teaching posts should be established between health service agencies and the educational centre.

Every student should be able to learn to care for individual patients in all aspects of health care. They should also learn to manage the nursing care of groups of patients. The student must learn to be a member of the health team in the fullest sense.

Additionally student status should constantly be reinforced by education in principles rather than excessive training in techniques, no matter how rapid the growth in medical technology may be. Discipline through responsibility, personal growth through understanding, the cultivation of enquiring minds are essential features in the development of the professional neophyte (Searle 1980b).

It can be seen from the above that there has been a long struggle for student status and for proper financing of student education and training.

Much that has been advocated over the years has now come about. The student enrolled in the new comprehensive course now pays a fee for formal education and training. Although some colleges implemented these courses in 1984, many of them have only offered them from 1986. It is expected that the implementation of the comprehensive course will prepare the student of nursing for her role in nursing tomorrow's patient in a balanced manner, which at the same time meets her needs for training and education.

Programme objectives (adapted from R425 of 22 February 1985)

(a) Such curriculum shall provide for the personal and professional development of the student so that, on completion of the course of study, he

- shows respect for the dignity and uniqueness of man in his social-cultural and religious context and approaches and understands him as a psychological, physical and social being within this context;
- is skilled in the diagnosing of individual, family, group and community health problems and in the planning and implementing of therapeutic action and nursing care for the health service consumers at any point along the health/illness continuum in all stages of the life cycle (including care of the dying), and evaluation thereof;
- is able to direct and control the interaction with health service consumers in such a way that sympathetic and empathic interaction takes place;
- is able to maintain the ethical and moral codes of the profession and practise within the prescriptions of the relevant laws;
- endorses the principle that a comprehensive health service is essential to raise the standard of health of the total population and in practice contributes to the promotion of such a service, bearing in mind factors from within and outside the borders of the country which pose a threat to health;
- is able to collaborate harmoniously within the nursing and multidisciplinary team in terms of the principle of interdependence and co-operation in attaining a common goal;
- is able to delineate personal practice according to personal know-

ledge and skill, practise it independently and accept responsibility therefor;

- is able to evaluate personal practice continuously and accept responsibility for continuing professional and personal development;
- evinces an enquiring and scientific approach to the problems of practice and is prepared to initiate and/or accept change;
- is able to manage a health service unit effectively;
- is able to provide effective clinical training within the health service unit;
- is acquainted with the extent and importance of the environmental health services and knows the professional role and responsibilities in respect of the services and in respect of personal professional actions where the services are not available;
- is able to promote community involvement at any point along the health/illness continuum in all stages of the life cycle;
- has the cognitive, psychomotor and affective skills to serve as a basis for effective practice and for continuing education.

7 Teaching nursing practice: Aspects of teaching and learning

7.1 SOCIO-AGOGIC ASPECTS: PAEDAGOGY AND ANDRAGOGY

Nursing is an interactive occurrence between humans as social beings. On the one hand is a human being, the nurse, the provider of a special form of social activity, nursing, and on the other is the recipient of nursing care, the patient or client. It was pointed out in chapter 1 that nursing care is not only concerned with the care of the sick person, but that it has a much broader dimension, that of keeping people well, preventing illness, rehabilitating persons into the community, helping them to make the best use of the potential left after illness or injury had struck, and accompanying them to the brink of eternity with care and concern.

The *social* part of the term 'social agogics' is easily understood for it is derived from the Latin *socius,* meaning fellow or companion.

The word 'agogics' is derived from the Greek *agogos*, leader, *agean,* to accompany.

The term thus implies the guidance of fellow human beings. In the nursing situation the nurse recognises human needs in a social interaction setting, and guides her fellow human beings along the path towards health or wholeness as far as is possible. She is primarily concerned with other people.

In nursing education we are concerned with preparing the student of nursing for this guidance function. We must prepare her to recognise the nursing needs of those human beings, well or ill, for whom she is caring, so that she is able to support, help and guide them in an educated, caring way.

In doing this, the nurse-tutor or lecturer is also concerned with social agogics, for she, as a human being herself, is charged with guiding other human beings, namely the students, towards professional adulthood. This is also an interaction situation, a social setting. She accompanies the student as a neophyte, and guides her right through her course of learning and study in order to assist her in fulfilling the desired social role of the professional or registered nurse.

The name is, of course, also applicable to the nurse-educator concerned with the preparation of the enrolled nurse. If nursing is a social activity, then the preparation of nurses for their social role is also a social activity – social agogics is thus involved in nursing and in teaching the practice of nursing.

7.1.1 Paedagogy

This is concerned with the guidance of the child (from the Greek *pais, paidos*) meaning a boy (child) and *agogos* a leader, *agein* to lead; *paidagogos* was the Greek slave who led a boy to school.

Human education is a phenomenon that exists; it is there! It will vary widely in different cultures, but it will always exist in some form. It concerns guidance by an adult, the teacher, the one who accompanies the educand along the path to responsible adulthood.

In nursing education the nurse-educator is faced with a dilemma. She will be involved mainly with the basic student of nursing, with the very young physical but not yet professional adult who may not yet be emotionally mature. Nursing education, where it concerns the young student or pupil and especially in the early stages of the basic course, falls between two stools – being an adolescent or a young adult, not yet a professional but in the process of becoming one.

Adulthood may be defined as a state in which the person has full control over himself and his actions, has moved from dependence to independence, accepts personal responsibility for his actions, can exercise judgement and make decisions, accepts the values and norms of the society (in this case the profession) in which he has his being, and is open to new possibilities and the changes that occur around him. He is capable of self-evaluation and is able to change what he feels to be wrong.

It goes without saying that this 'adulthood' cannot be achieved suddenly. It is a gradual process which is guided by the adult or adults, who act as mentors.

Professional adulthood does not mean being complacent and feeling satisfied that one has attained adulthood. The professional adult, indeed any adult, still has to travel through the rest of his life towards a meaningful fulfilment of his task as an adult, in the case of nursing, as a professional adult.

Searle (1975: 52) points out that 'not only must the tutors be able to transmit the scientific know-how of nursing they must be able to lead the students to an integration of their own spiritual, professional, aesthetic and social values into a coherent philosophy of service'.

It is thus obvious that the nurse-educator needs to be very sure of her aim and what subject-matter she intends to cover with her students. She is not only a disseminator of knowledge, but a person engaged in a vital social activity. A basic grounding in the natural and biological sciences is essential for the nurse-educator, but the human sciences are equally important.

For the nurse-educator, the professional adult represents the image of what the student nurse should become; the role model of the future professional nurse. In the same way, the clinical teacher and the professional nurse in charge of a unit represent the role model, the ideal on which the student nurse should model herself. This is an awesome responsibility. No one can prepare a student for all of the situations which she, as a professional nurse and a professional adult, will encounter – only a foundation can be laid, upon which the student can build in her future career. The student must reach a stage where she is able to accept responsibility for her own actions in her own professional practice.

7.1.2 Andragogy

The derivation of this word is from the Greek *aner*, with the stem *andr-* a man, and *agogos,* leading, literally leading a man, in this case a mature student.

Nursing students in basic courses progress further towards adulthood in their profession. Student nurses have to make some decisions and accept a degree of responsibility fairly early in their nursing careers. A successful nursing education programme needs to take andragogy into account in order to adapt teaching methods to incorporate andragogic principles to meet changing needs.

Andragogy is based on the belief that adults can learn. The adult has moved from a state of dependence to independence. Just as *paedagogy* is the art and science of *leading* and thus *teaching* children, so is *andragogy* the art and science of helping adults to learn. As has already been stated, the young student nurse reaches a stage between paedagogy where she is dependent on professional teachers, and independence where she is capable of independent, autonomous practice. The young student comes into the nursing profession already capable of directing a great deal of her own life, of a great deal of independent thought and action. This must never be forgotten.

The term *ephagogy* might well be used for this phase of becoming professionally adult. This word is derived from the Greek *ephebe*, a male citizen, aged between 18 and 20 years, who was given a special course of education, albeit mostly military. This prepared him for his future role in society, which is the aim of nursing education.

Malcolm Knowles (1971: 53, 54) actually states that in his observation, the child starts to be self-directing in many activities fairly early, starts accumulating 'experience on which he bases future learning', may prepare for social roles by taking on part-time jobs, and experiences the so-called 'adult-like' desire to know.

As the student nurse progresses from dependence to independence in professional practice, she needs to be treated as such. She can be encouraged to accept more and more responsibility for her own learning. This does not mean that the senior student nurse is left without guidance, but that the number of formal teaching sessions, formal lectures and the like should decrease, and be substituted by learning 'packages', 'modules' or other activities.

7.1.2.1 Commitment to learning

The adult learner feels a need to learn and wants to learn. She works towards a clearly-visualised goal. Career possibilities, many of which require post-registration qualifications, are becoming clearly defined, and future directions emerge.

A truly professional nurse, even when not motivated to undertake specific post-registration study, is always conscious of the need to keep up to date in her professional practice. This is seen to be necessary to the provision of excellent patient care, and forms a basis for learning, for searching for relevant reading material and for enquiring from experts and other members of the patient care team. All this provides motivation and the adult learner acquires a commitment towards learning, which may have been lacking previously. A professional nurse who is not committed to further learning, no matter how informal it may be, does not deserve to be called 'professional', nor is she truly professionally adult.

7.1.2.2 The environment for the facilitation of learning

The environment in which adult learners learn more readily is characterised by physical comfort, mutual trust and respect, freedom of expression, the ability and desire to help one another, and an acceptance of the fact that achievement levels in the group will differ.

The *physical environment* must be comfortable. This includes the seating arrangements; comfortable chairs and desks arranged in small groups so that face-to-face interaction is possible, and notes can be taken. The room temperature should be neither too hot nor too cold. Ventilation must be adequate. Lighting must allow all members of the group to see what is happening without straining, and to see what they themselves are doing. Facilities for showing and viewing video or film/slide presentations must suit the size of the group. It may be necessary to have a separate room for film shows. This must also be physically comfortable, including the seating, temperature and ventilation. Pleasant décor which is not distracting is also important.

The *psychological environment* includes ensuring an atmosphere of mutual trust with the 'teacher' of adults accepting the students as persons of worth and individuals, each with her own feelings and ideas. The student must feel free to express her views without fear. Calm debates should be encouraged when disagreements arise as individuals are bound to hold different viewpoints. Preconceived, judgemental attitudes should be discouraged. A general acceptance that some will achieve differently is fostered. Co-operative activities are encouraged and competitive striving is frowned upon.

7.1.2.3 Learning objectives

In the adult group learning situation, mutual determination of learning objectives is desirable. The 'teacher' of the group must encourage the adult students to consider the needs of the group members as a whole, the needs of the institution/s for which students are being prepared to work, or in which they are actually working, the knowledge and skill requirements of the course concerned, and above all the needs of the society which they will be, or are actually serving.

Goals need not necessarily be set too high. In many cases in adult education this is unlikely, unless the goals are to meet the requirements of a specific post-registration course. More importantly, students should realise that solid work is rewarded by the acquisition and retention of knowledge and skills.

7.1.2.4 Responsibility for learning

Adults can accept responsibility, in this case responsibility for learning. From having few responsibilities in childhood, adults progress to having many responsibilities in adulthood. A student nurse who is not properly prepared to assume the responsibilities inherent in professional adulthood, may become registered, but may resign – drop out – from professional nursing because she is given too much professional responsibility too soon. A recently registered nurse is *not* an expert in her field, and this must not be forgotten. Although the adult, the professional adult, must and will assume responsibility for her own future learning, she must be introduced to these needs slowly. A student nurse who, in her basic education and training during the period of preparation for professional adulthood, is gradually introduced to responsibility, will not feel the shock of one day being dependent, and the following day being expected to assume full responsibility. The term 'gradual' must be emphasised. Too much responsibility, too soon, will lead to student resignations, just as too little responsibility too late in student life will lead to resignations of registered personnel.

In post-registration learning experiences, the adult should accept a share of the responsibility for planning learning experiences, again within the framework of the available options, which should be pointed out by the 'teacher', the facilitator of learning. If adult learners are involved in assuming responsibility for planning and organising learning experiences, they become much more committed to it.

7.1.2.5 Focus on principles

Adults have the ability to focus on principles rather than on details, and their interests broaden. They are capable of creative, original ideas and are not concerned only with slavish imitation in the learning situation. Registered nurses must be capable of realising the principles behind their actions, and exercising educated judgement. If they cannot, they are not truly professionally adult. They should be able to sum up a situation, the principles behind nursing action, and to translate the principles concerned into nursing care plans and skills to meet the needs of those in their care.

7.1.2.6 Active participation in learning experiences

Adults do not enjoy 'passive' listening. Active listening is another thing. Asking questions and reacting to offered challenges constitute active participation. So too is involvement in organising groups into teacher-learning situations, co-operative learning projects, independent study, and sharing the results, with the aim of attaining mutual goals. Presentation of the material studied, role-playing and discussion are all examples of active participation. There are many more.

7.1.2.7 Learning based on past experience

Adults have accumulated many experiences. This fact must be exploited to the full so that there is mutual sharing of often very varied past experiences. All this will improve the quality of group-learning as well as individual learning.

7.1.2.8 Readiness to learn

In the adult this is increasingly orientated towards the need for development in a chosen career. If an adult can be roused out of the complacency which leads to obsolescence, then the offering of learning opportunities related to improving performance in the work area, and indeed to progressing up the hierarchy, if that interests him, will succeed. The adult is ready to learn what he feels is important to his area of work.

7.1.2.9 Progression from childhood

This is related to development from selfishness to tolerance, helpfulness to others and altruism. This change in the adult must be known to the facilitator of adult learning, so that it can be used to motivate groups towards mutual help in the pursuance of learning with an unselfish goal such as better patient care in mind.

7.1.2.10 Progression from childish impulsiveness to rational behaviour

The truly adult individual can be expected to behave rationally in the learning experience as well as in the work situation. This must be developed in the clinical situation where the application of theoretical knowledge occurs. As a professional adult, the professional nurse is concerned with guiding the student, and should not only show rational action of which she is capable, but should also lead the student to develop rational behaviour. This factor in the andragogic situation is of great importance to the facilitator of learning. If one expects people to behave like children then they are likely to do so. By expecting them to behave like rational adults and treating them accordingly, a firm basis for successful interaction in the learning situation will be established.

7.1.2.11 Change in time perspective

A change occurs in the progression toward adulthood from postponed application of knowledge and 'learning for future use', to immediacy of application. The adult's desire to learn is directed towards learning which can bring results which in turn is directed to obtaining immediate results. It becomes 'problem'-centred rather than 'subject'-centred (and often vague subjects). This must be emphasised in all ephagogic and andragogic education. If application to a real situation or problem is stressed when presenting subject-matter to the 'adult' or 'nearly adult', greater success will be achieved.

Evaluation, including self-evaluation is an essential part of learning. In dealing with andragogic students, allowances must be made for nervousness, fear of being ridiculed, changes in teaching methods since the student last undertook a course of formal education, and some physical and physiological changes, such as a lack of visual acuity, a somewhat lower reaction time and perhaps a reduction in energy levels.

The motivation underlying the need for learning, the acceptance and mutual trust between students and tutors, and the encouragement and mutual acceptance which can be built up in the group can compensate for all these.

The adult's ability to learn becomes more and more oriented to her expected social role. Thus a good role model in the person of the nurse-educator is essential, not only in the clinical field (the ward or other health service areas) but also in the more formal class-room setting.

7.2 EDUCATION

The word 'education' is derived from the Latin e = from, and *ducere* = to lead. It can be defined as a process of leading the person being e-duc-ated from a state of 'not knowing' or 'not being able to', to a state of 'knowing' or of 'being able to'. This 'being able to' is based on knowledge, and is not simply a technical skill which is applied without understanding the consequences of one's actions.

Education is aimed at the development of the whole person, and not just a specific aspect of his growth or progress. It is concerned with far more than the acquisition of knowledge, skills and the ability to think independently, for it is interested in the development of the entire personality of the person being educated. The nurse-educator would do well to think carefully about this fact. The young neophyte nurses, who are entrusted to her guidance for an important part of their nursing education, must be led to full development of their potential and their personalities.

Stunted physical growth is regarded with pity. Stunted emotional growth and personality development is just as deplorable.

Education is a social phenomenon which has existed since the beginning of time, when the first parents passed on to their children the knowledge that they had gained from life and the skills they had acquired to cope with a hostile environment. Education was and is necessary for the survival of the human race, and has continued to evolve from primitive times. Education began in the home and still does. Human progress throughout the ages, and especially the knowledge explosion of the past few decades, has made specialist education, as a preparation for a diversity of occupations, a fact of modern life. Thus, the nurse has to be educated in order to follow her chosen occupation.

It has been said that all education has a purpose, and is aimed at the attainment of a goal. The goal of nursing education is the preparation of young men and women to take a responsible place in the life-world of nursing, to prepare them to give educated, compassionate and personalised care of a highly skilled nature, on a continuous basis, to those in need of such care.

Nursing education is part of the main stream of education. The education of a professional nurse falls within the ambit of tertiary education, following on secondary or high school education.

Education occurs in a social setting, in a social situation. In nursing, the education of the student takes place in the world of health care. It is the task of the educator to make the life-world of nursing familiar to the student of nursing, and to guide and lead her along the path to professional adulthood.

Initially, the one being educated (the educand) is totally ignorant of the new world which she has entered. She has to master a bewildering number of skills in order to change her state of ignorance to one of knowledge and she

85

has to internalise the values and norms of the life-world of nursing to which she now has gained admittance.

Nursing education takes place largely in the caring situation, although a great deal of background theory is often acquired in a formal class-room-type setting. In the ward or unit situation it is the task of the person in charge of that unit to ensure that the student nurse becomes familiar with the world of nursing applicable to that particular unit. Thus, ability in medical nursing is acquired in a medical unit, surgical nursing in a surgical unit, and so on.

The registered nurse in the unit, by precept and example, by the presentation of a good role model, and by passing on her skill and expertise, has an important role to play. The nurse-educator or tutor should have free access to the units where students are being educated. There should be sufficient time and numbers of this category of nurse to make the correlation of theory and practice more real. Unfortunately, shortages have in many instances removed the tutor from the real life-world of nursing, which is to be deplored.

Education is a life-long activity. No one is ever fully or completely educated. No person can learn all there is to know about everything. No one subject has yet reached a state where all that could be known is known – in fact today's 'truth' often becomes tomorrow's fallacy.

Students are in a learning situation in the area of caring, and as educands they have a responsibility to themselves, to those educating them and to the recipients of their care to learn skills and judgement based on a sound theoretical background, so that they in turn can function as efficient, compassionate, fully competent professional nurses. Moreover, they must be able to hand on skills and professional expertise to future generations of student nurses.

Nursing education is deliberate, planned, purposeful, systematic guidance by the educator of the one being educated. It enables the educand to eventually accept full responsibility for independent action, and to exercise considered, educated judgement in decision making based on up-to-date knowledge in whatever situation she may face in her work. At the same time it must be remembered that nobody can possibly be prepared for every situation with which he may be confronted in practice. Education must lay a sound foundation upon which to build, so that those receiving that education are able to accept responsibility for their own actions based on this foundation.

So much has already been written on education that it would be superfluous to spend much time on it here. In studying education practice, students must read widely and assimilate from their reading what has meaning for them and for the course they are following to prepare them as nurse-educators. Students of nursing education should pause during their preparation as nursing lecturers to consider what their ultimate goal is. The personal deve-

86

lopment which must take place if the course of study is to have any value, is not merely to be seen in terms of gaining knowledge of the natural and biological sciences, the human sciences and the skills of teaching methodology, but should lead to the unfolding of the adult personality of the student nurse-educator so that she will become a more complete personality, and will thus in turn be better able to guide the young developing personality of the student nurse.

7.3 LEARNING

Educationalists have been concerned with how learning occurs ever since education emerged as a separate field of study. Many theories have been advanced to attempt to explain this phenomenon. The fact that every human being has the ability to learn, with the exception of those with severe mental retardation or severe brain damage, cannot be denied. But the manner in which learning occurs has been the subject of much research and of heated debate, and has given rise to various schools of thought.

The student nurse-educator must read widely, and synthesise for herself the thoughts from the various schools. There are, however, some aspects of learning which are basic to all schools of thought, and these will be elucidated.

7.3.1 Definition

Many definitions of this have been given, including the following:

(a) 'Learning is a relatively permanent change in a behavioural tendency that occurs as a result of reinforced practice' (Kimble & Garmenzy 1963: 133).
(b) 'Learning, in contrast to maturation, is a change in a living individual, which is not heralded by his genetic inheritance. It may be a change in insights, behaviour, perception, or motivation, or a combination of these' (Byge 1964: 1)'.
(c) 'Learning can be defined as the process of being modified, more or less permanently, by what happens in the world around us, by what we do and by what we observe' (Munn 1961: 372).
(d) 'Learning is a change in human disposition or capability which can be retained and which is not simply ascribable to growth' (Gagné 1970).
(e) 'Learning can be viewed as some form of change in the behaviour of those participating in the program, primarily cognitive behaviour' (Miller 1964: 18).

There are many explanations of how learning occurs that need not concern us here. For purposes of nursing education, learning could be defined as: *A relatively permanent change which occurs in the behaviour of a human being, both in the cognitive and affective fields, which is brought about by the individual's response to specific situations.*

This change may be the modification of present behaviour; it may be the acquisition of new knowledge and skills which have become part of the new response of the learner by internalisation, or by the elimination of an old response. Before this process can be regarded as learning, a degree of change must be *observable* not only in the practice of skills, but also in the cognitive elements which underlie the intelligent application of technical skills. The learner must be able to exercise judgement in the application of those skills, judgement which flows from knowledge acquired by learning. The change in behaviour must also be relatively permanent if it is to be regarded as learning. Insight, perception and motivation will be developed through learning, in response to what is done and observed in a situation. The situations for learning in nursing are provided by the practical life-world of nursing.

The learner, in the environment which is providing her with learning experiences, is subjected to a constant flow of experiences which impinge on her consciousness, and of which she becomes aware. She can perceive, pay attention, think, memorise and be influenced by suggestion. In order to promote or facilitate learning, the teacher points out possibilities, indicates relationships, makes suggestions, stimulates thought, and encourages the memorisation of salient points. In her guidance of the learner, she proposes changes in behaviour, in practice, and makes study material available. She motivates the learner, keeps learning objectives in mind and also points them out to the learner. Both the learner and the teacher strive towards the attainment of a definite goal. It must be pointed out, however, that *learning can only be done by the learner.* He can be helped and guided but, in the final analysis, *he must do the learning himself.*

In order for learning to occur, the person who is learning must of course have the mental capacity to learn. The response of the individual to learning situations will vary considerably, for each human being is unique. Some have very restricted mental capabilities, and will never progress very far along the road of learning. Although the nurses will have dealings with these human beings in the course of their nursing practice, the nurse-educator will not have them as students.

It is equally true that many who have the ability to learn do not do so and that many gifted people also waste their potential. The reasons are varied: many may not be willing or motivated to make the effort of learning. In the education of the nurse, the nurse-educator may be partly to blame, especially if she fails to make the student understand the relevance of some prescribed subjects to the 'whole', that is, the art and science of nursing. Studying the names of the 'knobs' on a bone may appear as dry as dust. If there is a demonstrable need for that knowledge, which may ensure the efficient nursing of a patient who has injured or fractured that bone or needs an operation, it will be studied with more interest as part of the 'whole'. And this is what nursing education is about.

Learning in itself also generates interest. The acquisition of knowledge leads to a demand for more knowledge. If the young learner can be guided towards acquiring enough self-discipline to make the initial effort to learn, interest will often be generated through mastery of the basic knowledge, and the student becomes so curious to discover more of what is, as yet, unknown to him, that studying, and thus learning, becomes a habit. 'A consummation devoutly to be wished', to quote Shakespeare.

Learning then, is the activity which is necessary to bring about a relatively permanent change in the thoughts and actions of the individual.

7.3.2 Types of learning

Educationalists have attempted to identify the various types of learning. The following is a synthesis of what is generally found in literature.

7.3.2.1 Classical conditioning

This is generally stated to be the simplest form of learning. Pavlov, in his work on the conditioning of dogs, was able to train the animals to show a response to a stimulus that would not normally have evoked that response.

By means of a special apparatus, Pavlov measured a dog's salivation when food was presented. This salivation was a normal physiological response. He then sounded a bell, immediately afterwards presenting food, then measuring the amount of saliva excreted. Later only a bell was rung, and the dog salivated as it had done when food was presented. This was a 'learned' or *conditioned* response. If this part of the experiment is continued, the dog eventually fails to salivate when the bell is rung, and then *extinction* is said to have taken place.

7.3.2.2 Stimulus-response learning (Gagné)

This type of learning is also called 'trial-and-error' learning by Thorndike and 'instrumental learning' by Kimble, and refers to the type of precise learning involving a skeletal muscle action that occurs gradually after a series of repeated performances of the action, until it is perfected. An example is showing a student nurse how to fold a corner when making a bed. The stimulus is the need or desire to make a neat corner. The student observes, attempts to carry out the action, which at first will be slow and clumsy, until through practice she becomes proficient.

7.3.2.3 Skill-learning chaining

This is a further development of stimulus–response learning, where a series of stimulus–response units build up to a skilled action. One action leads to another, until the total skill is acquired. The removal of sutures from a wound could be a case in point.

7.3.2.4 Verbal association

This is the response of the individual to language. It is similar to chaining, although it does not depend on observation but on the existing vocabulary of the individual, so that he learns through the building up of chains through sound.

The learning of anatomical terminology occurs largely through verbal association. In teaching nursing, the interrelationship of various aspects of the curriculum can be pointed out by verbal association.

7.3.2.5 Multiple discrimination

This goes a step further. The individual becomes able to differentiate between the signs and symptoms which distinguish a benign tumour from a malignant tumour. Learning the difference between two sets of symptoms needs discrimination as a mental activity of learning.

7.3.2.6 Learning of concepts

A concept is an internal process representing a common property of objects or events, usually represented by a word or a name. Some concepts are *concrete* and can thus be determined by observation, for example 'redness' or 'blueness' of an object. Objects can be classified according to their colour, shape, texture, etc. Thus, for example, fruit can be distinguished from flowers, and trees from grass.

Abstract concepts are formed by the individual upon recognition of common properties which cannot be seen, but which can be defined and understood. Asepsis is a definable state, as is contamination. Both are extremely important to the student nurse.

Some concepts may be concrete as well as abstract. It is possible to see (observe) when someone is physically lying down at rest, but peace of mind, security, etc are all necessary to achieve the *abstract* form of *rest*, which cannot be seen.

Conceptual learning involves the recognition of common attributes, which can be considered as possibilities. This allows the opportunity for discussion on an intellectual plane, without concrete examples being given to the learner.

7.3.2.7 Learning of principles

This is a further development of concept learning. It is the ability to define the relationships between two or more concepts, and to extract from them a rule or fundamental truth to guide reasoning and action.

Thus it is possible to learn the principles of asepsis and to practise a variety of techniques. The principle of asepsis underlies all that is done in nursing. How asepsis is maintained throughout, what is put where, whether gloves or forceps are employed, and other details are unimportant. Nurse-educators must be constantly alert to the need for the learning of principles. Details are of less importance.

7.3.2.8 Problem solving

This is a complicated form of learning, which occurs when 'two or more previously acquired principles are related or combined to produce a new capability, that can be shown to depend on a "higher order" principle' (Huckaby 1980: 12).

The learner, when confronted with a problem which requires a solution, either in reality or in a teaching format, brings to bear and integrates all the thoughts, concepts, previously acquired knowledge and established principles in order to solve the problem.

7.3.2.9 Social learning

This is a combination of other forms of learning, and is the means by which the individual acquires the social skills of interpersonal interaction.

This section may present a somewhat behaviouristic explanation of what many educationalists regard as types of learning. If they are considered in relation to the fact that the phenomenon of learning exists and that each individual, as a unique being, learns in his own way, in his own time and at his own pace, they are of value to the future nurse-educator. Nevertheless, consideration of the types of learning set out above has its use. A human being can control his response to many stimuli by the exercise of will, which makes him unique. Man will *not* learn if he does not want to do so. The nurse-educator can only guide, direct and point out factors of importance to the student. She can try to motivate, to encourage and make subject-matter available, but the actual learning is up to the student.

Related to learning are matters such as remembering and forgetting. The instance of being unable to recall a name, something recently read, or something that was 'known' a short while ago, is familiar to all. That the older person has a good memory for events that occurred a long time ago, while forgetting recent ones, is also well known.

Memory content may be *short term*, that is it is only retained for a short period of time, or it may be *long term*, which means that the knowledge is stored and can be retrieved or recalled when necessary.

Memory span will depend on many factors and differs from individual to individual. If he is interested, he is likely to remember for a longer period. If he is motivated, his learning ability is better. His state of health, the environment in which learning is taking place and distractions that may occur, all play a part. If it is necessary to telephone someone, a number can be found in the directory, memorised for a short period of time until the number has been successfully dialled, and then forgotten. If one wishes to retain the memory of that particular number for future use, it may be necessary to write it down and repeat it at intervals until it is memorised.

If one learns something thoroughly, relates it to other knowledge and stores it so that it can be recalled at will, long-term learning has been achieved.

7.3.3 Factors which influence learning

There has been much controversy concerning the correct terminology to apply to the factors that can influence learning. They have been called *principles* of learning, *laws* of learning, *conditions* of learning, *postulates* for learning, *processes* of learning and, no doubt, many more. There are many points of similarity, despite the different appellations.

The writer has summarised the common points and used the heading *factors which influence learning* as it seems to fit all the aspects which are mentioned without interfering too much with the theories advanced by the theorist in this field. Learning occurs; it is an accepted human phenomenon. It is also known that the span of memory varies. Various theories on the types of learning have also been touched upon. It has been stated that the learner must be presented with material and guided along the path of learning. Learning can be influenced and it is felt that consideration of those factors which can effect or influence the individual's ability to learn, will help the nurse-educator to plan the learning experiences which she offers her students, as well as to recognise and help iron out difficulties.

7.3.3.1 The individual

Learners are individuals, that is:
(a) Whatever the student learns, she must learn for herself. She is the only one who can do the learning.
(b) Every student learns at her own rate.

The factor of the individual is of vital importance to all learning. Every person who learns is endowed with different abilities which are the products of heredity and environment. It is very difficult to say where one ends and the other begins. It is quite unrealistic to say that primitive people would never make great pianists. If there is never any exposure to music and to pianos in their environment, how could they develop any knowledge of, or interest in, playing? A would-be ballerina needs innate ability. She also needs exposure to ballet from an early age, the will to achieve and the disciplined approach to her learning of the art, which must come from the environment.

Some learners have the good fortune to grasp things quickly and tend to become bored with their slower class-mates. They need a constant challenge to keep them functioning at their peak. The nurse-educator will have the so-called 'bright' student as well as many 'average' students. She must realise that an individual approach to those who need extra stimulus, as well as to those who are having difficulties, is essential for successful teaching. Lack of time and a shortage of tutors can cause problems, but recognition of individual differences can go a long way towards solving them.

There are students who are not deft with their hands and who take longer to acquire practical skills. These are not necessarily poor material. Many aspects of nursing require quite an advanced degree of technical ability, and it is possible to acquire this if the teacher is prepared to guide and to show patience. It is futile to make remarks like, 'Why are you so stupid? Nurse X learnt to do this in next to no time. Your fingers are all thumbs.'

A slow learner is not necessarily a poor learner and given time, may make a better performer than her quicker fellow-student. Her learning of factual material may take longer, but may be more thorough and better internalised than that of the so-called 'brighter' student.

When considering the factor of the individual, it must not be forgotten that individuals also vary considerably in learning prowess. Fatigue, temporary ill-health, emotional upsets, hunger, and many other factors may affect the individual's ability to concentrate, to pay attention and to practise, and his will to learn. A host of things such as very hot or very cold weather, raging toothache, a headache, or sunburn, may detract from learning.

The tutor must be aware of these variations, make reasonable allowances for them, and seek the cause when a student, who until then has been at least an average performer, starts to do consistently badly. Similarly, a bright student who suddenly becomes an under-achiever is exhibiting warning symptoms that something is wrong. The nurse-educator and, in the ward situation, the ward professional nurse, should also be alerted to warning signs. This might prevent unnecessary wastage. Previously energetic, interested students do not 'become lazy', to quote an often used phrase, without some reason. That state should be recognised as a subconscious cry for help, and the reason must be sought. The situation can then be remedied.

7.3.3.2 Motivation

Motivation is that which induces a person to do something, to act, and is necessary for learning. In order to arouse and maintain the will to learn, the student needs a spur, a purpose, an inducement, a *motive*. Motive implies action, physical or mental; it is a dynamic force. Motivation creates in the individual a need or a desire which prompts her to take action. The teacher must stimulate the individual so that she becomes a learner and, what is more, she wants to learn. Motives influence the way in which the individual reacts to a situation, in this case, the learning situation.

There are various methods by which motivation towards new learning may be achieved. They are all of vital importance to the nurse-educator, and are the following:

7.3.3.2.1 *Utilisation of existing motives*

No one, unless severely mentally handicapped or actually unconscious, is so devoid of reaction to the environment that there are no existing motives, which, if recognised and properly employed, can be used to stimulate learning. Some of these motives are:

- Interests
- Needs and desires
- Ideals
- Attitudes.

(a)   *Interests:* In seeking to utilise existing motives, it is necessary for the teacher of nursing to find out what *interests* the students already have. This can be done by discussion, by observation and by letting students write short essays on their hobbies, their extra-mural activities, the books they enjoy, and so on. This knowledge can be used as a background to stimulate interest in the job in hand: learning the practice of nursing. It is presumed that the majority of students of nursing are interested in alleviating the suffering of people who come to them, or will come to them, for nursing care.

The acquisition of new knowledge or skills or the performance of a seemingly tedious routine can become interesting if it relates to the process of nursing and to the care of people being nursed. Filling in countless 'intake and output' charts may seem meaningless, unless it can be seen against a patient's response to medication, for example the reduction of oedema, which brings him greater comfort.

If each 'intake and output' chart becomes a living part of providing nursing care, with a meaning that is intelligible to the student, her interest will be aroused. This interest will stem from her first interest, which was in helping sick people. Her performance in the accurate maintenance of a fluid balance chart will no longer be a boring chore. The original interest, which was a general one, will have obtained a specific interest and learning will thus occur.

(b)   *Needs* and *desires* of students should be determined and full use of them should be made in the process of teaching the student the practice of nursing. These needs and desires are the following:

- *She needs to be recognised as a person:* It is fashionable to talk of preventing *dehumanisation* or *depersonalisation* of a patient. Does this not also apply to a nurse, who is also a person? A nurse of course has to conform to certain norms, be able to put the patient before self, fit into the social role expectation of a nurse, but encouragement, praise when it is due and recognition of her as a person with needs, problems, difficulties and unique attributes, are often lacking.
- *She needs to learn – man needs to know:* He has come as far as he has along the path of knowledge and achievement as a result of searching for answers. Becoming a nurse does not separate the student from the human race. She will be curious, will want to know, will need to know. Questions are not impertinence – they are part of the need to know.
- *She needs job satisfaction:* The more skilled she becomes in handling people and their problems and the more adept at carrying out nursing techniques, the greater the job satisfaction. Learning to care skilfully and with understanding based on knowledge and compassion, is conducive to job satisfaction.

  Even where no cure is possible, job satisfaction can be obtained from the physical and emotional comfort brought to those for whom the nurse is caring.
- *She needs to succeed in what is being undertaken:* The student will want to pass examinations and eventually become qualified, but she also needs those successes which cannot be measured, obtained from knowing that a job is well done, that the person-in-care has benefited. Not only does the student need to succeed, she needs to know that she is succeeding. Many of the intangibles in nursing cannot be measured by the attainment of a diploma or certificate. Praise for achievement from those observing her in the clinical field and encouragement towards patient-care success are part of nursing education.
- *She must feel that what she is doing is relevant:* Tasks often do not seem to achieve anything or appear to have no bearing on patient care. This is also true of subjects studied in the nursing syllabus. It is thus the duty of those teaching nurses to bear this in mind and constantly to point out connections between knowing, learning and doing. Relevance is not always easy to grasp. The true educator makes of nursing education a

united whole, with each section related to the whole concept of quality patient care.

- *She must be confident in the performance of tasks:* No one wants to be unsure and inept, unable to handle people, equipment, records or situations. Guidance towards confident performance in all aspects is essential to good nursing education. No one is confident the very first time a technical procedure is performed. Practice, pointing out areas where improvement can be made, and encouragement at times of supervised practice are necessary. In the skills that are not necessarily technical in nature, guidance in and the opportunity to apply and test patient counselling skills, for instance, are also essential. Questions on how the student would handle a situation, what advice would be given to the patient, and on the whys and wherefores of a clinical condition, are a means by which confidence could be instilled. Here too, a word of praise, of encouragement and advice would contribute towards the achievement of confidence by the student.

- *She needs to feel part of a team – of belonging to a group:* Man is, after all, a social being. He does not live in isolation and nursing care is certainly not carried out in isolation. The student should not feel that her work is of no or only minor importance. Team spirit in the nursing team and in the health care team as a whole, must be fostered. The nurse-educator could also use this need to belong as a motivating factor.

- *She needs to reach her maximum potential:* No one wants to be an under-achiever. The teacher of the practice of nursing may have to help and guide some students more than others, so that, in the end, maximum achievement within the limits of potential is reached. Poor study methods, lack of direction, lack of encouragement, and much more can make the student lose interest. Motivation, to try again, to try harder and to employ different study methods, are all part of using motivation to reach maximum potential.

(c) *Ideals* are of special relevance. So often young students enter nursing filled with enthusiasm and ideals, only to have these decried and broken down, sometimes deliberately, often inadvertently, by more senior colleagues in the work situation. So often the idealistic young student is laughed at, told to 'grow up', that her ideals are 'unrealistic, stupid or unattainable'. The young student, with all the potential energy and force for achieving something for her fellow-man, is made to feel a fool. Instead of promoting idealism, using it and channelling it towards greater achievement, it is so often slapped down until the one who originally had high ideals either gives up or is miserable because those ideals cannot be attained or, even worse, is completely stripped of any idealistic thoughts and becomes as indifferent as the rest.

True, some ideals need the leaven of realism, but the striving for something better is always commendable and the nurse-educator should make use of whatever ideals students cherish so that they become motivating factors and not millstones around the necks of those who possess them. Indeed, ideals could well be fostered in those students who do not possess them or who have already learnt to repress them.

(d)   *Attitudes* are closely related to ideals. The student brings attitudes (settled modes of thinking) to nursing which have been inculcated by previous education and experience. Attitudes relating to values such as honesty, co-operation, loyalty, courtesy, sympathy, diligence, perseverance, fair-play and concern for others are all very desirable attributes in the nurse and should be fostered. The student may also bring less acceptable attitudes such as intolerance, impatience, laziness, casualness and negligence which, if a success is to be made of a nursing career, will need to be identified and eliminated. The teacher of the practice of nursing must seek the positiv attitudes and use them as motivating factors and endeavour to eliminate those which are less desirable.

7.3.3.2.2 *Formulation of objectives to be achieved*

The objectives must be clearly discernible by the students so that they will be motivated to learn in order to attain the objectives. The motives are thus based on these objectives. Objectives which are readily understood include the following:

(a)   Attaining a qualification for the purposes of
- obtaining work;
- earning more money;
- obtaining promotion;
- improving performance;
- attaining greater status.

(b)   Acquiring a new skill or improving on an old one for the purposes of
- obtaining more job satisfaction;
- being able to perform some special task;
- improvement in self-esteem;
- gaining the ability to pursue a specific hobby with greater enjoyment and satisfaction. This could include a very wide variety of subjects from flying to gardening; from embroidery to bricklaying.

The utilisation of motives can easily be integrated into teaching and therefore into learning. Definition of the end objective can be of inestimable value to the student of nursing or, for that matter, to any member of the health team, so that a motive on which to base learning, is achieved.

97

The use of the motivation factor can contribute a great deal to initiating and facilitating learning.

7.3.3.3 Totality

This means seeing the whole picture, and not just its component parts. It implies the learning of a *whole* as opposed to parts. A great deal has been written about this aspect of learning, and the question has been posed as to whether it is better to try to learn *all* (the total amount of) the material required, or whether it should be broken up into various parts, which are then mastered separately. Much has been said in favour of both methods. It is generally believed that seeing the *total picture* first and then breaking it down into parts for learning which must be continuously referred to the 'total' frame of reference, is acceptable and desirable. Where the material to be mastered is vast and can logically be broken into smaller sections, this must of course be done, provided that the student is constantly reminded of the 'wholeness' or totality of the material. Teaching a student of nursing basic sciences, whether natural or biological, without relating this to physiology and the necessity for being able to understand normal functions before proceeding to the study of abnormal functions and the care of the sick person, is a case in point. The sciences and physiology are usually presented to the student as separate entities, as are disease states. The totality of the picture must, however, be continuously emphasised so that the end result, the efficient, compassionate nursing care, based on the knowledge gained from the study of these and other subjects and synthesised by the student, is seen by the learner as the ultimate objective of any learning being acquired at that time. The subject-matter is broken down into meaningful units which can be mentally rebuilt constantly as in the case of a jigsaw puzzle but in more practical terms.

In order to make a jigsaw puzzle, a picture is transferred to a piece of board. This is then cut up into pieces or units, which have separate shapes and colours. These are then reassembled to form the original picture. Component units have been re-united in a composite whole: a total picture. Similarly the subject-matter of a nursing course can be broken up into separate units. They must, however, be seen as part of the composite whole, namely the art and science of nursing.

7.3.3.4 Satisfaction

Satisfaction as a reinforcement of learning is closely related to motivation. It is nevertheless considered separately by many educationalists and the same approach is followed here.

It has been said that man needs to learn. He wants to know. He wants to achieve. He wants to become someone and something. The satisfaction he gains from learning, knowing, achieving and becoming is vital to his continuing development. Job satisfaction is an important factor in any work situation. The student of nursing wants to learn nursing so that she can nurse effectively. Her particular satisfaction is derived from being able to help and support, from a position of knowledge, people in need of a special kind of help and support. The student of nursing needs to move towards the acceptance of responsibility for her nursing actions and towards the ultimate exercise of educated judgement in the provision of nursing care. The student needs the satisfaction of knowing what is being achieved, and of feeling that learning is occurring. Some of the learning will be *intrinsic,* such as the knowledge that the student as an individual has learnt, has become more observant and more dextrous or has contributed to someone's comfort or peace of mind. Other learning, particularly in the early stages, will be *extrinsically* engendered, and will come from the teachers.

Encouragement and judicious praise of work well done as professional independence is gradually attained, will do much to help the student learn. The need for speedy knowledge of results is well known in the educational field as a stimulus to further effort in learning. It also enables remedial action to be taken timeously when mistakes have been made. This is part of the satisfaction factor. To know that one has done well, or if one has not, to be able to correct errors before they become habits, ultimately leads to satisfaction.

This factor can and should be applied in the class-room. It is equally important in the clinical area. The ward or unit is the preformed field for the education of the student of nursing and should be properly utilised as a means of bringing satisfaction to the task of learning the practice of nursing.

7.3.3.5 Practice or repetition

An essential part of learning is the fact that, in order to perform a task or a technique skilfully, it needs to be repeated until it is mastered. A great deal of clinical learning involves the acquisition of technical skills, although technical skill which is not backed by knowledge and judgement is not sufficient. The factor of practice or repetition therefore merits consideration by those engaged in teaching the totality which is skilled nursing care.

Some acquire technical skills more rapidly than others. This is related to the first factor discussed, that of the individual. There is no hard and fast rule regarding the number of times a technical skill has to be repeated before it is mastered, or the length of time each practice session should occupy. Rest periods between repetitions often improve learning.

Once a technical skill is acquired it can be maintained by less frequent repetition. Even if a technical skill is not used for some considerable time, optimum performance would quickly be regained if it had been truly mastered in the first place.

Thus continual repetition of a skill, once mastered, is no longer learning, but simply the performance of a task which has to be done. It is often held up as an *example of experience* that someone has done a routine job for years. Experience of *what*? Of monotonous repetition, nothing more! Varied experience, entailing constant new learning, is more valuable and takes up far less time. A student of nursing who is sent to a specific ward for the purpose of furthering her nursing education and spends three months (or 480 hours) of so-called *medical experience* doing simple, routine, often housekeeping tasks, is not learning nursing.

Once a student can make a bed, she can make a bed. She may lose a measure of dexterity through lack of practice, but that is quickly regained. Learning to make a bed all over again is completely unnecessary. Granted, beds do have to be made frequently. As part of the care of the sick person who occupies the bed all the time or uses it for varying periods of time, this will be part of the totality factor of giving nursing care. Senseless repetition, by making many empty beds on a daily basis, teaches her nothing. Many other examples come to mind.

One wonders if, in our teaching of the practice of nursing, the whole point is not often missed. Should units not be staffed by a fairly stable group of enrolled nurses and enrolled nursing assistants, with fewer students, who could then really be involved in learning to nurse the patients, without the unnecessary repetition of routine tasks, that is repetition which is unnecessary for learning? No one would say that a student nurse, once bed-making had been mastered, should never make a bed again – but that bed-making should then become part of patient care in its totality, and not an end in itself.

The student must always be deeply involved with patient care, and should be part of the ward team, not supernumerary to the ward staff, but truly a *learner of nursing*.

7.3.3.6 New learning based on previous knowledge and experience

In all fields of learning, the learner is constantly building up knowledge and skill on the basis of what he has acquired in previous learning acts or events. The failure to attain more difficult and complicated knowledge or skills may be due to the fact that previous material was not thoroughly mastered. The whole technique of programmed learning, with its built-in aspect of remedial learning of previous material which was not properly mastered, is based on this evolving aspect of learning.

The fact that material that is learnt for examination purposes is forgotten immediately afterwards, is well known to nurse-educators. They are confronted with a group of students who passed their first examinations extremely well after a comparatively short period of crammed 'learning', and who then left college and returned to the wards or units for several months, usually with absolutely no follow-up teaching. On their return to college for the next 'block' period, previous knowledge of say, anatomy, has been forgotten because it was not reinforced in the meantime and new learning cannot be built upon what no longer exists. Thus re-learning has to be instituted. The basic problem is, however, that the knowledge was never really acquired in the first place, probably because the subject-matter was not seen in its totality.

It must also be remembered that reinforcement can be given in the unit situation, for if the learning acquired in the previous block is used as the basis for acquiring new technical skills, then the block 'learning' will become more permanent, and the skills will be mastered more rapidly. The link between previous knowledge, previously acquired skills, and new, desired performance must be clearly seen.

A better integration of theory and practice in the wards or units is urgently needed if learning only for examinations is not to be perpetuated. It is important that each ward or unit professional nurse must be aware of exactly what students are taught in college, and know the stage which each student in her ward or unit has reached in her nursing education, so that she can use this knowledge to build on when teaching in her unit.

Some training schools are using self-instructional modules for students to use between periods in college. These are all based on building on previous knowledge and experience.

It is of course absolutely essential for any nurse who is trying to guide the learning of anyone else to find out or pre-test the extent of previous knowledge before planning and implementing a learning programme. In this way the factor of new learning based on previous knowledge and experience can be integrated into teaching so that learning takes place.

7.3.3.7 The use of meaningful material

This factor is closely related to the previous one. The use of previous learning relates to what is now to be learnt in a meaningful manner, so that the student can see the relationship, and learning will be facilitated. It is simpler to learn a phrase that has some sense or meaning than to learn a jumble of unrelated words. It is also simpler to learn new material if *meaning* is given to it, meaning based on past material and on the total learning programme towards achieving the ultimate objective.

Man has the ability to use language, employ concepts and think. He has invented the words which make up his language and may use these to state a problem and work out a solution. He can see the relationship between things and is able to put together elements from previously acquired knowledge and experience to make something new. The material thus used must, however, have clearly discernible meaning in the new context, or it will be discarded. The teacher who can point out the relationships between old knowledge and experiences and that which still has to be acquired, will give the subject-matter meaning and the 'new' knowledge will be assimilated more readily.

The search for meaning in subject-matter, so that it can be presented to students in a way that will stimulate their interest is vital.

7.3.3.8 Active participation

It has already been stated that the *learner* is the only one who *can learn*, that the learner is an *individual*, who needs to be *motivated* to learn, needs *practice*, and needs to *base new learning* on old within a *meaningful context of totality*. The last factor influencing learning which will be discussed here, is interwoven with all these factors, which are in any case interdependent. This factor is that the learner needs to participate actively in her own learning. She learns by *doing* and not always in the physical sense, although this may be part of it. *Doing* can also include perception through the use of the organs of sense, such as sight, smell, touch and taste, or the perception of meaningful relationships by the use of thought. It has often been stated by the protagonists of 'teaching machines' that the learner needs to be physically active to be participating. This is a debatable point. If the learner is *actively listening*, she may actually be learning more than if she were physically pressing a button or writing down a fact. Watching attentively could be just as active as a more physical action. But it must be *attentive* watching: questions are to be asked when anything is not clear, and the 'watching' is not just standing around mechanically looking in the general direction of what is being demonstrated, without paying any attention.

An example is when a student of nursing is taught how to bath a baby. The technique is demonstrated with careful explanations being given of relevant points, details given of observations to be made, of pitfalls that can occur, and of how to avoid these. The learner then proceeds to practise the technique under the watchful eye of the teacher, until she can carry it out without assistance, with complete safety, and with the relevant background knowledge to enable her to deal with any eventuality.

The student has participated in learning throughout, from watching and listening to actual 'doing'. So many students, as well as teachers seem to think that learning 'just happens', and that if the students are physically present in a class they will somehow learn. This is not the case. If they do not participate actively, even if it is mental and not physical participation, they will not learn. No amount of 'teaching' will remedy this. The time which the student puts into learning, studying or attempting to master knowledge and skills is not measured in terms of the time passed with books or in a class, but in the time spent in active participation, mental or physical or both.

102

Without active participation in the act of learning, learning will not take place. The student should not only receive but must contribute and participate.

7.3.4 Some general comments on learning

Learning may occur in many ways, including:

(a) *Imitation:* This may be the conscious or unconscious copying of another's actions, skills or even manner of speaking. The importance of a good role model from the registered nurse is thus clear.

(b) *Trial and error:* This method could also be called 'trial and success'. The learner may be called upon to act in a situation of which he has no previous experience, in which case he may base his actions on theoretical background. But if he is called upon to act when confronted with alternatives, he will be forced to choose. It may happen that several attempts are made until the correct response is chosen. This would then be through 'trial and error'. A first correct response would be 'trial and success'. Hopefully the errors would ultimately lead to a correct response, namely success. It is a wasteful method of learning and in the sphere of nursing may even be dangerous.

(c) *Guided practice based on sound theory:* This is a more certain (and safe) method of learning, resulting in the achievement of co-ordinated, meaningful action. In this way new learning is based on previous knowledge and experience.

A few other points that merit consideration are the following:

- The student must be *ready*, physically and mentally, to learn. This readiness does not relate to motivation, but to physical development and intellectual abilities. It is especially applicable in the learning of young children. In more advanced courses, the student who has passed a basic course may be unable to proceed. Sometimes emotional maturity and experience may lead to readiness. The educator must exercise judgement here. Ill-health can also affect readiness. The ill student may be 'ready' upon complete recovery.

- The *emotional climate* in which learning must take place may affect the learner's ability to learn. Not only the emotional climate in the clinical area, but that of the home, the social scene generally and in the school of nursing may be relevant. Worries about health, parents, children, money and many other matters could affect learning.

- *Forgetting is part of learning:* Even that which has been thoroughly mastered will be forgotten if not used, but once the knowledge and/or skill is again required, re-learning will take place very quickly.

7.4 TEACHING

Thus far various aspects of education and learning have been considered. The teacher or nurse-educator has frequently been mentioned. It is now appropriate to look at the phenomenon of teaching itself.

7.4.1 Definition

At first glance a definition of what we all know exists appears to be easy. But is it in fact so? Dictionary definitions *(The Concise Oxford Dictionary)* include:

- Enable or cause person to do by instruction and training
- Give lessons at school or elsewhere in (eg nursing) or to (eg student)
- Give instruction to or educate
- Explain, show.

Chambers Twentieth Century Dictionary adds:

- To direct
- To guide the studies of
- To impart knowledge or art to
- To counsel.

Still others gleaned from various authors are:

- To facilitate learning (Guilbert 1977: 205)
- Creating environments in which learning can occur (James 1975: 1)
- Causing to learn (Hughes & Hughes 1959: 354)
- Concerned with helping a pupil to acquire knowledge and skills (Gunter 1977: 10).

A synthesis of these ideas seems to suggest that teaching involves helping, guiding and enabling a person to learn. It facilitates learning and creates an environment in which learning can occur. It is a social activity occurring between human beings. It may involve conscious activity by which a teacher tries to teach, or an activity from which a student learns, but which has not been consciously designed for that purpose. The registered nurse, by acting out her role model, unconsciously teaches. It is not a deliberately planned activity, but occurs as a result of a situation – by example – while nursing the patient.

Deliberately planned teaching activity also forms a considerable part of the education of the nurse for her future role. It is a human activity which requires interaction between human beings and if it is to be effective, that activity must take place by means of a two-way stream. The teacher who gives, creates an environment for learning, is actively involved. The same can be said of the learner. No one-sided activity this, with the teacher instructing and the learner receiving passively. If learning were a matter of absorbing like a sponge what is presented, then teaching machines that churn out facts in endless repetition would long ago have replaced the teacher.

The teacher is irreplaceable. It is only the teacher who can notice students' reactions and difficulties and who can test and probe to find causes for non-achievement, and for learning problems. The teacher who can find material and make it available, and constantly reviews and re-models presentation, at the same time constantly learns herself.

In teaching it is as well to remember that nothing is taught until it has been learned. The environment for learning created by the teacher will help the learner to identify strengths and make use of them, realise weaknesses and work on them and concentrate efforts towards a goal. Hyman (1974: 6) further says that teaching has three levels of meaning: the first level of meaning is an 'occupation' and the second the 'overall cluster of activities which we associate with a teacher, such as explaining, demonstrating, questioning, attending faculty meetings, advising students, and taking attendance', while the third level of meaning refers to a 'specific cluster of activities which includes such acts as explaining, questioning and motivating and excludes such acts as patrolling the hall, chatting, taking attendance, sharpening pencils, distributing textbooks, and collecting homework papers'.

The art of teaching is then a specific cluster of activities which assists the learner to learn.

7.4.2 Qualities of a teacher

In order to make a successful teacher, what qualities should be sought? Because teachers are individuals, these will obviously be varied, but some general guide-lines which should lead to success are the following:

The good teacher should be:

- Knowledgeable about his subject
- Up to date
- Interested in his work
- Enthusiastic
- Innovative
- Creative
- Interested in the wider world around him
- Intellectually gifted, yet able to discern the problems of others
- Able to bridge the gap between the world of the student and that of the adult (in the case of nursing of the professional adult)

- Possessed of
  - a sense of humour
  - patience
  - humanity and human kindness
  - a good memory
  - determination
  - emotional stability
  - motivation
  - communication and leadership skill
  - good health
  - the ability to use language well and clearly
- Personable.

An impossible catalogue of virtues? Perhaps. No one will possess all the qualities in full measure, but knowing what they are gives a guide to selection and a goal towards which the prospective teacher can strive. Perhaps some of the problems encountered in nursing education are caused by the fact that nurse-educators tend to be educated in isolation, away from the mainstream of other student activities, and that they are not really developed as well-rounded individuals, but rather as 'specialists' in the nursing field, who are being prepared to educate nursing students, also in an isolated environment. With the exception of students who attend university courses, diploma 'colleges' are colleges of nursing only, and students are not given the opportunity to mix with students following other courses. Their academic isolation is complete. Perhaps the value of the nurse as an independent professional worker in the broader society would be more apparent to other professions if her education took place where more cross-pollination of minds from students in other disciplines occur. Too much of the 'cloistered' person who has a 'vocation' clings to the public image of the nurse for her real contribution to society to be widely appreciated.

7.4.3 A few principles of teaching

The following are offered as guide-lines to successful teaching:

(a) *Good teacher-learner relationships* will facilitate teaching. The teacher who endeavours to know her students and to recognise their strengths and weaknesses, their previous knowledge and experience, and can create a climate for mutual trust, so that students are able and keen to ask questions and express problems, will go a long way. A teacher cannot afford the luxury of being prejudiced on moral or behavioural issues, or to have preconceived ideas about students, their background, language and possible reactions. Stereotyping, if applied to students, may sabotage the whole learning event.

(b) *The learning needs of students* must be determined. These are not based only on the curriculum, but on knowledge of students and their specific needs, as well as those of the health services for which they are being prepared.

(c) *Teaching and learning time* must be planned and co-ordinated. Impossible learning loads must be avoided.

(d) *Evaluation of results* both by the teacher and the student is important.

(e) *Effective communication* between students and all those who are concerned with their nursing education is vital.

(f) *Learning objectives must be clearly formulated* and known to students and teachers, so that these can be used as guides for evaluating results.

(g) *Teaching can be learned.* Practice, the use of guide-lines and the will to succeed will enable the teacher to achieve the goal. There are no 'born teachers'. Some have more natural abilities than others, but that is all.

(h) *The teacher should control the learning environment* so that the student has the facilities and opportunity to learn. This is part of the task of teaching, namely to facilitate learning. It may be necessary in the clinical field to seek for appropriate learning experiences. It may, in some circumstances, be necessary to use a simulation technique. If the student is to learn, she must not only be comfortable in the learning environment, but it must provide her with the opportunity to learn.

The education of the student of nursing should be under the direct or indirect supervision of educaton and *not* of service.

8 Systems used for teaching nursing

In order for teachers to teach and learners to learn nursing practice, some sort of systematic approach is necessary.

In chapter 2 the development of nursing education was reviewed, from the days of empirical learning, through learning from those in practice, through the apprenticeship systems, which today still bedevil the issue, to the nursing colleges and the modern practice of universities offering nursing education.

During this time many systems were developed and are still being evolved. Nursing education, like every other form of education, cannot be allowed to stagnate if it is to be effective. It must constantly seek to improve present means and find new and more effective means of preparing its practitioners so that its ultimate aim of providing the people in need of nursing care with the most efficient, up-to-date and humane care possible, may be attained.

Nursing practice has kept pace with medical practice, with developments in technology, with increased knowledge of man himself and how he thinks, feels and acts in various situations. It is not only medical knowledge that has bearing on the care of those in need of nursing care. Studying the humanities is of vital concern if man is not to be depersonalised, but is to be seen as a total human being with actual or potential health problems.

The South African Nursing Council has laid down minimum requirements for practica which students have to undertake in wards and units in the hospital setting, and also a minimum number of hours to be spent in the community. Minimum requirements for the presentation of theory are also laid down.

It is, however, particularly important that theory and practica be correlated. Systems of nursing education must therefore be devised according to which courses would be organised so as to meet all these requirements. The following points should then be considered:

(a) A balance between theory and practica must be maintained.
(b) Full use must be made of the time allocated for practica, so that the *education of the student* is promoted, and that appropriate practica is arranged at the appropriate level in training.
(c) Practica periods should be *evenly distributed* so that the service situation is not flooded with students at one time and completely without any at another. Haphazard allocation would not be conducive to good education of the student or to good patient care.
(d) Students must not provide the full work force of units. They should be

members of the team, but the purpose for which they are attached to the team is an educational one. They will give service in the process, but it must be planned service with a learning component, and not simply to get the work done. There should be enough other personnel, trained and assistant, to make this possible.

(e) Students must be prepared to write their examinations as scheduled. When they present themselves for training, the authorities have a responsibility to ensure that the students are able to complete the course within the specified time-limit. If students do not contribute their share and fail their examinations, they themselves lengthen their period of training. A lengthened training period should never be the fault of the authorities.

(f) Students must be reasonably able to cope with both the theoretical and practical amount of work required of them. They are *students* (and must be seen as such) and thus learners in the practical and theoretical areas.

(g) The organisation of the course must allow the student sufficient time to do *independent work*, as well as to make use of the library.

(h) It must be possible for students to consult with teachers regarding problems with their studies, or anything else for that matter.

(i) Time should be available for students to practise various nursing techniques, if necessary under supervision.

As far as teachers are concerned, the organisation of the course must leave teachers time

- to read, study, attend updating lectures, and generally keep up to date;
- to spend in the clinical area to observe present patient care;
- to spend in marking tests, examinations or assignments;
- to give guidance in the preparation of projects;
- to spend with students who have problems;
- to devote to clinical teaching;
- to prepare and update lectures and teaching programmes in general;
- to prepare audio-visual material;
- to try out new teaching methods;
- to discuss teaching programmes with other members of the teaching staff.

Factors which will influence the organisation of courses will include the following:

- The time allocated to theory
- The time allocated to practica
- The number of trained tutors available

- The availability of outside lecturers
- The number of clinical teachers available
- The time available to unit professional nurses to teach
- The ability and willingness of unit professional nurses to teach
- The support available from nurse-administrators in the allocation of students according to their educational needs and educational background and insight of these nurse-administrators into the education of students
- The number of students at various levels of training
- The policy regarding the intake of students per annum
- The language media of courses and number of students in each group
- Student attrition rates
- Policy regarding keeping service running by filling student posts with pupils and nursing assistants so that students can use their time productively from an education point of view
- The minimum requirements, theoretical and practical, laid down for the course
- The proximity of class-rooms to practical areas
- The policy regarding duplication of lectures, etc
- Whether the nursing college serves one or several hospitals, and if the latter, how far they are from the college
- Availability of facilities such as class-rooms, adequate libraries, etc. Project work and assignments cannot be used as teaching methods under any system if there are too few books and periodicals to which students have easy access
- Prescribed examination dates and portion of course which has to be completed before students are eligible for examination
- Other entrance requirements, including internal examinations or assessments which have to be met
- Availability of clerical staff to deal with record-keeping and other organisation details.

8.1 THE BLOCK SYSTEM

This system is probably most generally in use in the RSA, and the one with which most nurses are familiar.

The word 'block' has many uses in the English language. The sense in which it is used in the connotation of 'block system' is that of a 'section or portion', in this case 'of the course of nursing education'. The manner in which the system is applied, causes one to wonder whether another meaning of the word block, that is 'obstruction', 'making inactive' would not be more appropriate, for many of the features of the block system as presently implemented obstruct rather than promote true nursing education! The block system owes its origins to technical education, where blocks or sections of theoretical instruction are interspersed with blocks or portions of practice.

As it was originally devised and expected to be implemented, it was a good system, for the theoretical instruction was only planned to give a grounding in the basic principles, and follow-up work was expected to be undertaken throughout the practice periods. It was never intended that the system should divide the indivisible into separate compartments.

The system was first used in nursing education in Sweden, and was introduced into South Africa in 1943 by Miss EM Pike, then matron of Groote Schuur Hospital in Cape Town, in its full form.

In practice the block system divides the syllabus into sections. Students are then removed from the practice situation for a varying period of time, and attend a nursing college or the lecture department of a hospital or nursing school full-time. During this time the section of the syllabus allocated to that particular block is covered.

The time spent in the class-room may occupy from one-fifth to one-third of the total period of the course. Thus, if the three-year diploma in general nursing is taken as an example, from 7½ to 12 months may be allocated to college or class-room attendance in the three years (for practical purposes it would actually be from eight to 12 months in 36 months). This time would be divided between the first, second and third years of training and blocks would be so arranged that students would complete the relevant subject-matter in preparation for the first-year, second-year and third-year examinations of the South African Nursing Council. During the intervening time, the students do full-time clinical or community health practica.

An example of how the block system may be implemented, is as follows:

FIRST YEAR

Subjects
General Nursing Science I (Fundamental Nursing Science)
Anatomy
Physiology
Applied Sciences I (Chemistry, Biophysics, Microbiology, Parisitology, Nutrition, Pharmacology)

Practica
General nursing science
Community nursing science (Introduction only)

Examinations
General Nursing Science I (Fundamental Nursing Science)
General nursing practica

111

Anatomy
Physiology
Applied Sciences I (Chemistry, Biophysics, Microbiology and Parasitology)

SECOND YEAR

Subjects
General Nursing Science II
Applied Sciences II (Nutrition and Pharmacology)
Social Sciences I
Midwifery I
Psychiatric Nursing Science I
Ethos and professional practice

Practica
General nursing science
Community nursing science
Midwifery
Psychiatric nursing science

Examinations
General Nursing Science II
General nursing science practica
Applied Sciences II (Nutrition and Pharmacology)
Social Sciences I

THIRD YEAR

Subjects
General Nursing Science III
Social Sciences II
Ethos and professional practice
Community Nursing Science II

Practica
General nursing science
Community nursing science
Psychiatric nursing science (Principal component)

Examinations
General Nursing Science III
Social Science II
Psychiatric Nursing Science II
Psychiatric nursing science practica

112

FOURTH YEAR

Subjects
General Nursing Science IV (Ethos and professional practice)
Community nursing science
Midwifery II

Practica
General nursing science
Community nursing science
Midwifery

Examinations
General Nursing Science IV (Ethos and Professional Practice)
General nursing science practica
Community Nursing Science
Community nursing science practica
Midwifery II
Midwifery practica

The actual periods of class-room attendance and practica must be determined by the colleges and institutions providing practica in accordance with Government Notice R425 (1985) and anything appearing in directives issued by the South African Nursing Council from time to time, and curricula approved by that body.

In order for the block system to be successful, it is essential that when the student is away from the class-room, correlation of theory and practica takes place, that clinical instructors, ward personnel and tutors continue the theoretical instruction, and that there is compulsory project or assignment work by students throughout. This is one of the greatest weaknesses of the block system as presently implemented, for without continuous motivation for the student to study and learn, it can become a glorified 'cram system', with very little benefit being derived from the clinical practice. When it is realised that the longest period of the student nurse's education is spent in the area of clinical practica (24 to 21 months), then the importance of organising this to promote *education* cannot be overlooked. *Teaching and learning* the practice of nursing *cannot* occur in nursing colleges or class-rooms only.

The block system can be applied to one hospital and its lecture department or college, or to a group of hospitals with students attending a central college. The continuation of their nursing education outside the college is of equal importance in both cases.

113

As with any system, the block system has its advantages and disadvantages.

8.1.1 Advantages

8.1.1.1 Facilities

In a central college or class-room unit, provision can be made for

- enough class-rooms of appropriate size with all amenities;
- good audio-visual materials and equipment;
- a well-stocked library;
- study areas;
- laboratory facilities; and
- hiring extra facilities when necessary.

8.1.1.2 Personnel

- Fewer tutors can handle more students (this is no excuse for a reduction in the number of tutors, but by centralising, better use can be made of them than by spreading them thinly over many small schools).
- Suitably qualified personnel can be more readily obtained in larger centres.
- Teaching personnel can keep up to date more readily in large centres, with access to developments in the health sciences as well as trends in education.
- Teaching time can be regulated and vacation time arranged so that the workload of tutors is evenly distributed.
- Tutors have time for preparation, including the preparation of audio-visual material.
- Outside lecturers for specific subjects can be obtained more easily by larger centres.
- Use can be made of specialist nurses to give lectures within the range of their expertise.

8.1.1.3 Students

- Students are freed from the stresses of the ward situation.
- The medium of instruction can be chosen.
- Supervised study periods can be arranged.
- Group student projects as well as other group activities can be undertaken.
- The library and other learning aids such as tapes and slides, are readily available.

114

- An atmosphere conducive to study can be created, away from the disturbance of other students who do not wish to study in the evenings. Those in college are all there for the same purpose at the same time.
- Tutors are readily available to deal with problems in learning or lack of understanding of subject-matter.
- Weekends are free for a specified period each year.

8.1.1.4 General

- Field trips can be readily arranged.
- Experimentation and research in teaching methods and other areas are facilitated.
- Programmes, which include the part to be played by clinical instructors and unit professional nurses, can be worked out and tutor time in units with students can be organised.
- Wards know exactly what personnel are available for the whole month.
- Smaller hospitals can continue to train in association with a college.

8.1.2 Disadvantages

- Block periods could become cram periods, which is educationally unsound and leads to easy forgetting.
- Shortage of tutors could lead to classes which are much too large. This imposes an added burden on tutors:
  - There are more papers/tasks/assignments to mark.
  - There is no time for keeping up to date.
  - There is little time for preparation.
  - Pressures cause frustration.
  - Tutors cannot practise in the units and lose touch with nursing reality.
- If carefully planned extension work and follow-up between blocks is not followed, students do not see clinical practica as a learning time, but simply as a job to be done.
- A student who becomes ill during a block period will miss lectures and catching up may not be possible. Such a student would then have to attend a later block which could lengthen the training period.
- Slower students may be left behind.
- Long hours of continuous lectures, can produce poor learning if not broken by other activities.
- Thirty-four percent more student nurse posts are required under this sys-

tem than under the old daily lecture release system, which makes it more expensive.

- Correlation of theory and practice can easily fail.
- Unequal numbers of students at different levels of training can be withdrawn from the wards at different times of the year, depending on intake and whether or not blocks are duplicated. This could lead to too few students or senior students at one period, and too many students at another.

8.1.3 Implementation

In order that the block system may be successful, the following are essential:

- Careful planning
- Clear statement of objectives
- Co-ordination of teaching and clinical instructors and unit staff
- Regular consultation as well as close liaison between all categories of personnel responsible for the education of the students in the class-room, ward and unit
- Allocation of students to units according to their learning needs
- Sufficiently trained teaching personnel with a promotion structure that will draw them to teaching
- Correct nursing practice in the clinical situation so that theory and practice are actually correlated
- A planned programme of extension work based on reality and student needs, and which is properly implemented
- Provision of learning material such as relevant, up-to-date textbooks and other literature in the wards and units so that students have the opportunity to look up relevant points as they occur when caring for patients *then and there*, and do not need to wait to go to the hospital or college library
- New material should not be provided just before an examination
- Theory must run parallel to what is required in the clinical situation
- Theory blocks must be planned so that students obtain the maximum benefit. They must not be postponed because of service requirements. Proper planning should prevent this
- Clinical teaching must also be done on night duty.

8.2 THE STUDY-DAY/S SYSTEM

This is a system which sets aside a specific day or days each week for work in the class-room, library and study time, field trips and testing.

This method might be applied to the three-year diploma in general nursing, as follows:

FIRST YEAR

Class-room attendance: Two days per week for 40 weeks
Subjects: As for the first year of the block system
Clinical practica: Three days per week for 40 weeks; four to eight weeks' full-time night duty (four weeks' optional night duty)
Leave: Four weeks
Examinations: The same as for the block system

SECOND YEAR

Class-room attendance: Two to 1½ days per week for 40 weeks
Subjects: As for the block system
Clinical practica: Three to 3½ days per week for 40 weeks; four to eight weeks' full-time night duty (four weeks may be optional full-time day practica if only four weeks are spent on night duty)
Leave: Four weeks
Examinations: The same as for the block system

THIRD YEAR

Class-room attendance: 1½ days per week for 40 weeks
Subjects: As for the block system
Clinical practica: 3½ days per week for 40 weeks; four to eight weeks' full-time night duty (four weeks may be optional full-time day practica if only four weeks' night duty is worked)
Leave: Four weeks
Examinations: The same as for the block system.

This system does require a great deal of careful planning and co-ordination, and can be combined with short blocks as well. It can be adapted to any course.

8.2.1 Advantages

- Study time, as well as time for project work, can be provided during 'study days'.
- Students are away from ward stress because they are released for full days (or half days in later years).
- Theory is presented more slowly so that the slower student can keep up with the class.
- Regular, spaced testing is possible.
- Time is available for the repetition of material that has not been grasped in the first instance.

- Time is available for the student's self-activity.
- Interest is stimulated throughout by constant, continuous exposure to both theory and practica.
- Many varied teaching strategies can be employed.
- Student illness does not cause disruption of the course.

8.2.2 Disadvantages

- Organisation and administration are much more difficult.
- The tutor may have different classes at different stages of training during the week, which could make preparation more difficult.
- Class-room facilities must be near the clinical practica area. Thus it is an unsuitable system for smaller hospitals, which need to send students to a centralised college.
- Wards have to be more alert to student study days and off-duty planning is more complicated.

8.3 DAILY LECTURE RELEASE SYSTEM

This is really the 'bad old system' according to which students attend lectures during the week on release from the wards. The release should, of course, be in duty time but lectures may have been arranged in off-duty periods, although the student can be compensated in terms of time by being given a longer off-duty period. An off-duty period which is interrupted by a lecture is not very satisfactory.

8.3.1 Advantages

There are very few advantages:

- Theory and practica can be correlated more readily.
- Subject-matter can be presented gradually and regularly.
- Students have time to assimilate gradually.

8.3.2 Disadvantages

- Duplication and even triplication of lectures is necessary every day.
- Organisation is very difficult.
- Wards are constantly disrupted by different students being released for lectures at different times.
- When the ward or unit is very busy, it may not be possible to release the student when the lecture is due. She may thus arrive late or not at all.

118

- Students are subject to stress. Their minds wander back to the situation they have left, and attention is not given to the lecture.
- No time is provided for study, library work, etc, except when off duty, which is not conducive to good learning.
- Tutors' time is not used to maximum advantage, and their preparation time, time for updating and time for clinical work are reduced to a minimum.

8.4 DAILY CONCURRENT THEORY AND PRACTICA SYSTEM

In this system the student attends lectures either in the morning or the afternoon, and does clinical practica for the rest of the time. It is a system that is in use at most universities. The theoretical work is usually presented during the term when the university is open and full-time practica is undertaken during university vacations, except for the *leave* period allocated each year. Night duty can present problems, depending on the number of students.

Good organisation is essential and the ratio of theory to practica should be 1:1½. That is, in a week of 40 hours, 16 hours (or two days) should be allocated for theory, including study time, and 24 hours for practica. The difficulty arises when students follow courses from other disciplines, as timetable arrangements may make it impossible for study days to be arranged, and students may have to be released daily for varying periods. In one university it has been possible to arrange lectures so that the students spend full days on the campus and full days in the wards, and this is really what a true study-day approach entails.

8.4.1 Advantages

- Good correlation of theory and practica is possible.
- If properly planned, study time as well as time for project work, assignments, etc, can also be fitted in.
- If students are away for half-days, ward professional nurses know and can make arrangements accordingly.
- Student illness does not cause too much disruption.
- Students can be stimulated and motivated by what they are learning in class, or experiencing in clinical practica.
- It is possible to expose students to a variety of lecturers and teaching techniques.

8.4.2 Disadvantages

- If this system is not properly organised, students are subject to a great deal of stress as they may have to miss lectures or arrive late.

- Wards may have to release students at crisis periods or at odd hours which can be disruptive.
- If students attend classes most mornings, and only do practica in the afternoons, they never experience the ward at peak periods, and therefore do not have a realistic picture of ward work.

Organisation is of vital importance if this system is to succeed.

8.5 THE MODULAR SYSTEM

This is a system of training that is increasingly finding favour in various countries. In order to understand what a module is, it is well to go outside nursing for an example. Advertisements are found daily in our magazines and newspapers for 'modular' furniture. By buying appropriate modules of different sizes and with different functions, which can all be linked together, it is possible to build up a wall fitting, a series of kitchen fittings, a room divider and other useful composites. Each module forms a unit and is designed for a specific purpose, such as a cupboard, a desk surface, shelving of varying widths, areas for storing bottles, glasses, and many more. Each unit or module is in itself functional, but linked together, makes a composite whole. Extensions can be made, modifications brought about to meet changing needs, and the time taken to reach the end result can be spaced according to requirements.

If this concept were then to be applied to nursing education, careful thought and some imagination would produce units of work which

- belong together;
- can be related to others; and
- are extensions or modifications of those previously used.

Shore (1973) describes a module in the following way:

> The term 'module' is used in at least three contexts in education.
>
> In secondary education, particularly in North America it often refers to a block of time from 10 – 50 minutes within a school's daily timetable. These modules of time are combined in various numbers to provide class sessions of different length and study periods for students. A much less common use of 'module' is to describe a small group or cell of students who work together. A third meaning of 'module' and one assumed here is a unit of instruction, usually self-contained.

Goldsmid and Goldsmid (1973) define a module as 'a self-contained, independent unit of a planned series of learning activities designed to help the student to accomplish certain well-defined objectives'. They also maintain that 'while differences in definition exist, it seems to be generally agreed that a module is a curriculum package intended for self-study'.

Shore (1973) maintains that there are four different types of modules:

- *Modules based on complete existing courses:* Sequential presentation of units of work.
- *Modules based on parts of existing courses.*
- *Supplementary course modules* which can be used
  - to fill in gaps in existing knowledge
  - for remedial work
  - to supplement laboratory work
  - as preparation for further study.

- *Modules on general topics:* Those which are not compulsory components of a course.

If one is to use modular instruction in teaching the practice of nursing, then those planning modules must study the course as a whole, and ensure that the overall objectives are achieved.

Nursing requires the acquisition of theory, and practical skills based on that theory. In all the systems discussed previously, the necessity for correlating theory and practice has been stressed. How then could a modular system of nursing education be devised?

It is realised that this course is being phased out, but studying the example given will demonstrate how a modular system of nursing education can be planned and implemented.

The work, or rather the syllabus and related clinical practica would need to be divided into units, such as the following:

Diploma in general nursing – three years

Module/unit

		Weeks
1	Basic theory units of introduction to the natural and biological sciences, including laboratory work	4
2	Introduction to the social sciences	4
3	Anatomy consolidation	2
4	Medical Nursing 1	12
5	Medical Nursing 2	12
6	Surgical Nursing 1	12
7	Surgical Nursing 2	12
8	Physiology consolidation	2

9	Paediatric Nursing 1	8
10	Paediatric Nursing 2	8
11	Community health nursing	8

The specialised departments

12	Intensive care	10
13	Urological nursing	5
	Gynaecological nursing	5
14	ENT nursing	
	Ophthalmic nursing	10
	Orthopaedic nursing	
15	Operating theatre	10
16	Out-patient department and casualty	10
17	Out-patient department and casualty	10
		144

52 weeks per annum × 3   = 156
− 12 weeks' leave   = 144

Modules 12 to 17 can also be divided into smaller units.

The first two units or modules will be largely class-room-orientated, although a certain amount of daily exposure to the clinical situation would be possible after the first week.

Another unit of two weeks should be allocated during the first year to prepare students for the South African Nursing Council's first-year examination. Theory for this examination will be included in the modules taken during the year.

The rest of the year can be divided between medical nursing (module 4) and surgical nursing (module 6).

Commencing at the first intake of students, modules could be allocated as follows:

YEAR 1

Weeks	1	2	3	4	5	6	7	8	9	10	11	12	13
Modules/units	1	1	1	1	2	2	2	2	4	4	4	4	4

Weeks	14	15	16	17	18	19	20	21	22	23	24	25	26
Modules/units	4	4	4	4	4	4	4	6	6	6	6	6	6

Weeks	27	28	29	30	31	32	33	34	35	36	37	38	39
Modules/units	6	6	6	6	6	6	9	9	9	9	9	9	9

Weeks	40	41	42	43	44	45	46	47	48	49	50	51	52
Modules/units	9	3	3	LEAVE				13	13	13	13	13	13

YEAR 2

Weeks	1	2	3	4	5	6	7	8	9	10	11	12	13
Modules/units	5	5	5	5	5	5	5	5	5	5	5	5	12

Weeks	14	15	16	17	18	19	20	21	22	23	24	25	26
Modules/units	12	12	12	12	12	12	12	12	12	7	7	7	7

Weeks	27	28	29	30	31	32	33	34	35	36	37	38	39
Modules/units	7	7	7	7	7	7	7	7	10	10	10	10	10

Weeks	40	41	42	43	44	45	46	47	48	49	50	51	52
Modules/units	10	10	10	13	13	13	13	8	8	LEAVE			

YEAR 3

Weeks	1	2	3	4	5	6	7	8	9	10	11	12	13
Modules/units	11	11	11	11	11	11	11	11	14	14	14	14	14

Weeks	14	15	16	17	18	19	20	21	22	23	24	25	26
Modules/units	14	14	14	14	14	15	15	15	15	15	15	15	15

Weeks	27	28	29	30	31	32	33	34	35	36	37	38	39
Modules/units	15	15	16	16	16	16	16	16	16	16	16	16	17

Weeks	40	41	42	43	44	45	46	47	48	49	50	51	52
Modules/units	17	17	17	17	17	17	17	17	17		LEAVE		

This is roughly how units could be divided. They could be interchangeable and should be correlated with South African Nursing Council examinations.

Each intake is divided into groups and, beyond units 1 and 2 and at the appropriate time, 3 and 9, some could be allocated to medical units while others go to surgical units.

The basic theory given in units 1 and 2 must be built on and integrated throughout all the other units, and units of different years must be interwoven, so that wards always have their full quota of students. One large master plan would have to be drawn up for every training school wanting to make use of modular training.

Each unit, except 1, 2, 3 and 9, would then consist of the following:

(a) A period of one week for introducing the theory of the module
(b) A period of six to eight weeks, depending on the length of the unit of practica with related theory given daily, every second day or twice a week throughout
(c) A period of one week for revision, consolidation, and examination in the lecture department.

Clinical assessments and projects are allocated to each module. Failure of a module requires repetition.

The tutor and clinical instructors are responsible for the theoretical instruction throughout the time spent on the module, and they accompany students into the clinical area, liaise with the ward staff, and help with the correlation of theory and practice, clinical practica and clinical assessment.

Students thus know their module tutors and instructors and vice versa, which will ensure that problem areas are identified and dealt with timeously.

This system requires a great deal of organisation, adequate teaching staff and excellent liaison with clinical areas.

The programme must make allowances for the following:

• Covering the portion of the syllabus at the required time

124

- Night–duty allocation, which can be done on a system of internal rotation within the module
- Meeting leave requirements
- Meeting service requirements
- Proper allocation of tutors and clinical instructors, either on a specialist or a rotation basis, depending on the policy and capabilities of personnel.

This is an idea of the way in which physical planning of the modular system could be applied to the diploma course in general nursing for registration with the South African Nursing Council. A similar pattern could be drawn up to include the additional time and subjects of the new comprehensive course. It must be emphasised that each module designed, except for the introductory one, is a combination of theory and practica, and that the tutors are closely involved with their students in both the class-room *and* the clinical situation throughout the module for which they are responsible. In a comprehensive course this would necessitate work in the midwifery, psychiatric and community nursing areas.

A more modular arrangement is the following:

A tutor or clinical teaching professional nurse should be allocated to each group, and be concerned with the teaching of clinical nursing practica and the integration of theory and practica, so that these become one 'whole'. The tutors and clinical teachers should move in and out of college with their groups. Those offering other sections of the syllabus should do follow-up work where this is applicable. The whole course must be approached on an integrated basis.

FIRST YEAR

4 weeks	*Orientation*
	Selected theoretical instruction and clinical practica in fundamental nursing science
12 weeks	*College attendance*
	Divided into three periods of four weeks, spread throughout the year
28 weeks	*Clinical practica and guidance*
	General nursing science divided between college attendance periods
4 weeks	*Consolidation*
	Theory
	Study periods
	Examinations
Four weeks	*Leave*

Subjects to be covered
Fundamental Nursing Science (General Nursing Science I)
Anatomy ⎱ could perhaps be combined as Anatomy and
Physiology ⎰ Physiology I and II
Applied Sciences I

SECOND YEAR

8 weeks	*College attendance*
	Divided into two periods of four weeks spread throughout the year
4 weeks	*Leave*

Subjects to be covered
General Nursing Science III
Social Sciences II
General Nursing Science IV (portion of syllabus)
Community Nursing Science
Midwifery II

THIRD YEAR

8 weeks	*College attendance*
	Two periods of four weeks, spread during the year
16 weeks	*Clinical nursing practica* in general nursing science, divided during the year, with guidance throughout
4 weeks	*Community nursing science practica*
	Students, when allocated to community nursing science practica combine theoretical instruction with clinical learning experience under guidance
16 weeks	*Midwifery*
	Students, when allocated to midwifery practica, combine theoretical instruction with clinical learning experience under guidance
4 weeks	*Consolidation*
	As in first year

FOURTH YEAR

30 periods	Theoretical instruction, planned withdrawal of students from the clinical situation as required
20 weeks	*General nursing science practica,* with special attention to ward management and professional practice (This latter aspect will

	have been stressed throughout, but will be given practical application in the clinical situation.)
16 weeks	*Psychiatric nursing science practica*
	Students, when allocated to phychiatric nursing science practica, combine theoretical instruction with clinical learning experience, under guidance throughout.
4 weeks	*Consolidation*
	As in first year
4 weeks	*Leave*

There have been many variations on the scheme proposed above, but the one outlined here, combining as it does a good deal of the modular system – which could be further adapted – would be one way of completing the syllabus, and ensuring the spread of clinical learning experiences under the continuous guidance and assistance of tutors and/or clinical teaching professional nurses.

20 weeks	*Clinical practica* with tutor and teaching professional nurse guidance throughout
8 weeks	*Midwifery practica*
	During this period theoretical instruction is also included
8 weeks	*Psychiatric nursing practica*
	During this period theoretical instruction is also included
4 weeks	*Consolidation*
	As in first year
4 weeks	*Leave*

Subjects to be covered
General Nursing Science II
Applied Sciences II (Completion of syllabus)
Social Sciences II
Midwifery I
Psychiatric Nursing Science I

Once units or modules have been identified and a time span allocated to each, the detailed planning of each module must be undertaken. The steps to be followed in designing each module, or for that matter in the initial planning stage, are the following (from Kurtz & Klingstedt, and Goldsmid & Goldsmid):
(a) Determine and state objectives.
(b) Arrange the objectives in the sequence in which instruction should be given.
(c) Draw up a pre-test for students. This will
  • tell what students already know;

- enable matching with what students *should* know before tackling the relevant module;
- enable supplementary remedial work to be undertaken; and
- place students with the same level of knowledge in one group.

(d) State why the *content* is important for the particular course of study.
(e) Design the necessary activities to be undertaken. In a course of nursing this will include reading and mastering study material, the acquisition of technical skills based on a sound theoretical foundation, and clear observation of those for whom care is provided so that care is based on educated judgement. Learning experiences must be available and selected for their suitability.
(f) Establish a resource centre, with library facilities, audio-visual aids, resource persons (tutors), and technical assistants to control resource material. That resource personnel are available to help and guide students throughout their programmes, is essential.

The construction of learning packages in module form, to be done between block periods, if properly planned and implemented, could make the actual block periods less of a 'cramming' event. By supplementing the material covered in the block period with properly constructed follow-up work, by the use of learning resources, including resource persons, and the planning of proper time available for completing learning packages, much of the disadvantages at present experienced in the 'block' system could be eliminated.

A modular system of instruction has much to be said for it. Advantages for the student could include:

- Knowledge of objectives so that the reason for studying material is seen and the total picture is clear
- Knowledge of the results of evaluation
- Motivation to achieve
- Self-pacing, as students can plan their study time to meet the limitations of their own abilities
- Opportunity for repetition and remedial work according to individual needs
- Opportunity to study in greater depth if special interest in an aspect is aroused
- The development of self-discipline regarding study habits
- Availability of personnel in resource centres at all reasonable times, who can assist with individual learning difficulties.

The teachers or in this case nurse-educators, might well find the following points to their advantage:

128

- Greater job satisfaction as students, in studying and producing better work, give them a sense of achievement
- The opportunity to give individual attention to students
- Time to keep up to date; in fact, the enforcement of continued study to plan, design, evaluate, re-plan and re-design modules on a continuous basis
- Freedom from routine, repetitive lectures. Contact periods could include group discussions, tutorials and special, but not routine lectures
- Mental stimulus, as the mind is not constantly bogged down with keeping to rigid time schedules in the class-room setting.

The success of the modular system will depend on

- the overall planning;
- the meticulous planning of each unit;
- the interest and enthusiasm of those involved in the implementation thereof;
- constant revision to meet changing needs;
- the acceptance of the system by all concerned with the education of the nurse;
- the underlying sound *educational* basis for all planning;
- the acceptance of the student as above all a *student of nursing*, and a provider of care only as it forms part of her learning. She is a *part* of the team and a cog in the wheel but not the *largest* part of the work force, nor the *only* cog in the wheel of nursing care.

8.6 TEACHING BY OBJECTIVES: A SYSTEMS APPROACH

According to *The Concise Oxford Dictionary* (1961), a system is a 'complex whole, set of connected things or parts, organised body of material or immaterial things', while *Chambers Twentieth Century Dictionary* defines it as 'anything formed of parts placed together or adjusted into a regular or connected whole, a set of things considered as a connected whole, a full and connected view of some department of knowledge, a method of organisation', and *Websters Encyclopaedia Dictionary* (1969) says a system is 'any assemblage of things forming a regular and connected whole, things connected according to a scheme, . . . a plan or scheme according to which things are connected into a whole'.

Objective is defined by *The Concise Oxford Dictionary* (1961) as a 'Point aimed at', and by the *Chambers Twentieth Century Dictionary* as 'The point to which quotations are directed'. *Websters Encyclopaedia Dictionary* (1969) defines it as 'the aim of an . . . operation or manoeuver, ultimate purpose'.

In chapter 3, objectives were seen as markers along the way to a goal. A summary of these definitions is the following: *An objective* is the point aimed at, the point towards which all activity is directed, a marker along the way, while *a system* is an organisation of connected parts to form a whole according to a scheme.

In order to use a systems approach in teaching the practice of nursing, the relevant parts must be identified, a scheme worked out for the presentation of the different parts so that they are seen as an interrelated whole, the objectives for the whole activity or the main objective must be defined, and the intermediate and the specific objectives clarified. Chapter 3 has dealt with the basic principles of setting objectives, or markers along the way. More attention will now be given to the systems approach as such. A systems approach provides the framework for organising an educational programme, it provides the skeleton which can then be given flesh by the educators concerned with each part. It defines:

- *What* the course is aiming at, for example preparing the registered nurse
- *Where* to begin
- *How* to proceed (listing the stages)
- *What* should be accomplished
- *How* to evaluate the end product, both at the intermediate stages, and at the end of the course.

In other words, it breaks the syllabus down into manageable units, with subsystems as required, and sets the overall objectives, the intermediate objectives and the objectives for subsystems, which relate to the *whole*, that of the education of the registered nurse for the practice of nursing.

In order to do this, it takes into consideration the functions which the registered nurse (the enrolled nurse or the enrolled nursing assistant, as the case may be) is expected to fulfil.

Rautenbach identified these functions as follows:

The role and function of the registered nurse

- The ability to make decisions
- Assisting in toilet care
- Carrying out highly complex technical skills
- The ability to carry out all aspects of health care
- Capability in the evaluation of what is relevant for today and necessary for learning tomorrow's technology
- Proficiency in the drawing up of new priorities
- The capability to function as enabler in care

- Demonstrating professional competence
- Carrying out ward based practical assignments
- Supplying routine bedside care
- Skill in carrying out the caring aspect of nursing
- Ability to perceive the patient as an individual
- The capability to empathise with individual health problems
- Supervising nursing care
- Assisting the students to appreciate the need of the human being
- The ability to apply scientific principles underlying nursing therapy
- Developing the necessary appreciation of the importance of preventive, curative and rehabilitative health services in the community
- The ability to recognise signs and symptoms and mastering the diagnostic, therapeutic and technical skills in nursing
- The ability to appreciate their role and responsibility in the health service of the community
- Providing personal health-care service working interdependently with physicians and others to keep people well and care for them when they are sick
- The ability to function as a responsible member of a health-care team by interpreting and carrying out the instructions of others.

The role and function of the enrolled nurse

- Supplying nursing care under the supervision of a registered professional nurse or physician
- Assisting the registered nurse in the carrying out of complex nursing functions
- Carrying out less technical nursing procedures
- Performing selected tasks and responsibilities within the framework of maintenance and promotion of health, prevention of illness, care and rehabilitation of the sick and disabled, achieving a dignified death, and such additional acts not requiring the skills, judgements, and knowledge of an independent nurse or the registered nurse
- Responsibility for implementing direct nursing service to people in a range of settings under the direction of an independent nurse or a registered nurse.

The role and function of the enrolled nursing assistant

- The ability to carry out nursing duties in a hospital under the supervision of a qualified nurse, mental nurse or midwife
- The ability to function as a backup for a trained nurse

131

- Performing specific functions that require considerable less use of judgement
- The ability to relate well to patients
- The ability to function adequately in any basic nursing situation.

These form a guide-line for future planning. They are valid for the 1980s, and the planning when using a systems approach must undergo constant revision to meet changing needs. It sets criteria against which evaluation at various levels can take place.

The systems approach in teaching the practice of nursing can be used to plan the programme, to organise

- the subject-matter;
- the physical facilities, including equipment, library, resource centres, audio-visual aids;
- the human resource persons, lecturers, tutors, teachers, theoretical and clinical;
- the necessary learning experiences, clinical as well as theoretical;
- the combination of theory and practica;
- evaluation
- remedial or re-teaching where necessary into a meaningful whole.

The systems approach allows enough flexibility to adapt to changing needs as it is essentially dynamic in character. Searle (1979) has combined the systems approach to nursing education and the setting of objectives under the following headings:

Step 1
Identify *community needs:*

- whether local, regional or national
- extent of the needs
- role, scope and functions of the proposed practitioner
- support services available
- specific community problems in the overall provision of health care.

Step 2
Identify *specific professional competence* required.

Step 3
Describe the *category of worker* required. Who must do what, when and where (RN, EN, ENA)? Is the necessary number of people to be trained in these categories available?

Step 4

(a) Identify *instructional objectives and activities needed to* equip practitioners. This depends on the educational background of the prospective student or pupil.

(b) Identify *amount of time* required to master essential scientific content.

Step 5

(a) Identify *instructional activities and resources, develop the syllabus.* The student must be able to

- relate subject-matter to pre-knowledge;
- understand importance of a personal philosophy of service and involvement;
- understand interrelationships of various parts of course;
- study in the real-life situation;
- receive feedback on progress throughout.

(b) Ensure that *methods and media* are related to the course content and objectives and student potential.

(c) Arrange *units* (or sections) in logical sequence.

Step 6

Set up the course, in other words, implement the plan.

Step 7

Evaluate student performance and educational objectives and activities. The criteria used for evaluation must be valid, consistent, and directed to all aspects of learning, cognitive, affective and psychomotor.

Step 8

Evaluation of newly qualified practitioner performance, including

- observation sessions;
- interviews;
- work performance and checks on participation in the work situation;
- checks for errors of judgement;
- analysis of complaints;
- inspection and other reports,

with remedial action where necessary.

The role played by clinical practica in the education of the nurse must not be forgotten. A student of nursing is being prepared to *nurse.* Action based on sound theory has to be fostered. In designing a systems approach with the setting of objectives for the course and subsections thereof, this fundamental fact must be kept in mind.

The learning of students must be directed towards the following:

- Acquiring technical skills and clinical judgement
- Acquiring a sound theoretical base upon which to act
- Gaining skill in caring for all categories of patients/clients in all spheres where nursing care, as health care, is given
- Acting as a full member of the health team, with definite independent functions and responsibilities
- Individual development towards excellent performance in clinical practice
- The ability to evaluate the results of actions, including self-evaluation
- The ability to manage nursing care of individuals and groups
- Skill in clinical assessment, critical thinking, nursing care planning, and the transmitting of nursing knowledge and techniques to neophytes in the profession
- Developing an acceptable role-model image
- The ability to establish priorities, based on sound knowledge and judgement based in turn on experience in the real-life laboratory, ward or unit in which clinical competence is gained.

The systems approach requires the nurse-educator to identify the specific unit objectives within the overall objective. These objectives are descriptions of definite student competence which must have been achieved at the completion of a unit of work. A clear description must be given in each section or subsection of what a student must know, and be able to do, and under what specific conditions, that is, clearly worded criteria for the evaluation phase must be provided, and should be available to the student. The ultimate consumers of nursing care and their specific needs must always be at the fore, for the student nurse is being prepared to meet the health-care needs of patients and clients. A person being prepared to practise nursing is not being educated for some imaginary role. It is a *real* role, based on the *real needs* of real people.

In literature on the systems approach to education, reference is frequently made to *cybernetic* systems, these being communication and control mechanisms. Odorne (1970) describes it as: 'Identification of training needs, training effort, evaluation, feedback, back to identification, and so on'. A cybernetic system sets goals, supplies training (or education) techniques, assesses whether goals have been achieved and gives feedback to trainers (or students) and employers (those using 'trained' students), with communication taking place throughout. The trainer (or tutor) is controlling the trainees (or students) and their course/s by means of the programme designed to meet their needs. He controls materials presented and manner of presentation, and participates in evaluation. In has great value as long as it does not become an automatic 'closed' type of system.

The tutor who plans to use the systems approach should, according to Searle (1980) acquire the skills to

- state educational objectives in behavioural terms;
- plan a curriculum and select learning activities;
- construct tests and other measurement devices;
- see the relationship between professional training programmes and subsequent practice;
- see the relationship between principles of learning and the role of the teacher;
- identify role objectives in educational planning;
- see the underlying principles and methods of curriculum planning;
- understand the principles and practices of evaluation of educational performance.

The systems approach has much to offer in nursing education. Its study is commended to all potential nurse-educators.

9 Teaching strategies in nursing education

The strategies which may be used to teach the practice of nursing are very varied indeed. They can be used to great advantage, or they can be used in such a manner that the so-called learning event becomes a non-event. The use of the various strategies, alone or in combination, depends to a large extent on the individual's choice and abilities. All that will be done in this chapter is to describe various teaching strategies, point out factors which may lead to success or failure, and indicate the obvious advantages and disadvantages. It is then up to the nurse-educator to choose the strategy or strategies which are most appropriate to the teacher and to the individuals who will be the recipients of the guidance of the teacher, with the ultimate object of enabling them to learn.

It must also be mentioned that nursing has two distinct aspects, namely clinical (or practical) and theoretical. Successful nursing education must blend these two so that practice is based on theory, and theoretical knowledge gives direction in the clinical field – one cannot exist without the other. Although a special section of this work will be devoted to 'clinical' instruction and others will deal with the presentation of 'theory', they cannot, and *must* not, be seen in separate compartments, but as a basic whole, the so-called 'separate' units merging in the totality which is nursing practice.

9.1 THE LECTURE

A lecture is a formal presentation of subject-matter by the lecturer. It is not necessarily a teaching method; a simple lecture or the presentation of a paper before a large group may possess an element of teaching, but the lecture method of teaching is more specific, planned and aimed at *teaching* or enabling the members of the group to learn.

A formal lecture is given to a captive, seated audience by a lecturer or teacher standing in front of the group. The lecture, as a teaching strategy, is a prepared presentation in which the lecturer talks more or less continuously for a specified time to members of the audience, who listen and may take notes which they feel are particularly important. The lecture is a formal occurrence. There is no real discussion, although students are often encouraged to ask questions, either at the end or at specific times during the lecture. These questions usually centre around the clarification of points.

136

A lecture is not meant to simply re-state facts or to repeat what various people have written in books. A student can look up and learn facts, and can read far more widely on the subject than the lecturer can present in one lecture or even in a course of lectures. Almost verbatim regurgitation of material which others have organised and written or stated, is a waste of time.

The lecture as a teaching method should incorporate the following:

(a) The information presented should aim at explaining relationships or stating general principles. These will of course express the personal viewpoint of the lecturer, but different opinions should also be highlighted.

(b) Material should be presented in an original manner so that interest in the subject is stimulated and the student is motivated to find out more.

(c) The presentation of new, as yet unpublished material and new discoveries.

(d) The explanation of the aim of the portion of the curriculum being studied at that time in relation to the total objectives.

(e) The statement of a problem, which it proposes to investigate, so that students can see it in perspective and be guided to a further search for what is not known.

(f) The establishment of contact with students, so that the lecturer focuses on being *understood* by the students, not merely heard and seen. Contact has not been established when a class is dull and lethargic, nor is tacit agreement with what the lecturer says, sufficient.

(g) The offering of a challenge to students, by arousing curiosity, stimulating the imagination, engendering the spirit of enquiry, and leading to the use of creative thought.

(h) The clarification of difficult points, including seeking out problems which students are encountering, and attempting to iron these out. The larger the group, the more difficult this is to obtain, but it is nevertheless important. It is amazing what eye contact can do, even in larger groups.

9.1.1 The lecture as a teaching method

9.1.1.1 Advantages

(a) *It makes economical use of time (for the teacher) and of resources:* If properly prepared, a lecture can present a great deal of relevant material in a short period of time.

(b) *Large groups can be reached.* The lecture method can be used to present the relevant material, introduce subject-matter or suggest interpretations to a very large number of people at the same time, the number being limited only by size of the room and the efficiency of the public address system.

(c) *The teacher is present:* Interaction is thus possible. A tape recording of a lecture, played back, does not provide the same opportunity for interaction. Teaching and learning are human events, and as such need the presence, at some stage, of teacher as well as learner.

(d) *Clarification and interpretation are possible:* A good lecturer can explain and interpret facts and point out different points of view, for which the student, left to his own devices, might have to spend a great deal of time in searching. Study of a particular textbook is not the answer either, as it usually presents only one point of view, namely that of the author.

(e) *Orientation to a whole programme is possible:* The good lecture which has been well prepared, can be used to orientate the student, pointing out what he will be expected to know (objective) at the end of the course, and the relevant basic knowledge necessary for success.

(f) *Exposure to authorities:* A lecture given by a well-known authority on a certain subject, who is able to convey his own enthusiasm to others when detailing first-hand experience, can make a lasting impression and inspire students to previously unknown heights.

(g) *Use can be made of special attributes of the lecturer:* The experience, enthusiasm and ability to present an organised body of subject-matter in an inspirational manner, and special skills when delivering the lecture, are attributes which some lecturers possess. These should be capitalised on.

(h) *Timing can be flexible:* A lecture can be scheduled for any time during a course of study.

(i) *Combination is possible:* A lecture can be combined easily and effectively with many other methods of instruction.

9.1.1.2 Disadvantages

(a) *Passivity of student:* A student may feel that attendance is all that is required, and that no other activity, such as preparation before a lecture, is necessary.

(b) *Regurgitation of subject-matter:* A lecture may be nothing more than a regurgitation of facts presented in a textbook. This is, of course, more the fault of the lecturer than of the lecture as a teaching technique. To convey information which is readily available elsewhere, without adding anything to it, is a waste of time.

(c) *It may be boring:* This again will depend on the lecturer. An unenthusiastic, ill-prepared presenter who speaks badly or inaudibly in a droning, monotonous voice will be boring, even soporific, and should not lecture.

(d) *The lecturer gets little feedback from the group:* This can to some extent be obviated by the judicious use of questions, and by an alert lecturer watching the reactions of the audience.

138

(e) *It does not facilitate learning problem-solving:* A large group prevents discussion and large-scale interaction, which are better in smaller groups.

(f) *There is little possibility of assesing the progress of learning except by formal testing:* Again a small group, such as in a tutorial, can achieve more.

(g) *It does not allow for individual learning rates:* A course of lectures proceeds willy-nilly, and slow learners, or those with unrecognised problems, are left behind.

(h) *Low retention:* Only about 20% of what is said during a lecture is likely to be remembered as no reinforcement takes place.

9.1.2 When lectures should be used

Bearing in mind the abovementioned advantages and disadvantages, lectures should be used:

- To introduce a programme to students, pointing out the objectives, the procedures to be followed and the learning resources available
- To give specific information which is not readily available elsewhere
- To introduce a subject and indicate to the students its importance and scope
- To create a learning climate for the subsequent use of other techniques
- To present basic information on which subsequent learning activity is to be built
- To review, clarify, or summarise what has already been covered in a specific course.

9.1.3 The requirements of a good lecture

There are several points that go to the making of a good lecture and these might be stated as follows:

- It must stimulate group interest throughout.
- It must be well planned.
- It must have a clear purpose.
- It must develop in a logical manner.
- It must be relevant to the needs of the group.
- It must be well presented, that is clear, audible, with a good sentence construction and verbal or other illustrations to suit the level of knowledge of the group, with variation in tone and pace.
- Unnecessary and irritating gestures must be avoided.
- All visual aids must be integrated into the whole.
- It must be interspersed at planned intervals with the judicious use of relevant questions.

- It should not be longer than 20 minutes without a break for questioning, the use of some visual aid such as the overhead projector, or perhaps a chart, diagram, poster or even slides. No lecture, even when interrupted by these methods, should last longer than one hour.
- Notes should be used to guide a lecturer, and not be read word for word.

9.1.4 The preparation of lecture notes

As lecturing, because of large classes and a shortage of tutors, still forms such a large part of the formal teaching event in nursing colleges and schools, some time must be devoted to the preparation of lecture notes or teaching guides.

Preparation must of course not only centre around the lecture as such, but should include an outline of the total teaching programme set against a time schedule. This must be flexible enough to allow for modification when particular difficulties are encountered with students, in case of illness and with equipment or other presentation difficulties, but rigid enough to ensure that the total programme is covered within the desired time schedule. The proposed time schedule must also be approached from a realistic standpoint.

What is really required is the following:

- Establish overall objectives.
- Decide on the subject–matter to be covered, that is a detailed syllabus.
- Determine a realistic time schedule, that is, what must be covered in each 'block' of instruction. Under the block system of education these will coincide with each specific block. Under the study–day system the subject–matter will be divided into periods of time such as months, quarters or semesters.
- Detailed planning can then be undertaken, including provision for testing, study time, library work, etc. This further divides the programme into subject–matter for each session with, if possible, appropriate methods for teaching and other details.
- The individual lecture can then be prepared.

The individual lecture plan should include the following aspects:

- A clear statement of the topic to be covered
- An indication of the level of education already attained by students
- The objectives which the lecturer is striving to achieve by the lecture
- Time available
- An orientation of the students to the topic, that is, summarising what has been done in previous classes or placing the topic in an overall scheme

- The teaching technique to be used, that is, whether it will be a straight-forward formal lecture, whether discussions or questions will be incorporated, etc
- Teaching aids to be used, that is, overhead projectors, films, charts, models, diagrams, chalkboard, etc
- Subject-matter, which is then divided into headings in the form of an outline – phrases or key words are sufficient In this outline clear indications should be made as to
  - what must be placed on the chalkboard (or overhead projector)
  - what will be illustrated by chart, slide, etc – all clearly numbered
  - any learner activities to be used, that is, distribution of notes, pamphlets, diagrams
  - questions, if any, to be put
- Summary of the lecture, including possible use of the chalkboard or overhead projector transparency for this purpose
- References for further reading
- Closure.

An example of a lecture guide might be the following:

Subject: Anatomy of the heart
Learners: First-year student nurses, Xth week of anatomy block (9th month of training)
Objectives: To guide students to a clear knowledge of the basic anatomy of the normal human heart, so that functions can be understood and that later presentation of pathology will be seen in relation to the norm
Time available: 8 am to 10 am (break will be necessary)
Orientation of students: Open textbooks – relation to material already studied in this block/course
Technique: Formal lecture, illustrated by charts, diagrams and blackboard work, as well as the use of transparencies and a model

Teaching aids:
Frohse chart of heart
Model of heart
Chalkboard and white, red and blue chalk
    and/or
Prepared transparencies which overlap, so that the total picture can be shown, and then portions removed in layers as the presentation proceeds

Subject-matter:
Size and position: chart
Layers: model, chart
Chambers: chart, transparencies, model of heart

Valves: model of heart
Vessels entering and leaving heart: chart, model, transparencies
Internal structures: model of heart
Blood supply to heart muscle: chart, model, transparencies
Conduction system: model of heart, model, chart, transparencies.

Time for questions at various levels can be interspersed in the plan, also the time schedule, that is, what must be covered in the first, second, third and fourth quarters. Time should be allowed for a break (a two-hour lesson is too long).

The following method is to be used for summarising the lecture.

9.1.5 Overall chalkboard scheme

The following scheme should be drawn up on the chalkboard:

The heart
Size
Position
Relations

Layers of the heart
Pericardium
Myocardium
Endocardium

Septum

Chambers
   Atria: Right atrium
       Left atrium
   Ventricles: Right ventricle
        Left ventricle

Valves
Between chambers
   Right side: Tricuspid valve
   Left side: Bicuspid valve (mitral valve)
From chambers
   Left ventricle: aortic semilunar valve
   Right ventricle: pulmonary semilunar valve

Vessels entering and leaving the heart
To right atrium: superior and inferior vena cavae
From right ventricle: pulmonary trunk
To left atrium: four pulmonary veins
From left ventricle: aorta

Internal structures
Chordae tendinae
Papillary muscles

Blood supply to heart muscle
Coronary vessels

Conduction system
Sinoatrial node
Atrioventricular node
Atrioventricular bundle (bundle of His)
Purkinje fibres

This scheme can be built up as the lecture proceeds. More details than the bare outline will, or course, be given. When it comes to revision, the more detailed sections can be erased and only the underlined sections (here italicised) left on the board. The details can then again be supplied by means of response to questions put to the class.

If the lecturer involves the students in the course of the lecture by stimulating their interest and asking questions judiciously, then the lecture can be as good a means of teaching as any other. Students who are listening attentively and are intellectually stimulated, and who are considering issues raised by the lecturer, are not passive sponges, simply absorbing what is said. Lectures have a definite contribution to make towards teaching if judiciously and effectively used.

9.2 THE DEMONSTRATION

This is one of the best-known teaching strategies used in nursing education, especially in teaching the basis of practical skills. The origin of the word is the Latin *de-monstrare*, meaning to show, so that demonstration is a means of 'show'-ing something, and in the nursing context, of 'showing how'. It is a visual presentation of a nursing technique using actual equipment for the purpose of showing how something should be done. However, in teaching the practice of nursing, it entails much more than the mere demonstration of a procedure, and it cannot serve much purpose if it is presented in a vacuum. It is very important to know *how* to carry out a technical procedure, but it is equally important to know *why* the procedure is being carried out, and also to realise the dangers inherent to it.

Demonstrations are employed for the purpose of 'showing how to do' various actions as in the following cases:

(a) Showing students or pupils how to carry out a nursing technique, which, to them, is completely new

143

(b) Illustrating the application of fundamental scientific principles to the process of nursing. How many nurses, in teaching the art of giving an intramuscular injection, remember to point out that a thick needle actually causes less pain to the patient than does a thin one? (This is due to the physical fact that fluid injected through a large needle is under less pressure, and thus causes less pain than when the fluid is forced through a thin needle. In the latter case far more force has to be exerted to inject the same amount of fluid.)

(c) For the purpose of demonstrating techniques which are to replace those currently in use; this may or may not include the use of new equipment

(d) Showing students, in a practical manner, how to achieve a sound nurse-patient relationship when carrying out patient care

(e) Showing students or pupils how to do something which is concerned with the total care of the patient, but which does not *require* his physcial presence. Testing of urine is one example of this.

9.2.1 The essentials of a good demonstration

These are the following:

- A demonstration shows how things are done.
- Everyone attending should be able to see what is being demonstrated, thus groups should be small to facilitate interaction.
- The demonstrator must be able to carry out the technique competently.
- Equipment should be assembled and tested prior to the demonstration.
- The setting should be as true to life as possible. If a patient is used, then he must be informed of the purpose of the demonstration and his consent obtained beforehand.
- Where possible, without prejudice to the patient, the demonstration should be accomplished by a step-by-step elucidation of the procedure.
- The demonstration should be preceded by a briefing session, and followed by a discussion.
- Learners should be given an opportunity for practice sessions following the demonstration, so that they may become proficient in the technique.

Many students, having seen a demonstration carried out by a competent practitioner, or having seen a film demonstration of a technique, may be most frustrated when they find themselves clumsy and awkward. This is a point that should be remembered when teaching the practice of nursing to young students.

Another point that must be remembered is that some people are naturally more dexterous than others and that it takes time to master skills even if the learner is reasonably dexterous. No one will perform perfectly at the first attempt and some will take longer than others to master it. This does not mean that they will not ultimately be good practical nurses.

Demonstrations are carried out daily, formally and informally. Helping a student nurse to make a patient comfortable in bed is an example of informal 'showing how'. However, in the context of this book we are more concerned with the formal demonstration.

9.2.2 Disadvantages and advantages

One of the most vital questions to be answered is *where* should the demonstration take place? Ultimately it is essential that the demonstration be given in the real–life situation, using patients in the ward or unit on whom various procedures have to be performed as part of their nursing care. This produces the necessary realism, but it naturally has drawbacks, a few of which are listed here:

(a) It is an encroachment on the privacy of the patient and therefore his consent and co-operation must be obtained.
(b) The number of students who can benefit from such a demonstration is limited, which means a good deal of repetition to cater for all students.
(c) Questions and answers, except in very general terms, are not possible.
(d) It is not possible to stop a procedure or to repeat part of it in order to clarify a point. The care which is being given to the patient is of paramount importance, and should be done in the way it would have been if the demonstration was not carried out.
(e) The necessary correlation of theory and practice will have to be undertaken away from the real situation. This problem is not insurmountable, but may make the planning of teaching more difficult as patient care cannot always wait for the time required to ensure that this is done.
(f) It takes longer to demonstrate than to give patient care, and thus it may be more tiring for the patient.
(g) Procedures which must of necessity be taught to students, may not be readily available.

The alternative, which despite many objections does have certain merits, is to plan and carry out a demonstration without patients, using as realistically simulated a situation as is possible.

The advantages of this method are:

- It allows discussion and questioning to take place while it is carried out.
- Repetition – or stopping to illustrate a point – is possible.
- More students are able to watch the demonstration.

- It can produce a practice area where students can become more familiar with handling equipment before actually attempting to carry out a technique on a patient.
- The atmosphere may be more relaxed and thus students will ask questions there and then.
- It is possible to demonstrate procedures which are not readily available in the real-life situation.

The one thing that must be emphasised is that simulated situations *must* be followed up by a demonstration in the 'real' situation, that is in the ward or unit. It is here that the teaching role of the ward professional nurse must be used to the maximum.

9.2.3 Basic requirements

No matter where the demonstration is carried out, there are some common basic requirements:

9.2.3.1 Preparation

- Plan the procedure so that steps follow logically.
- Select the patient simulation situation.
- Assemble and test the apparatus.
- Practise the technique.
- Determine objectives.
- Determine the number of students who will benefit.
- Ensure that students have the necessary knowledge of procedure – presentation of underlying theory must be part of preparation. Students must be aware of points to be observed.
- Explain how specific apparatus works and allow students to handle apparatus before attempting to use it. Injecting fluid with a syringe looks very simple when handled by a competent practitioner, but handling that syringe for the first time has many pitfalls. Similarly, handling a clamp during the administration of a nasogastric feed also looks so easy when the demonstrator, almost without thinking, opens or closes it. Does she ever think of the first time she used such a piece of equipment herself?
- Plan summary and questioning sessions.

9.2.3.2 Procedure

(a) The demonstrator must be competent and must understand the underlying theory.

146

(b) Before commencing, the objective, as well as what is to follow and the special points to be observed must be explained to the students. If the demonstration is to be carried out on a patient, they must be told to remember or make a note of any queries so that these can be dealt with at the end of the demonstration, away from the patient.

(c) Students must be warned not to make remarks or observations which may cause anxiety or distress to the patient. Similarly, the demonstrator must refrain from remarks which would upset the patient.

(d) The demonstrator must observe essential safety precautions throughout 'live' demonstrations.

(e) The demonstrator must work efficiently, quietly and demonstrate the essential good nurse–patient relationship in the 'live' situation. Her adaptation, without panic, to any unexpected occurrence in carrying out the procedure will be a lesson in itself. A student, by observing the teacher's reaction to the situation and the patient's response to treatment, may learn a great deal that will be of practical value to her in her future practice.

(f) The skill to be demonstrated should first be performed at the normal rate of working. The demonstrator sets a standard of performance which the students or pupils must later emulate. Once the skill has been demonstrated, it can be broken down into logical parts so that the student can practise what has been shown, away from the patient if need be, and master areas which present special difficulties to her. It may seem easy to handle a syringe until faced with the reality of doing so. By drawing up and injecting fluid into some innocuous object such as an orange, the student will acquire a certain amount of dexterity, which will then be transferred to the 'real' situation.

9.2.3.3 Follow-up

After a demonstration, if the objective is to be realised, the following points are vital:

(a) Review of the procedure, again emphasising the theoretical background.

(b) Inviting and answering questions, stimulating discussion and clearing up problem areas.

(c) Evaluation of the success or otherwise of the demonstration.

(d) Organising supervised practice and enabling students to eventually demonstrate their competence to a group or to an individual. As part of her patient care function, the ward or unit professional nurse needs to be assured of the competence of her students to undertake nursing care. She must also be assured that the future professional practitioner of nursing can, in turn, teach others. Thus she should arrange for more senior students to demonstrate in their turn to more junior students or pupils. By this means her teaching role is fulfilled and it is not only the 'clinical sisters' or instructors who demonstrate. Tutors and other nurses competent in techniques, as well as in the teaching strategy of a demonstration, can be employed for this purpose.

Demonstrations concerning practical techniques which do not require the physical presence of the patient, may quite conveniently be shown to larger groups outside the 'real' situation. However, they should also be translated to the actual practice situation for reinforcement. Testing urine on a demonstration table with all the equipment ready to hand, and in a small corner of a sluice-room or a special 'testing-room' will, although the test procedure is in each case the same, present different problems to the person carrying out the test. These can only be understood and solved in the actual situation. Although a class demonstration in front of a large group at a table will include the theory and emphasis will be laid on the necessity of locking away reagents, the reinforcement that this receives in the ward or unit where keys have to be obtained and returned, makes it much more likely that the student will remember it.

Demonstrations are used in teaching not only nurses, but also patients, relatives and friends of patients and clients in general. A very good example of a demonstration commonly given is that to a group of expectant mothers (and even fathers) on how to bath a baby.

The basic principles of such demonstrations remain the same. The group being taught, their home conditions and their level of education must be taken into consideration, so that realism is always uppermost at the demonstration. This applies equally to a person-to-person demonstration where one mother is taught how to bath her baby, or one patient is taught how to test his urine. Many such examples are part of the nursing world and occur daily. They are all demonstrations – 'showing how'. They are all part of teaching the practice of nursing, albeit to those not conventionally part of the nursing team.

9.3 THE LECTURE DEMONSTRATION

This term states what the strategy is, that is, the combination of a lecture and a demonstration. It is longer and somewhat more formal, and requires more preparation than the simple explanation which precedes the demonstration proper.

The lecture/s which leads up to the demonstration must be as carefully planned as every other lecture.

An example would be a series of lectures on the anatomy, physiology and pathology of the lung, an explanation of the procedure and the reasons for it being carried out, with special reference to the patient in question, followed by a demonstration of postural drainage.

This would, in the same way as would a demonstration, be *followed up* by review, a session of asking and answering questions, discussions, evaluation of the amount of knowledge gained, and the organisation of supervised practice.

9.4 ASSIGNMENTS

According to *The Concise Oxford Dictionary,* an assignment is 'a task allocated to a person', while Tracey (1971:200-201) defines an assignment as 'a method where the instructor assigns readings in books, periodicals, manuals or handouts, requires the completion of a project or research paper; or prescribes problems and exercises for the practice of a skill', and Heidgerken sees it as 'the chief means of directing learning activities outside the classrooms' (1965: 357).

An assignment includes the allocation of guided learning activities to individuals or groups of individuals in order to

(a) prepare students for a subsequent lecture discussion or other group activity;
(b) ensure that the background knowledge of students is similar. It can be used to remedy poor learning or inadequate knowledge as a pre-course preparation;
(c) prepare, during a course, for a subsequent section;
(d) cover a specific aspect of the study material which is not to be presented formally;
(e) supplement material presented in formal lectures; and
(f) guide and direct individual study and research.

An assignment usually requires the completion of a written report. The individual carries out his own learning activity which can be seen as a form of programmed learning.

9.4.1 Advantages

(a) A far greater amount of material, which can also be studied in greater depth, can be covered in a shorter period of time than is possible by any other means.
(b) Assignments can be used as a substitute for lectures.
(c) Assignments can make lectures, demonstrations and clinical practica more meaningful.

149

(d) Students are able to read the material assigned for study as it appears in the original writing and context, and do not receive it second-hand.

(e) Assignments can be given to individuals to remedy their own deficiencies in knowledge or skills, without revealing these to others. This obviates the holding back of a whole group, because of the deficiency in knowledge of a few.

9.4.2 Disadvantages

(a) Possible lack of motivation on the part of the students.

(b) Assignment assessment is very time-consuming for teachers.

(c) Students may not know how to consult and use resource material effectively.

(d) Assignments may not be clearly stated, leading to confusion.

(e) The material assigned may be beyond the capabilities of the students concerned.

(f) The tutor may require too many reference books or other resources to be consulted.

(g) Students can delay starting work on an assignment until it is too late to undertake a worthwhile study.

(h) Students' work may not be thorough enough to bring about learning.

9.4.3 Characteristics of a good assignment

(a) Students are motivated to produce good, thorough work.

(b) Objectives are defined clearly and concisely.

(c) Objectives must meet the learning needs of individual students, as well as of the course as a whole.

(d) The student must know exactly what she is expected to do and the time allocated in which to complete it.

(e) The assignment is carefully planned with regard to

- its relevance to the course and/or to the individual;
- the time available;
- reading references and resource materials suggested; and
- availability of resource material.

Once completed, an assignment must be marked with due care, comments made which will assist the student to remedy errors and improve future learning, and handed back to the student with as little delay as possible. If this is not done, wrong information may be reinforced in the mind of the student, or a valuable teaching/learning experience may be lost.

9.5 PROJECTS

A project entails the investigation of some problem which leads to learning activity and usually requires a visual presentation of the findings which may take the form of a scrapbook, when it is individual work. It may also entail a whole display or exhibit combining several forms of visual presentation, in which case it is a group project.

A student or group of students may select their own project, or the nurse-educator may allocate a project to a group or to an individual student. The project must fit into the programme or section of the programme of nursing education being offered. It must have educational value and be relevant to the course.

Project work is designed to bring students face to face with reality, and can correlate subjects where appropriate. Subject barriers can be broken down by the use of this method.

In group project work the students, having selected a project or having been allocated one, break it down into component parts. The preparation of the visual presentation is planned and tasks are allocated. Different members of the group then undertake the necessary research work for their part of the project. The whole group, who should have appointed a group leader, meet at stated intervals to assess progress, assist one another with ideas or resource material, and plan the final presentation. It is a good idea for two or three people to work on a component part of a group project at a time. Each one's talents and knowledge supplement those of the other, and they act as a stimulus for each other.

The nurse-educator who has allocated or approved the project must always be available to assist, guide, encourage and criticise when and where necessary.

When the group decides on its own project, within the boundaries prescribed by the subject-matter to be covered, the plan must be submitted for approval to the responsible nurse-educator.

Students can be encouraged to initiate a subject for project work; whatever is selected must have the approval of the instructor and must receive co-operation from all involved. Students who are well motivated can produce very good individual or group projects and the knowledge thus acquired can be considerable and is likely to 'stick'.

After selecting the topic, the student/s should present a detailed plan of procedure for approval. Points to be considered include:

- Does the project have educational content?
- Is it practical?
- Is is suitable for the needs and the level of learning of the student/s?
- Can it be completed within the allocated time?

- Is it realistic from the point of view of costs, available material and other resources which are needed?
- Does it pose enough of a challenge to the student/s without being so much of a burden that its learning potential is negated?
- Does it allow for creative thinking rather than repetitive exercise?

Projects can be allocated by the unit professional nurse in the unit teaching situation, but they may also be allocated by members of a clinical teaching department. In this case the time factor might be less limiting as it could be extended over a longer period. Even in this latter situation, it will always require the co-operation of the registered nurses in charge of units if their patients or clients are the subject of study. Indeed, in this case they may be of tremendous value by contributing their knowledge and experience to the student or group of students engaged on such a project.

Project work involves a great deal of participation from all concerned who, by the very nature of their involvement, learn not only from their own research, but also from that of others participating in the project. Participants learn to use independent thought and action, and yet to co-operate as a group. They also learn to evaluate their own efforts, as well as those of others.

It is difficult to allocate projects to students being educated by the block system, except when there is a teacher available for follow-up work between blocks, when it can be most successful.

Some suggestions for project work include the following:

- *Mothercraft:* The investigation of the needs of a prospective mother in preparing for her first baby.
- *Surgical nursing:* Causes and prevention of wound infection.
- *Medical nursing:* Patient education for discharge of a patient with diabetes mellitus.
- *Nutrition:* Dietary deficiencies and their prevention.
- *Ward administration:* The essential elements in the administration of a medical ward.

The inventive, innovative, creative nurse-educator can constantly add to this list according to the available time and the educational needs of students.

Good projects should always be open for viewing. This stimulates students to greater effort in future project work.

It may be difficult for the unit professional nurse to see project teaching as part of her function. If she herself has not been exposed to project teaching, she may need guidance. If ward or unit teaching has been properly presented in the learning experience of the student nurse, then projects should have been included.

In the unit situation projects will necessarily have to be short because of the changes in personnel. Nevertheless, it is a worthwhile method of stimulating interest and encouraging purposeful background reading, literature research and discussions.

A simple project, such as the methods used in a unit for nursing care of patients suffering from a specific ailment, can be very useful as it will entail a revision of anatomy, physiology and pathology. The considerable variation in methods of treatment and the response of the individual in each case can be compared. Apply a project method of studying the nursing care of several paraplegic patients in a special unit, or to coronary care, to babies with gastro-enteritis or any type of disease condition which necessitates treatment in a unit, and the idea will begin to seem less strange. A 'case study' is really a form of project, although the method employed in this particular instance may be more structured.

Another project might be the preparation of health education material for waiting patients in an out-patient department, an antenatal clinic or some other area where patients or clients are congregated together.

Project methods provide for purposeful activity and are student-centred. Again the project must be seen through to its logical conclusion and be judged. This evaluation can be concurrent, step by step, or it can be terminal – that is, on completion of the project – or both methods of evaluation can be applied. If projects are approached with thought and are well planned, their use as a teaching strategy can be invaluable.

9.6 GROUP DISCUSSION

A group discussion is a valuable teaching strategy, especially when dealing with more senior students. The emphasis is on *participation,* which means that the group must not be large, the average size suggested being between ten and 15. The larger the group, the more talking will be done by the same few persons.

The aim of the group discussion technique is to encourage an exchange of views. For this, face-to-face contact is desirable. Sitting around a table which should preferably be circular, or placing comfortable chairs in a circle, is ideal. This type of arrangement prevents one person from dominating another.

Group discussion is not teaching *per se.* It is particularly useful in stimulating extension of knowledge and developing critical thinking. It encourages the student to think for herself, and to develop confidence in her ability to come up with ideas and to express them to others. It can form part of the socialisation into the nursing profession, by learning to co-operate with others, to look at problems in a non-judgemental way and to interact with colleagues in active problem solving. It helps to clarify vague thoughts.

For a group discussion to be successful it must have a successful leader. In the early stages this can be the nurse-educator, but at a later stage other members of the group could be initiated into group leadership, which will stand them in good stead in their future careers.

The leader must have a good background knowledge of the subject under discussion, so that she can act as a resource person when needed. The leader should pose the problem clearly and then invite opinions, after which discussion should be allowed to flow freely, except when one person tends to dominate the group by 'holding the floor'. The leader must then be ready to intervene and redirect the flow of the discussion, and also to draw the more reticent members into the discussion. The leader may have to focus or refocus attention on the subject or problem being dealt with. This may be done by simply saying 'let's get back to the subject', or more subtly by repeating what a participant has said, and then asking a question which redirects the line of discussion. It may occasionally be necessary for the leader to recap or summarise what has already been said. A member of the group could also be asked to do this. This play often puts things back into perspective.

Group discussion could well be used in portions of the basic course dealing with ethical problems, with problems of management of patient care, with basic ward administration, and with student problems *per se*.

Organised, planned use of group discussions as a teaching technique holds many possibilities for the nurse-educator.

Problem solving in a unit situation can also be tackled by means of group discussion among members of the unit personnel. The actuality of a real problem will have great meaning for the student. Discussions of actual cases in the unit provide valuable group discussion material.

The posing of hypothetical problems by the nurse-educator can stimulate interest and improve the potential skills of future unit professional nurses. It is also a very useful tool in in-service education.

9.7 CASE HISTORY

A case history – or a nursing case history – is a collection of data centred around a patient. It details

- the history of the patient, medical as well as relevant social data;
- the nature of the complaint;
- signs and symptoms;
- the provisional diagnosis;

- the physical assessment of the patient;
- the tests used to establish the diagnosis;
- the final diagnosis;
- the anatomy, physiology, and pathology associated with the illness;
- possible complications;
- the prescribed mental treatment;
- the nursing care plan, including identification of potential problems;
- the progress of the patient;
- comments.

It is a collection of factual evidence obtained from the real-life situation. The student has to collect, organise and present the data herself. It should present a well-rounded picture of the patient before he entered hospital, and give information of his home circumstances, previous illnesses, and treatment prior to illness. It describes his actual nursing care plan and medical treatment as well as his response to that treatment and care.

The section allowed for comment may be used to evaluate the nursing care plan used and suggest alternatives where appropriate.

In nursing education the case history emphasises the person who is a patient, the *nursing case* of that person, and the management of nursing problems. Medical data are only included when they are relevant to *nursing care*. A nursing case history that concentrates on medical rather than nursing treatment does not achieve the learning of the practice of nursing.

Case history exercises can be given to students at different levels of training. Early case histories will concentrate on collecting information, and observation. Students will need a great deal of guidance and must be able to work according to a structured pattern. As their nursing knowledge and skills improve, the 'comment' section will become increasingly important.

Hypothetical case histories which present salient information and require students to draw up their own nursing care plans are also useful teaching tools. These require the student to exercise judgement and go beyond the collection of data.

Case histories which pose a health problem situation and require a detailed description of the course of an illness and its effects on a patient, the nursing and medical care and possible complications, as well as methods to prevent or deal with them as and when they arise, is a valid method for the evaluation of nursing students.

Clinical workbooks for various areas of nursing can be designed, based on a hypothetical case history, which builds up incidents along the course of the progress of the patient's illness, and which requires the completion of various questions. This is another method of guiding and learning based on the case history technique.

An example of this technique would be the following:

(a) Description of the situation at the onset of the illness
  - Diagnosis
  - Medical orders.
(b) Definition of condition
  (To be completed by student)
(c) Factors predisposing to condition
  (To be completed by student)
(d) Signs and symptoms
  The signs and symptoms of the clinical picture are *listed*, and the student is required to explain each one, giving reasons for their occurrence, including the pathophysiology. The student is also required to describe nursing actions which could be taken to deal with each.
(e) Treatment and nursing care
  This includes the rationale behind medical tests, the significance of readings, and the nurse's handling of the patient at various stages. This would depend on the nature of the illness and whether intensive care, such as cardiac monitoring, was necessary. Also included are:
  - A detailed nursing care plan;
  - A list of the medications given; the student would be required to complete a table of physiological average, route, side-effects, nursing responsibilities, action and dosage.
(f) Possible complications
  The reasons for their occurrence and significance of findings, as well as means of dealing with them, should they arise.
(g) Preparation for discharge
(h) Follow-up care required

An ingenious nurse-educator could find many applications for such a technique in teaching the practice of nursing. It can stimulate independent learning, create interest and bring reality to otherwise dry-as-dust presentation of learning material.

Another format which could be used for the compilation and presentation of a case history is the following:

(a) Personal data
  - Age
  - Sex
  - Marital status
  - Children
  - Occupation
(b) History
  - Complaint on first presentation for care

- Medical history
- Social history
- Nursing history

(c) On admission
- Signs and symptoms
- Provisional diagnosis
- Nursing observations
- Emotional state
- Medical care plan
- Nursing care plan

(d) Theoretical background

Everything is done against background reading of relevant theoretical knowledge: keep a bibliography of works consulted. The following aspects must be covered in reading:

Relevant

- Anatomy and physiology, especially of affected organs
- Disease condition
  - Pathology
  - Causes, including any relevant microbiology, social causes, trauma, etc
  - Epidemiology
  - Signs and symptoms
  - Usual course
  - Treatment, including:
    (i) Pharmacology related to drugs used
    (ii) Surgical procedures
    (iii) Nursing techniques
    (iv) Medico-legal hazards related to any form of treatment
    (v) The necessary observation and preventive measures, as well as measures to be taken in an emergency.

(e) Treatment of patient and progress report
- Special tests carried out and the interpretation of results
- Final diagnosis
- Medical treatment and its effects on the patient and on the disease state
- Nursing treatment and its effects on the patient and on the disease state
- Mental state – any changes occurring during treatment
- Social problems and methods of handling these
- Special observations
- Rehabilitation

- Outcome of illness
- Any follow-up care recommended and methods of achieving this, for example referrals to community health care, etc.

(f) Assessment of case
This should include assessment of medical and nursing care, follow-up care and any relevant facts which could point to improvement in the management of care, ward management, equipment used, allocation of staff, ward teaching, health education, education of patient and relatives, etc.

The information required for this can be obtained from various sources, such as:

- Background reading
- Studying case notes and charts
- Personal observation
- Laboratory reports
- Queries of
  - patient
  - instructor
  - medical officer
  - nursing colleagues
  - other members of the health team.

The important aspect is that the student nurse should have an open mind and be ready to participate to the full in the total care of the patient. It affords the opportunity to integrate subject content which has perhaps until now been seen as separate compartments of required study material, without much relevance to the work in hand. Physical science (especially medical biophysics), chemistry (especially biochemistry), anatomy and physiology, microbiology and pharmacology, psychology and sociology, the art and science of nursing, and other subjects, if applied to the particular 'case' being studies, assume new meaning.

The problems which occur, the interaction with the patient and the support and help necessary in giving patient care, are all part of the case history. Active participation in the care of the patient and follow-up are vital. A case history simply written from notes, is not nearly as valuable. It may be a form of intellectual exercise and as such will have some learning input, but it will not teach as much as a case history where the student is actively involved – at least at some stage during the illness – in the case of the person whose case history she is writing.

Case histories may be presented by a student to other members of the group so that all will benefit.

9.8 WORKBOOKS

These are designed to ensure that certain aspects of the work are covered and to guide learning activities. They are actually a form of programmed instruction, although they do not give as much detailed information as do programmed learning guides, nor do they have built-in evaluation mechanisms to assess the progress of learning.

A workbook can, for instance, be designed to guide students through observations which should be made, and activities which should be carried out in ward administration or while undertaking community health practica. It is a means of guided self-instruction and can be applied to many fields of nursing, including general as well as specialist areas. Simple, well designed workbooks could, for instance, guide the student through all aspects of the care of the patients who undergo different forms of surgery, the care of the terminally ill, persons in intensive care, and many more. Workbooks are carefully designed teaching tools, which have to be completed by the student and submitted for scrutiny and comment, and usually for the allocation of marks or symbols.

The workbook must point to areas which must receive attention in the live situation. Relevant questions, which focus the attention of the students on aspects of work related to patient care which might otherwise be overlooked, must be posed. The completion of workbooks should be simple and not too time consuming. The wording of the text must be unambiguous and relevant. Too many demands must not be placed on the student.

Workbooks must be explained to students, who must be motivated to use them properly. Complete honesty is necessary. If any problems present themselves, these should be dealt with in consultation with those teaching the course. The student should be quizzed about the data recorded in the workbook and the underlying scientific principles. By this means the nurse-educator can ensure that the student gains the maximum benefit from the workbook, and obtains insight into the application of the process of nursing to the patients for whom she is caring.

The workbook must never be seen as an end in itself, but as a means to the end of learning the practice of nursing so as to be able to care for people with health-care needs.

9.9 FIELD TRIPS

Field trips in nursing are generally thought of in terms of visits to outside agencies. This is largely true, but there is no reason why they could not also be understood to mean visits to other departments or to other fields of activity within the nursing context in the organisation in which the nurse is em-

159

ployed. As part of nursing education programmes, planned visits could be arranged to departments such as the

- nurse teaching department or college
- clinical teaching department
- central sterilising department
- out-patient department
- operating theatres
- paediatric units
- X-ray department
- dispensary
- supply stores
- kitchen and dietary department, etc,

to name but a few which would be extremely valuable.

These internal field trips must be very well planned. They must not simply take the form of a conducted tour, where one is a few hours away from one's own place of work, and suffers from sore feet!

In planning a field trip, care must be taken to define the objective and then to get all the resources needed to make it a true learning experience. After taking part in an internal field trip, the participants should have a clear idea of the aims and objectives of the department visited, the measures taken to achieve these objectives, the manner in which the work dovetails with that of other departments, and how their own field of nursing activity fits into the total picture.

Internal as well as external field trips form part of basic nursing education, though again, they may take the form of time-consuming expeditions which, because of inadequate preparation of the participants, very large groups who can neither hear nor see what is happening and a general lack of planning, achieve very little.

9.9.1 Preliminary planning

This entails the following:

(a) Making a survey of learning needs of the group of students.
(b) Identifying ways of meeting these needs. Here the use of internal or external field trips might well meet a class or group need.
(c) Surveying the existing facilities, both internal and external, in the community which would meet these needs. Which are suitable, where are they located, what transport facilities are necessary and available?
(d) A preliminary visit to the agency if it is external, or to the department if internal.

160

(e) Discussion with the agency or department head which will clarify the
- objective of the proposed field trip;
- type of information and learning experience required;
- probable size of the group;
- level of knowledge of the group;
- length of time available;
- agency or department staff who are available to impart knowledge, conduct a discussion or answer questions.
(f) Mutual agreement as to the date and time of visit. This must be confirmed in writing.
(g) Making the necessary transport arrangements.
(h) Where it is necessary to get permission for the group to visit the agency or department, this must be done in writing.
(i) Preliminary planning for the type of information and manner of presentation to course participants prior to the field trip. The necessary arrangements must then be made.
(j) The preparation of a printed handout for course participants stating
- the date, time and place of trip;
- the objectives of the field trip;
- the observations which should be made;
- any special dress required for the occasion;
- any safety regulations which must be observed.
(k) The organisation of some sort of card file system which gives resources available and makes future planning easier. The cards must of course be kept up to date and a note made on each card, after a field trip, stating its suitability or otherwise.
(l) Making arrangements for the course tutor to accompany the group in order to act as a resource person, to direct attention to pertinent points and to be on hand to deal with any problems that may arise.

9.9.2 Follow-up activities

These are extremely important as the whole purpose of the trip may be lost if the learning experiences are not consolidated. These include:
(a) A letter of thanks to the agency or department in question
(b) Discussion with the whole group involved regarding the field trip. This discussion must relate to
- objectives
- observations
- evaluation of learning experience
- application of observations to the participant's own field of nursing activity

- suggestions for the future.
(c) A short objective-type test which may be given to the group to determine whether and to what degree any learning took place as a result of the trip
(d) Evaluation by the staff of the nursing education department as to the effect of the field trip/s and any improvements which could be implemented in future planning.

The field trip should be seen as a carefully planned visit or tour to a place away from the area where the course is being presented. It has a definite aim or objective which allows for personal observation of objects, methods and care activities which cannot easily be brought into the teaching area or reproduced there. These activities could, of course, be shown by means of a film or slides, but this is not a 'real' situation, which is what a field trip affords. A film can only show part of the whole, and the surroundings are left out.

The field trip may take up quite a short space of time, such as an hour, when it involves a visit to another department, the college or, if the course is run for persons in extra-institutional agencies, the hospital. It may take a day or even two. Longer field trips can also be arranged though the organisation of these is more difficult.

Field trips can do much to stimulate students' interest. All the senses can be involved in the learning activities, learners being able to see, touch, smell, hear, feel and in some cases, even taste.

During field trips, learners can assess the different effects that varying conditions may have on the health of the individual, can come to realise what frustrations can develop, and how patients are adversely affected by incorrect preparation for operation or for X-ray investigation.

They can become aware of the complexities of the central sterilising department, the need for correct ordering, prompt return of used material and a thousand and one aspects of interdepartmental work which had never previously occurred to them.

An outside field trip can bring to the attention of learners, the factors in the community which contribute to ill-health, the difficulties people experience in caring adequately for their families, and the relationship between what presents in the wards and what occurs in the community.

Interdisciplinary hospital field trips are also valuable education experiences, for so many nurses working in a general hospital have never seen the inside of a psychiatric hospital. Yet this is a hospital to which they send and from which they receive patients.

Field trips are also fruitful sources of material for assignments, exhibits, projects and other learning activities. Learners get to know one another in a fairly informal way, and they also get to know members of their profession in other fields of nursing. They act as a link between the community services and the hospital services.

There are disadvantages. Field trips can be time consuming and expensive. They must be planned carefully and followed up if they are to be of real value.

They are an excellent teaching method if carefully pre-planned, well administered and integrated into the full learning programme. The nurse-educator would do well to give them careful consideration when deciding upon the activities of her department.

9.10 SEMINARS

The word seminar comes from the Latin *seminarium*, meaning a seed plot. *Chambers Twentieth Century Dictionary* defines it: 'Originally used in German, meaning a group of students working in a specific subject of study under a teacher.' It is a method of organising a class so that guided discussion can take place on a specific topic or problem.

The students are allocated a subject to prepare. Each one in the group, which of course cannot be too large, will prepare an aspect of the subject for discussion. This must be clearly defined, and the preparation by each student must be thorough. Students must clearly understand what is required of them.

Each student then in turn presents the aspect of the subject which she has prepared. These presentations must be clear and concise.

After the presentation of all aspects free discussion by the students is allowed. The tutor in charge of the group may briefly add an aspect which has been omitted, or give a different point of view, after which her role is only to keep the discussion flowing, to prevent dominance of the group by one member and to keep it to the point. Students must be led to provide their own answers to the questions posed.

It is a technique which requires a certain degree of knowledge and clinical experience, and is therefore more suited to senior students. The seeds which are sown must be given the opportunity to grow and develop to full maturity, assisted by the efforts of a good gardener (the tutor conducting the seminar), and must not be allowed to wither and die.

Another method of introducing the seminar may be for one or two members to prepare a short paper for discussion. Students must be forewarned so that they can do background reading and formulate ideas which can contribute to the subsequent discussion. The student involvement which occurs in seminar teaching gives them practice in expressing themselves, assessing the thoughts of others and determining relationships between various aspects of the subject-matter presented. It affords opportunity for summarising material, is student-centred, and gives the opportunity for the practice of interpersonal relationship skills.

9.11 TUTORIALS

This form of teaching is an old technique which is used a great deal in tertiary education. It is particularly suitable to senior students who have the capacity for individual work.

The course is presented in the form of lectures, during which individual reading is allocated and guide-lines are offered for the study of material. Students are free to consult the instructor (tutor) in the intervals, but the groups come together regularly (say weekly) to discuss individual reading and draw conclusions. Large lecture groups are divided into small units and different meeting times are set aside for the various smaller groups. The tutor or instructor asks questions relevant to the assigned reading. Students answer questions which are designed to show whether the students have grasped the subject-matter, and will show up any gaps in the students' mastery of the material. The tutor or instructor then guides them further, and suggests further reading or other means of acquiring the relevant information. Problems can be discussed and difficult points clarified. A great deal of individual work is required, but participation in the tutorial sessions is encouraged, and students who are keen to learn can benefit greatly from this form of teaching.

9.12 SYMPOSIA

This is another form of group activity although it can be used with bigger groups, and there is less individual participation.

The word 'symposium' comes from the Latin form of the Greek word *symposion, syn,* meaning with and *posis,* meaning drinking. It therefore technically means 'a drinking together'. In the sense in which it is used today, perhaps 'drinking together of knowledge' would be a correct interpretation.

The method of presentation is for two or more speakers to present important facets of the same general theme or topic, with some time at the end of the scheduled session provided for questions from the audience. In the nursing context, a symposium dealing with the care of the aged could be arranged, and experts from medicine, community health nursing, social work, social services and geriatric nursing might present their aspects or specialised knowledge of the subject.

The topic is divided into different phases and presented in the form of a lecture, one speaker following the other. A chairman introduces all the speakers and may make transitional statements. The chairman must see that speakers keep to their allotted time, usually ten to 15 minutes. At the end the chairman briefly summarises what has been said and opens the discussion, directing questions to the relevant speaker. When the time available has expired, the chairman closes the proceedings with a short word of thanks to the speakers, or calls upon somebody previously designated for the task, to do so.

A symposium can bring experts together, it can be presented to a large group of people, makes economical use of time and is varied by the change of speakers. It often broadens the perspective of those taking part in the presentation, as well as those listening.

Senior students can also be encouraged to present their own symposium on some aspect of the subject-matter. This can be an interesting and rewarding teaching/learning experience.

9.13 SIMULATION TECHNIQUES

According to *The Concise Oxford Dictionary*, to simulate means 'to feign, to pretend, to have or feel, to resemble, to mimic' (derived from the Latin *simulare, similis*, meaning like).

These techniques can be used to make physical forms resemble the real thing very closely, and are used in clinical teaching where wounds can be simulated, and techniques like removing stitches, clips or drains can be demonstrated and practised before the student attempts to carry out the technique in the live situation.

Simulation can be used in the teaching of first aid where feigned or simulated injuries from accidents can be produced, even to the pumping of blood from cut arteries.

Stitching can be practised on pieces of fresh meat, which gives the student the chance to 'feel' what it is like to insert stitches, and episiotomies can be practised on the external genitalia of a slaughtered cow.

Manikins have been developed for the practice of cardio-pulmonary resuscitation, for the practice of urinary catheterisation and many more. Practising giving an injection into an orange is a simulation technique. The ingenious tutor/clinical teacher can devise numerous examples.

9.13.1 Role play

Role play is also based on simulation techniques. This method of instruction requires the spontaneous acting out of a situation by two or more participants under the direction of the nurse-educator.

The situation to be acted out is described to the group, the students are allocated roles to play and given a briefing as to individual characteristics, details that are not necessarily shared by the other participants. The 'playlet' is then enacted, each person playing the role as he feels it would or should happen. The other members of the group form the audience, making notes if necessary. When the action is concluded, a general discussion follows. Roles can be reversed, so that members can feel what it is like to be the receiver of information, of complaints or of other people's problems instead of being the giver of information, the complainant or the one with the problem. Other members of the group can be asked to act out the same roles, particularly if they are critical of the interpretation given to the situation, by stating that 'it wouldn't have happened like that'. More discussion follows. Often very different reactions to the same scene are acted out and valuable ideas can be brought out.

Success lies in the original scripting of the scene to be enacted, the briefing or scene setting. Participants may be briefed separately, so that they do not know details about other participants, but have to determine it during the playlet. A planned scenario could have a registered nurse, a houseman and a student nurse, with the doctor complaining to the sister about some real or imagined negligence on the part of the student. This would give the student insight into the handling of such a situation in real life. Roles to be played could include more than one student, enrolled nurses, patients and their relatives, even more senior personnel, or non-nursing staff such as housekeepers, dispensary staff, messengers, secretaries and so forth. A little imaginaton in the scripting of the situation is all that is required. By playing the roles of others, students can become aware of what is can feel like to be in another person's shoes. Also, because the situation is not real, the playlet can be re-played and another approach tried, which is not possible in a real-life situation.

Competent leadership is essential to the success of this method. Students may 'dry up', or they may become aggressive if criticised by the group and the situation has to be carefully watched and guided. It may be necessary to defuse a potential confrontation and some students may not want to role play, while many others relish the limelight.

It is an ideal method for teaching students to undertake health education. As a teaching method it can be very rewarding, if properly controlled, and it usually holds the attention of the group to whom it can be a welcome break from more conventional teaching techniques.

Role play should be built upon carefully structured situations which are based on real-life situations. It must be in the hands of those who understand the technique and student nurse-educators should be given practice in the technique during their training.

9.13.2 Learning games

These are also a form of simulation technique. They were originally developed in the business world and in military training, but they can be equally effectively applied to other forms of education. Learning games can be very complicated and may even require apparatus which is costly and difficult to operate, but others are relatively simple, and once the basic materials have been assembled, perhaps at the cost of time and trouble but very little else, they can be re-used for different groups.

A test of how students would organise their time and establish priorities could be presented in the form of a learning game.

A list is made of the types of situations which confront a professional nurse in charge of a medical (or surgical, paediatric or any other) unit during her first hour on duty. This list could then be duplicated and handed to each member of a student group. Each learner is then given a set time to organise the work and state briefly what she would do with each item on the list. The group then discusses how each member has dealt with what was presented and lively debate which has a distinct learning component, can ensue.

Another game could be built up around a nursing care situation, where the care is described and students are asked to list briefly what nursing care should be given to that person. Again discussion follows and lively participation will ensure success of learning from the simulated situation. Handling of crisis situations might provide material for other games.

The design of a simulation game will force the nurse–educator to think clearly about what is to be achieved. A real-life situation must be translated into learning elements. Suitable and feasible inputs, such as problems, complications, reactions or other events suitable for the level of knowledge and experience of the students for whom the game is designed must be posed. Reality must be a guiding principle. The material's relevance must be considered. Questions such as whether the game is to be conducted on a points basis, or whether it is simply to serve as a basis for discussion, must also be answered. Practice and subsequent revision are important. No game will be perfect the first time it is devised.

Whatever simulation technique is employed, the following aspects should be remembered:

- Simulation can only imitate the real situation, it cannot duplicate it.
- It can only measure, not teach all aspects of performance.
- It is possible to cover a wide range of situations which might be difficult to experience sufficiently in real life, to build up appropriate responses.
- Learning can be increased by good feedback.
- It can be used as a form of assessment.
- It can be used to develop clinical judgement.
- It can shorten the time needed to experience and gain mastery in handling a variety of nursing care situations. The care of a patient who has had a lifetime of treatment for a chronic disease can be condensed into a

short space of time and appropriate nursing intervention at each stage can be studied.

- Professional skills and attitudes can be built up and reinforced by the use of simulated situations.

9.14 PROGRAMMED LEARNING

Programmed learning or programmed instruction is a method of helping or guiding the student to learn by providing material according to which the student follows a specific study guide, and can learn by himself.

It may be presented in book form, by means of tapes, slides and other visual or audio-visual material and study guides, or by the use of teaching machines.

Programmed learning was first devised by the American psychologist BF Skinner, and was based on three principles:

(a) To learn something correctly the first time is better than to make mistakes which have to be corrected later. This necessitates re-learning whereas correct responses 'reinforce' learning whilst errors are minimised.
(b) Immediate knowledge of results is conducive to learning.
(c) Every student should be able to respond to each point and thus be an active participant in the learning event. This does not occur in a conventional class-room setting.

9.14.1 Advantages

The protagonists of programmed learning quote the following advantages:

(a) Students work at their own pace.
(b) It permits mass teaching, and can reach groups otherwise cut off from learning centres.
(c) The sequential steps to be followed in the learning event can be small and designed for orderly and controlled development of a student's knowledge and skills.
(d) Immediate feedback to the students is possible.
(e) Students participate actively.
(f) Students are not afraid of making a response. In a large group they may be unwilling to respond to a question for fear of being embarrassed by a wrong answer.
(g) There is high availability of programmes.
(h) Programmed learning can be used to supplement teaching in times of staff shortages.
(i) Programmed learning can be used to help students who have had to miss class due to illness.

(j) Programmes can be designed to provide revision of work covered some time ago, before tackling new material which requires that specific knowledge upon which to build.

9.14.2 Disadvantages

The disadvantages include:
(a) Preparation time is long and thus expensive.
(b) A great deal of skill is required to draw up good 'teaching programmes'. Special educational competence is necessary.
(c) The absence of the teacher-student interaction may lead to a lack of stimulation of the student.
(d) The mechanical nature of the process may be boring to the student.
(e) There is no opportunity for group interaction. Group dynamics as an integral part of teaching is overlooked.
(f) A student may skip through the programme if the self-evaluation required at each step is omitted or remedial learning is not undertaken when necessary.
(g) The correct conclusion may be reached by guessing or without grasping the significance of the whole. In other words, the programmer has done all the thinking and not the learners.

9.14.3 Production

The production of a programme necessitates the following steps:
(a) Analyse the subject-matter to be studied.
(b) Divide the subject-matter into a sequence of small steps, each of which could be grasped even by a slow learner.
(c) Provide very clear instructions in the study guides to lead the student through each step or 'frame'.
(d) Plan tests of learning achieved at the end of each frame. This is done by posing questions.
(e) The student then checks the results of learning by consulting the answer given in the programme. A correct answer reinforces the learning; a wrong one can be corrected immediately.
(f) If the answer is correct the student passes on to the next frame, but if not he can again work through the appropriate section of the guide, and try again.

In the preparation of a successful programme, the following principles must be observed:
(a) The programme must suit the level which the learner has reached in his studies.

(b) Testing and revising programmes is essential if they are to be valid, clear learning guides.

(c) The learner must be required to make an active response by answering test questions.

(d) The second frame must be built on knowledge gained in the first frame, and so on.

(e) General revision and testing should occur regularly during the process of working through a programme, so that the frame or part can be seen in the context of the whole.

(f) Revision after testing must also take place until the majority of students are able to respond correctly to the questions the first time. This will entail very careful writing of the material used in the frame.

(g) In programme production and printing, the learner must be prevented from seeing the correct response immediately. He must first supply a response himself and *then* be able to check it. Various devices exist such as a vertical series of frames, with the correct responses given in the right-hand margin of the page which is hidden from the learner by a piece of paper, or some other material which slides down to uncover the correct answer as required.

(h) Pre-testing of a learner is often necessary to determine whether he is ready for a particular programme.

(i) Post-testing of the whole section of subject-matter must occur at the end of the programme. If the score is unsatisfactory, the student must work through the entire programme again.

If programmed instruction is to be used, it must be introduced with care to students, so that they understand what it is all about and are motivated to participate. Those who are unfamiliar with programmes often think that the work presented in the frames of a programmed book are too easy because there appears to be little chance of the learner making the wrong response. There may also appear to be too much repetition. This may be because they are already familiar with the subject-matter. Programmes are designed to guide *learners*, and the aim is to make the minimum of errors, as this reinforces correct learning. A good programme will always be found to be easy by some students, the majority will find it more difficult but still respond correctly most of the time, and a few will find it really difficult, but will, although it may take longer, eventually pass the 'post test'.

There are two types of programmes:

(a) *Linear programmes:* Each step is so small and each response so short that all learners follow the same route or *line.* If a student gives an incorrect response he simply returns to the frame he has just studied, thus backing up, as it were.

(b) *Branching programmes:* In this type provision is made for the student who makes an error because of faulty background knowledge or some such reason. His attention is then shunted on to a *branch* line, and the error explained in detail. Remedial work is given and a new test taken. He is then branched back to the stage at which he has left the line. If no error is made the student proceeds to the next frame in line.

Excellent programmes can be developed using tapes, slides, a study guide and built-in tests. In teaching the practice of nursing, sounds such as heart beats and abnormal breathing can be supplied by a tape, with a slide at the same time showing the student where to place the stethoscope. The tape and/or study guide can direct the student to a textbook for study, and test questions are set at the end of each section. All these can also be combined with short films or film strips. Programmes can be drawn up which would make the learning of nursing care of infectious diseases interesting and possible to large numbers, who might not have the opportunity to nurse such cases. The written word is supplemented and made more alive.

Teaching machines are similar to this type of programme. Frames are presented visually and the student presses a button in response. Otherwise the programme is the same. Teaching machines are expensive, however, and are more liable to break down.

Written programmes are often presented in the form of books, which can also be expensive for students, and they may not always meet the specific needs of a group of students or of a particular course. Other written material can be typed and reproduced easily and relatively cheaply. Such material is also relatively easy to amend in the event of changes in treatment or new knowledge.

Any learning package which sets out definite objectives, which guides the student through the material, and which achieves the desired learning, which is then confirmed by some form of post-testing, is an example of programmed learning. A programme may be long or short, and provided it has been tested and validated, has many applications in learning the practice of nursing.

9.15 LEARNING BY DOING

This method, or the concept of learning by *trial and error*, is not only wasteful of time and resources, but it may in fact be dangerous. Of course students learn by practice, but it must be guided, supervised practice which is based on sound knowledge. There is no such thing in learning the practice of nursing as trying something out on a patient. Such actions would deny the person who is a patient the right to safety at the hands of those caring for him. No registered nurse in charge of nursing care can be so irresponsible as to delegate care to a student or pupil without satisfying herself that the student or pupil is competent. 'In-service' or 'on-the-job' training is a misnomer for nurse education. Student nurses are students who must be guided to professional adulthood by a series of planned learning experiences based on theoretical background which is reinforced and brought to reality in the practical situation.

In order to teach the practice of nursing in the clinical or live situation, the following teaching strategies could be employed.

9.16 PRECEPT AND EXAMPLE

Precept derives from the Latin *praeceptum,* meaning instruct and example, something to be imitated, thus teaching or instruction by means of a pattern to be imitated; the acting out of a role model of professional practice in nursing which is worthy of imitation.

The unit professional nurse, other registered nurses in the unit, the teacher from the clinical teaching department, the tutor, the clinical nursing specialist and the 'matron' are all role models upon whom neophytes base their image of professional practice. It is a very demanding role, but an infinitely worthwhile one. The actions and attitudes of those filling these role models are often the determining factor in shaping the future attitudes of students and pupils towards patients, clients, relatives, friends and colleagues in the health team and all categories of workers in the caring situation.

The actions and attitudes displayed by those fulfilling the role model actually shape the professional practice of those looking to them as an exemplification of true professional nursing. It is the manner in which the teacher in the clinical setting sees and uses herself and her philosophy regarding the practice of her profession which are communicated to those within her sphere of influence.

Nurses are trained to nurse, and to nurse *people*. Registered nurses interpreting their role models must continue to nurse people. They must not be seen to withdraw from active nursing when they complete their period of training towards registration. As role models it is essential that they continue active participation in nursing care. They must remain active, interested and ready to continue their own nursing education, even if only by enquiry and reading. By doing so they serve as an inspiration to students with regard to future patient care activities, to the unstinted participation in nursing care and to a positive attitude towards patient care. The unit professional nurse must function as a living example to her students.

The fact that the good ward professional nurse does teach, must be emphasised. Care and consideration for the comfort and safety of patients and clients, heed for their feelings and for those of other members of the health team are often taught by precept and example. Negative teaching plays a

172

part in formulating attitudes in students and pupils, though it is certainly not a technique to be recommended. Bad examples which are blatantly obvious may cause a student to reject them completely for herself, but other attitudes and practices which are less obviously the cause of patient or client anxiety or distress, may come to be accepted as the norm. Therefore the registered nurse needs to be constantly on her guard against such occurrences. The passing on of bad habits or negative attitudes is to be deplored and avoided at all costs.

The use of the effect of a poor performance by a registered person can provide a 'teachable moment' if done constructively, in the interest of patient care and not in the spirit of carping criticism of a colleague. However, it needs to be handled with tact and understanding. The quality of care that the professional practitioner of nursing renders and which she insists upon from her personnel, is also part of teaching by precept and example. The upholding of standards must not only be demanded, it must also be practised by the person in charge of a unit. She must be regarded by her colleagues and students or pupils as a sympathetic person, with a sense of personal integrity in all she undertakes. She must show enthusiasm and interest. She must be knowledgeable and professionally competent.

The basic elements of teaching by precept and example may be summarised as follows. The person, be she unit professional nurse or her deputy must always present an image which exemplifies:

- A philosophy of service
- Professional and personal integrity
- Professional competence and knowledge based on practice, study, enquiry, an open mind and realism
- Dedication to her task
- Enthusiasm and interest in all she does
- Sympathy and empathy in her dealings with patients, clients, their relatives and friends and all co-workers
- An understanding of the problems of patients and clients
- An understanding of the problems of learners
- An ability to cope with crises and unexpected occurrences with calmness, confidence and competence
- The ability to guide and teach, to communicate and to engender good interpersonal relationships
- Fairness in all her dealings
- A respect for the human dignity and worth of all men
- An appreciation of the sanctity of life.

No one person will measure up to all the expectations of a role model at all times – human beings are fallible. An imperfect role model must be helped to recognise and remedy her imperfection as far as possible.

Students and pupils must be guided towards presenting a good role model. They must be encouraged and not discouraged, for an imperfect role
model can be improved. Students will be heartened if they are helped to
realise this.

9.17 USE OF THE 'TEACHABLE MOMENT'

The 'teachable moment' can be described as that moment when something
occurs during nursing care where immediate intervention is desirable and
which can be used there and then to impart knowledge to those involved in
the particular caring incident. It is this moment in the practice situation
which, if seized upon, can be of inestimable value in the teaching strategy of
a unit.

'Teachable moments' occur many times during a nursing care day. Many
are wasted, but many more are used, often subconsciously. A teachable moment occurs in a real-life situation. It occurs without serious planning. No
preparation is necessary beyond that acquired in daily practice and by keeping up to date. It is one of the teaching tools much more readily available to
the trained staff in a unit than to the clinical teacher or tutor from outside. To
negate the importance of the teachable moment would be to negate the unit
professional nurse's responsibility for patient care and thus the possibility that
teaching will achieve that quality of care which should be her ultimate objective. All occurrences which arise in the nursing care situation, whether they
have professional, administrative, technical care, patient/client needs or emotional or psychological implications, are potential teaching situations. Many
such situations have in fact more than one such implication. The action taken
by the unit professional nurse, or other member of the health team, may in itself have teaching content.

How much more value would it not have if its teaching potential were to
be perceived by an alert unit professional nurse, senior nurse or other member of the health team so that the potential is immediately recognised and the
opportunity grasped.

The recognition of the teachable moment whenever it occurs and the use
made of it is one of the best methods which the competent, interested, up-to-
date unit professional nurse has of passing on the expertise which she has acquired over the years, to those preparing to follow in her steps.

9.18 THE NURSING ROUND

A nursing round is a teaching strategy which nurses seem to feel applies only
to medical students and their tutors. Yet it can also be employed satisfactorily
in teaching the practice of nursing.

A nursing round is in fact a planned, organised visit to the patient, be he in bed or out of it, for the purpose of assessing the nursing care being given to that patient, discussing his progress and making the necessary adjustments or changes in his care. The 'ward round' that the professional nurse does as a routine to her patients is a nursing round. Its extension to include other members of the unit team could make it one of the most valuable teaching strategies in teaching the practice of nursing. It also brings the person in charge of the unit, or her deputy, into more frequent and intimate contact with the nursing care of the patient, which is her prime responsibility.

The nursing round can be used in several ways as a teaching strategy:

(a) By the *head of the unit* conducting a round with other members of the nursing personnel. The inclusion of junior members of the team in such a round is invaluable, as patients so often talk to such members of staff and thus valuable information can be obtained which might otherwise be lost. Cognisance must be taken of the total picture of the patient, his treatment and response to treatment, his mental attitude, background and community resources available on discharge. Of course care must be taken, as is the case in medical teaching rounds, to avoid discussions in front of the patient which may cause anxiety. Nevertheless, the patient should, where possible, be involved and his opinion sought. Some of the teaching may be done in the 'sister's office' or the clinic room; it is a method which presents opportunities for a 'real', 'live' correlation of theory and practice.

(b) By the *clinical teaching department* as a means of demonstrating specific points of nursing care. It would, of course, be a prerequisite for the clinical teacher to have the required background knowledge and skills to deal with the treatments involved, and that the necessary arrangements had been made with the head of the department prior to the nursing round, and her co-operation obtained. Again it is an ideal opportunity for correlating theory and practice in the 'live' situation.

(c) By members of the *college, lecture room or other teaching staff,* again after having obtained the necessary permission and co-operation from the person in charge of the unit. It would serve well to bring 'theoretical' teachers into the 'practical' situation to the mutal benefit of both theoretical and practical training. A shortage of tutors may make this difficult to achieve, but it is worth striving for.

A great deal of material can be covered in the course of one teaching nursing round. The variety of diseases from which the patients are suffering, and the methods being used to treat them as well as the unique plans developed by the personnel of the specific department to cope with nursing care problems, are all teaching points. The head of the department, even if she does not conduct the round, can be present on the round conducted by 'clinical teaching' or 'college' personnel. It must never be undertaken without her knowledge or consent.

It is not suggested that teaching nursing rounds be carried out daily, but they should be planned and co-ordinated so that they are carried out at least weekly, and that all members of the nursing personnel are involved either in conducting the rounds or in participating in them. Nursing care cannot stop while rounds are being made, therefore all staff cannot be involved at the same time. With proper planning though, all members of a unit's nursing personnel can be incorporated in such a round at least once a week.

9.19 NURSING CARE PLANS

These are nothing new; they have been with us from the beginning of nursing. Their more precise formulation and use may be somewhat unfamiliar to many nurses.

Nursing care plans should be well thought out and the manner in which they are used should be of the utmost simplicity so that they are readily understood by all and easily become part of the routine practice.

A nursing care plan is a plan of nursing action which includes a summary of a patient's health problems, an assessment of his present state and nursing needs and should include a statement of both short-term and long-term objectives. It should be flexible and may include alternative nursing actions.

The planning should be the concern of the team nursing the patient. The medical practitioner will initiate the medical treatment and he is a valuable source of information, but nursing care is ultimately the responsibility of the nurse in charge of the unit and must have her sanction.

A nursing care plan which involves a great deal of writing will not be easy to adhere to and lends itself to failure. Something in the form of basic data and a checklist is much more likely to succeed. It may be necessary to evolve different nursing care plan forms for different departments. The following is given as an example of a basic health history and the formulation of a nursing care plan based on this – many variations are possible.

UNIT

Form A
BASIC HEALTH HISTORY on admission to hospital – To be completed by the nurse.
Mark as many as possible with an X only. Only fill in applicable sections.

1 PERSONAL DETAILS

Name.................................... Hospital registration number ....
Age... Sex..
Employment...
Family composition...
....
Area in which patient lives ....
....

2 DIAGNOSIS

Provisional..
Final...

3 TEMPERATURE..

4 PULSE RATE?.............................. Regular ....
                                            Irregular ....

5 RESPIRATORY SYSTEM

Respiration rate...

Respiration distress
YES	
NO	

If YES, indicate type:

Dyspnoea
Orthopnoea
Asthmatic wheeze

Cheyne-Stokes
Very shallow
Stridor

Cough

None
Dry
Productive
Crouplike

Epistaxis...........................
Haemoptysis ....

6 BLOOD PRESSURE

Systolic...

Diastolic...

Ever had: Hypertension?
           Hypotension?

7 STATE OF CONSCIOUSNESS

Fully conscious ....

Unconscious ....

Able to respond to stimuli only with difficulty ....

Able to communicate ....

Unable to communicate ....

8 MENTAL ATTITUDE

Co-operative...

Unco-operative..

Anxious...

Aggressive...

Passive...

In a highly tense state..

Disorientated...

9 PUPILS

Both react to light..

Neither react to light ....

Only one reacts to light..

                L R

Both fixed ....

Left fixed...

Right fixed ....

Equal ....

Unequal...

10 DEFORMITIES/DEFECTS IN MUSCULAR SYSTEM

Paralysis

                                                                  L R

Hemiplegia   Hand only

Quadriplegia   Arm only

                                          Leg only

                                  L R

Shortening of leg

Shortening of arm

Muscle wastage: Arm
                Leg

Limp
Joint stiffness
Amputations: Arm   Leg
           Hand   Foot
           Finger   Toe

	L	R

11 SIGHT

	L	R

Appears to be able to see...
Appears to have difficulty in seeing ....
Appears to be unable to see ....
Wears glasses for reading ....
Wears glasses all the time..

12 HEARING

Appears to be able to hear ....
Appears to have difficulty in hearing....................................
Appears to be unable to hear..
Wears a hearing aid ....

13 SPEECH

Clear..
Slurred ....
Unco-ordinated ....

14 WEIGHT

Normal weight...
Present weight...
Recent loss..
Recent gain...

15 URINARY TRACT (mark abnormalities with an X)

Urine test
   Alb
   Sugar
   Ketones
   Cloudiness
   Blood
   Specify: High SG
            Low SG

Other
   Oliguria
   Dysuria
   Frequency
   Abnormal odour
   Incontinence
   Haematuria

16 SKIN (mark any of the following which are present with an X)

Rash	
Pallor	
Lumps	
Jaundice	
Peeling	
Decubitus ulcer	
Redness over sacrum	
Burn	
Petechiae	

Coldness	
Sweat	
Dryness/dehydration	
Oedema: Localised / Generalised	
Ascites	
Blue lips	
Cyanosis	
Ruddiness	
Ecchymosis	

17 DIGESTIVE TRACT (mark any of the following abnormalities present with an X)

Anorexia	
Nausea	
Vomiting	
Haematemesis	
Abdominal pain	
Distension	
Colostomy	
Caecostomy	
Gastrostomy	
Mouth: Dry / Cracked / Sores	

Constipation	
Diarrhoea	
Melaena	
Frank blood in stool	
Green	
Incontinence	
Difficulty in swallowing	
Ileostomy	
Tongue: Dry / Cracked / Furred	

18 PROBLEMS IDENTIFIED BY ECG

....
....

19 GYNAECOLOGICAL HISTORY (mark any appropriate with an X; complete others)

Age of menarche	
Age of menopause	
Number of pregnancies	
Number of full-time births	
Number of miscarriages	
Infertility	
Menstruates regularly	
Menstruates irregularly	
Dysmenorrhoea	

Amenorrhoea...
Menorrhagia...
Metrorrhagia...
Leucorrhoea..
Cystocele ....
Rectocele..

Family planning methods:
    Never used ....
    Pill ....
    IUD..
    Depo...
    Sterilised ....

20 OTHER HEALTH ABNORMALITIES (mark with an X)

Tremor ....
Convulsions ....
Epilepsy ....
Hyperthyroidism ....
Hypothyroidism..................................
Diabetes mellitus................................   Site
Fatigue...
Pain..
Prostheses ....
Paraesthesia ....

Allergies: Hay fever
           Asthma
           Contact dermatitis
           Rhinitis
           GI tract allergy
           Migraine

Emaciation
Gout
Arthritis
Obesity

21 PREVIOUS ILLNESSES

....
....

22 PRESENT COMPLAINTS

....

....

23 PRESENT MEDICATIONS

....

....

24 INVESTIGATIONS ORDERED	RESULTS
....	....
....	....
....	....
....	....
....	....
....	....

25 MEDICAL TREATMENT ORDERED

....

Basic forms of this nature could be printed. Much of the information has to be recorded in any case, so that presents little hardship. The rest is quickly dealt with by filling in the odd figure or making an X in the appropriate place.

Attached to this history is Form B which selects the problems, lists the nursing care needed to deal with the problem and marks progress. A page lasting for a week or less could then be employed. An example of Form B is given below.

Form B

Patient's name:.. Unit:..................... Reg no:.................

Problem identified	Nursing care plan (including objective)	RESPONSE				
		Day 1	Day 2	Day 3	Day 4	Day 5

An example of the use of such a nursing care plan in the nursing of an elderly male patient admitted with congestive cardiac failure is now given:

INFORMATION OBTAINED FROM FORM A

1 Mr John Jones
   76 years   Male
   Retired farmer
   Wife aged 70
   Two sons   38   42
   Three grandchildren
   Port Elizabeth
2 Diagnosis: Congestive cardiac failure
3 35,5°C
4 86   Irregular
5 26   Distressed
        Dyspnoea
        Dry cough
6 $\frac{180}{110}$ Has had hypertension

7 Fully conscious
8 Mentally anxious
9 Pupils both react to light
10 Deformities, etc NAD
11 Sightreads with glasses
12 Appears to have difficulty in hearing
13 Speech clear
14 Recent gain of 6 kg
15 Urine: Alb
            Highly concentrated SG, 1020
            Oliguria
16 Skin: Dry   Oedema
            Lips blue
            Redness over sacrum
17 Anorexia
   Constipation
   Mouth: Dry
18 ECG presents evidence of right-sided failure
20 Fatigue

The nursing care problems identified are:

Irregular pulse

Nursing care plan: Administer antiarrhythmic
drugs as ordered
(name of drug)

Day 1	Day 2	Day 3	Day 4	Day 5
Rate: 76 Less arrhythmia	Rate: 68 No arrhythmia	Rate: 70 No arrhythmia	Rate: Stable	Stable

Dyspnoea

Nursing care plan: To relieve dyspnoea
(a) O$_2$ by nasal catheter

Day 1	Day 2	Day 3	Day 4	Day 5
Some relief	Intermittently only	Discontinued	—	—

(b) Prop up in bed

Day 1	Day 2	Day 3	Day 4	Day 5
Some relief	Better	Able to reduce pillows	Fewer pillows	Stable

(c) Reduce activity to prevent physical distress

Day 1	Day 2	Day 3	Day 4	Day 5
Full wash	Passive movements	Passive movements	Allow to wash face	Increase activities $^a/_c$ response

Raised blood pressure

Nursing care plan: Monitor and give drugs ordered

Day 1	Day 2	Day 3	Day 4	Day 5
$\dfrac{160}{100}$	$\dfrac{150}{95}$	$\dfrac{145}{95}$	$\dfrac{140}{90}$	Stable

Mental anxiety

Nursing care plan: To relieve anxiety

(a) Establish a good relationship
(b) Bell always at hand: make sure that the patient knows how to use it
(c) Respond promptly
(d) The patient is somewhat deaf: be sure he can hear and understands what is said
(e) Locker must be within easy reach with all requirements at hand

Urine

Alb in urine
High concentrated SG
Oliguria

Nursing care plan

(a) Daily urine test
(b) Measure and chart fluid intake and output

Day 1	Day 2	Day 3	Day 4	Day 5

Under these list SG, albumen, and fluid intake and output

Skin dry, lips blue, oedema, redness over sacrum

Nursing care plan

(a) Limit fluid intake according to output
(b) Administer diuretic (name) as ordered
(c) Restrict sodium intake
(d) Put on sheepskin. Watch reddened sacral area. Attend to toilet of the area. Change position if possible. Use ripple mattress. Lift out of bed into armchair

Day 1	Day 2	Day 3	Day 4	Day 5

Report the results of nursing intervention under each day column in each listed area, (a) to (d)

Anorexia, constipation, dry mouth
Nursing care plan
(a) Small frequent feeds: low bulk, low calorie. Avoid gas-forming foods, restrict sodium
(b) Prevent straining at stool. Give laxatives as required (state type)
(c) Oral hygiene as required. Keep mouth moist

Day 1	Day 2	Day 3	Day 4	Day 5

Report the results of nursing intervention under each day in each listed area, (a) to (c)

General care instructions
(a) Promote rest and sleep
(b) Help with feeding as necessary; patient must not be made too dependent
(c) Passive exercise at first
(d) Commence health education as part of a normal routine, for example diet, exercise, medication, avoidance of excess, weight reduction, regular checks, signs of incipient problems

Day 1	Day 2	Day 3	Day 4	Day 5

Report the results of nursing intervention under each day in each area listed, (a) to (b)

The object of this section is to point out the use of the nursing care plan as a teaching aid. While many nurses are familiar with written nursing care plans on the kardex record of the patient, where instructions such as full wash; care to pressure areas; intake and output chart; blood pressure four-hourly; passive exercise; four pillows; salt-free, low-calorie diet; etc, are listed, this method of writing a nursing care plan has less teaching value than the one detailed above. It is clear that in discussing a patient, a complete though brief assessment of his day-to-day progress is given in the plan suggested, which makes the whole rationale of care easy to understand. If the student is taught to use nursing care plans in this manner, it will facilitate her learning and her correlation of theory and practice. The example given is by no means the only possibility, it is only a guide.

A hospital may, by means of committee investigations, trial, evaluation and revision, eventually come up with a means of writing nursing care plans which are not only simple and easy to implement, but present valuable permanent records of patient care, and at the same time serve as excellent teaching material in learning the practice of nursing.

9.20 CLINICAL CONFERENCES

These may be described as conferences held by people involved in giving health care to people. There are two types, namely the team conference and the nursing care conference. Both present excellent teaching and learning opportunities.

9.20.1 The team conference

A team conference is one in which various members of the health-care team come together to discuss patients for whom they are caring jointly. It could include a medical practitioner, who is usually the leader of the health-care team, members of the nursing staff, physiotherapists and occupational therapists, a dietician, social worker, or specialist in some field of medicine, etc. The conference then discusses various patients and their physical problems, including diagnosis, treatment, response to treatment, changes made and specific problems, medical, nursing and social. A total picture of care is obtained. While it may not be possible for everyone to actually participate in such a conference, there is no reason why only the practising nurse in charge should participate. Other nurses including students, must have the opportunity to learn to state the nursing point of view as part of their learning experience. They can be guided to make a meaningful contribution. Similarly, if such a conference is seen as a true learning-teaching mechanism, it can be set up so that nurses and students or members of other disciplines can at least listen to the discussions at the conference.

For team conferences to be successful, it is necessary that full records, including nursing care plans, results of tests, progress reports, etc, are available for conference participants. Sometimes team conferences can actually include a visit to the patient being discussed, so that he becomes part of the whole; he may be examined, asked for his opinion and generally consulted. This could take the form of a conference ward round. In more sophisticated centres, the visit to and examination of the patient could be put on video-tape which could then be included in the team conference. Similarly, in suitably equipped centres, closed circuit television could make the team conference available to a much larger group of students of all disciplines. The possibilities for teaching and learning are exciting.

9.20.2 The nursing care conference

This can form the central point of both nursing care given to patients or clients and of the unit teaching programme. All members of the nursing care team, except those immediately involved in urgent nursing care, should be included in such a conference which should be organised on a regular basis. They should be planned, organised teaching-learning sessions where selected patients are discussed in detail. The aim is *nursing care,* given to patients in specific ways *by the nurse.* Of course, medical background to the patient's care is necessary, but it should not be the only aspect discussed. The structuring of a nursing care conference as a teaching mechanism is important. It can be planned in the following way:

(a) *Time:* A suitable time must be chosen – say visiting hours on Friday afternoon between 15h00 and 16h30. (This will depend on the unit and other factors such as urgent patient care needs.) If, for example, the ward is 'on intake' on Fridays, then another suitable day is chosen.

(b) *Participants:* All nursing staff, except those urgently needed for patient care, must participate. This means that no students or pupils should be off-duty on the selected day, that as many trained staff as possible are available, and that shifts should be organised in such a way that all potential participants are available for the conference.

(c) *Selection of patients:* As this is a 'teaching patient care' conference, the selection of those patients whose nursing care is to be discussed, should ensure that the diagnoses of those selected are varied, or present special nursing care problems so as to maximise learning. The number selected should also be limited to those problems which can be discussed in reasonably sufficient detail to enable the conference to be a real teaching-learning situation.

(d) *Selection of a team leader for the conference:* While the leader may be the professional nurse in charge, or her deputy, it could also be part of the exercise of preparing students for future leadership to give them the opportunity to organise and conduct a nursing care conference under guidance. In a teaching conference, the leader could also be a tutor or a member of the clinical teaching department staff.

(e) *Method of presentation:* Some sort of system is necessary and the following is suggested as a guide:

- A *brief* review of anatomy, physiology and pathology related to the specific case
- A *brief* review of medical findings, including results of investigations and the significance thereof
- A *brief* summary of medical treatment

- An assessment of *nursing* care problems related to medical treatments
- A detailed review of the nursing care plan, eliciting participation from *all* members of the nursing staff who have been concerned in giving nursing care to the particular patient whose nursing care is the subject of the conference.

(f) *Identification* of any new problems in nursing care.

(g) *Evaluation* of the patient's response, favourable or otherwise, to both medical and nursing treatment. Although the emphasis is on *nursing care* it is essential that medical information which contributes to the understanding of the patient's nursing requirements is made available and included in the conference.

(h) *Discussion:* General fruitful, constructive discussion, aimed at identifying means of improving patient care. Students should be encouraged to take an active, creative and constructive part in discussions which can become one of the most fruitful and enjoyable aspects of their learning experience. A conference of this nature should challenge the students to think. The conference leader must guide and encourage. Dominance by one or two members of the group *must* be prevented. A formal teaching nursing care conference not only serves to reinforce theoretical knowledge obtained in a class-room or from books, but also to correlate theory and practice, stimulate wider reading, introduce and reinforce positive constructive attitudes to patient care and to develop a lively questioning mind that is always seeking means of improving patient care.

Care must be taken to avoid discussing only the negative or problem aspects of care. It is equally important to the teaching-learning aspects of such a conference that compassionate, skilful care is also mentioned. Although problems must be solved, good care and the response of the patient to such care must be pointed out. A balance must be achieved between praise and blame, between sudden dramatic occurrences and the very necessary routine long-term type of care which forms the basis of most nursing care. Dealing with a cardiac arrest has drama, nursing a patient in mild cardiac failure has not. Yet skilful nursing of the latter is as important as of the former. The correct attitude to all forms of patient care can be emphasised in a skilfully conducted nursing care conference. Again the good conference leader has an obligation to see that students and less skilful members of the personnel are given the opportunity, under guidance, to develop their skills in conducting such conferences.

189

Informal nursing care conferences which take place while providing that care, are also excellent methods of teaching and learning. The learning is available to fewer people at a time, in fact it may be on a person-to-person basis, but it is none the less valid as a teaching strategy. The student who approaches the ward professional nurse with a statement, 'Mrs Jones seems to have so much difficulty in taking her prescribed medication (or diet, exercise, etc), what can I do to help her?' is initiating an informal nursing care conference. Many more examples come to mind. Two or three nursing personnel in a unit might start up a discussion as to why certain patients appear to do better than others. This might promote enquiry into whether there is any difference in the specific nursing care given which could develop into a fruitful informal nursing care conference.

It has already been stated that a great deal of teaching and learning in the unit situation is informal. The above remarks serve to emphasise this point.

9.21 NURSING CLINICS OR PATIENT-CENTRED DISCUSSIONS

This method can be used in the unit situation with proper planning, although it is also useful for a clinical teaching department, or even a tutor from the college.

A nursing clinic differs from a nursing care conference in that the presence of a selected patient or patients is necessary for at least part of the time. It differs from the nursing round in that the patient is removed from his usual place in the unit and brought to a separate room, where disturbance of other patients is avoided and a teaching-learning atmosphere can be created. A nursing clinic is always directed towards the nursing care of a patient or patients and is not concerned with the medical management of a disease, except in so far as this affects nursing management. This might well occur when medical treatment includes the administration of intravenous therapy. Such a treatment might well pose nursing problems, not only in the maintenance of the therapy, recording and watching for side-effects, but it might affect such points as the positioning of the patient, his mobility, his ability to carry out certain actions for himself, his anxiety and that of his relatives, to mention but a few.

The planning of a nursing clinic, whether in or outside the unit, is vital and includes the following:

- Determining the objective of the clinic, for example studying the nursing care of patients with similar diagnoses or undergoing similar treatment
- Selecting the appropriate patient or patients

190

- Securing the consent of the patient/s
- Securing the setting to be used
- Collecting all the data pertinent to the nursing care of the patient, his care plan, nursing care record and other relevant information
- Selecting the time suitable to patients, ward routine and personnel.

A nursing clinic could be arranged for a specific time of day, on say the second and fourth Wednesday of each month and all personnel must be aware of this as part of the teaching strategy in the unit. It can also be conducted more frequently.

The clinic is run on fairly formal lines and the patient or patients are not present all the time.

The person conducting the clinic introduces the topic, defines the purpose of the clinic and points out specific features to be observed. The nursing care already given could be sketched and any problems already encountered could be mentioned. The patient/s could then be presented in person. Relevant questions could be asked and a physical examination could be made. The patient/s could then be returned to their normal care area. After this, opportunity is afforded the group for discussion, for suggestions regarding care and for observations.

This method needs competence on the part of the person conducting the clinic. Again, though, opportunity must be created for neophyte professional nurses, at least in their final year, to gain experience in conducting nursing clinics as part of their preparation for practice. The person conducting the clinic must be aware of or sensitive to the needs of the learners as well as those of the patients, and be up to date regarding current trends in nursng and medicine.

Nursing clinics in the unit may be a way of identifying areas where care can be improved and also potential problems identified before they actually occur. Such identification could lead to preventive measures being taken so that the problems, in fact, do not arise. They thus contribute to patient care by saving unnecessary suffering and discomfort and could also save valuable nursing time which might be required if preventive measures were not instituted timeously. Participation by students in such clinics can provide invaluable learning opportunities.

9.22 PROBLEM-ORIENTED NURSING RECORDS

These are really an extension of writing nursing care plans which are continued and altered over a space of time. Problems are identified in the nursing care of a patient according to his diagnosis and signs and symptoms. Nursing treatment is then listed and a record is kept of the response to treatment for each problem.

The teaching component is related to the use of the record to show the student how the patient has responded to medical and nursing treatment. It is a continuous teaching tool as well as one that could be employed after discharge as part of a teaching programme.

Recording as a teaching strategy, no matter what form the record takes, should be mentioned. The methods used for keeping patient records and for charting have to be demonstrated to students and they have to become proficient in using them. Not only do the methods need demonstration, but the reasons for keeping such records, the progress or otherwise which can be seen from charts and the legal aspects of record-keeping must be explained. The 'theory' of this, if not related to the practice situation, is sterile. Effective use of patient records, whether problem oriented or not, in the nursing care situation makes the whole process 'come alive'. Personnel have to be instructed as to *what* must be charted, but even more important, they must know *why*, and what observations there are which require immediate action. The necessity for checking at the change of shifts or more frequently, must be clarified.

Every student or pupil must be made aware of the fact that correct charting involves the safety, if not the life of the patient or client and reflects on the professional reputation of the nurse and even the doctor. Accurate record-keeping is one of the best safeguards there is against potential hazards, negligence on the part of health-care personnel and malpractice. It forms the basis and is fundamental to all good nursing and medical care. Therefore, teaching the importance of record-keeping in the real-life situation is of paramount importance. The effects of failures in record-keeping can be stressed where they will have the most impact.

9.23 WARD ROUNDS

This implies the use of various types of ward rounds which already take place as a means of teaching. They include nursing service manager's rounds and doctor's rounds, whether the latter are merely rounds where the physician visits his patients and assesses progress, and makes any necessary changes in treatment, or whether they are more formal 'teaching' rounds such as occur in medical training hospitals.

9.23.1 Nursing service manager's rounds

These can be invaluable teaching situations if properly employed. They should be approached systematically, the aim being more than a check on patient care. The educational development of the student should also receive consideration and nursing service managers, all of whom also have a teaching component in their functions, should make a point of conducting ward rounds with students and not only with the nursing practitioner in charge of the unit. They should conduct on-going checks, and will expect the student to be able to give a knowledgeable account of diagnosis, treatment and response to treatment. Nursing care plans could be inspected and discussed. Knowledge of medico-legal hazards could be tested. The variations are endless.

A nursing service manager's round is concerned with checking whether the person in charge of the unit is conversant with her teaching responsibility and that she does, in fact, teach. Her teaching programme should be inspected and some formal teaching sessions could be attended.

The 'matron' doing the round should ensure that the unit 'sister' is conversant with the syllabi of the students and pupils who are assigned to her unit, and that she is fully aware of the stage reached by the various members of her personnel in training.

9.23.2 The doctor's round

As already mentioned, this can be the usual visit of doctors to their patients, or it can be a specific teaching round. Whatever the case may be, a doctor's round can be an extremely valuable teaching strategy. The person in charge of a unit has to ensure that students are taught how to do rounds with the doctor, what reports or queries she must put to him about the condition of *his* patients who are also *her* patients. The manner of assisting the doctor with his physical examination of the patients or his diagnostic procedures has to be demonstrated. Respect for the patient's privacy and dignity could again be emphasised. Verbal or written prescriptions for treatment must be dealt with and the student must become competent in this as well as in the manner of handling telephonic prescriptions. She has to be taught what to do in the following problem areas:

- Overdose prescriptions
- Illegible or unsigned prescriptions
- Illegal directives
- Directives that are contrary to institutional policy.

The student also has to be taught how to incorporate medical prescriptions in nursing care plans, treatment or medicine lists or kardex forms, whichever method is used in the specific unit or institution. She must also learn how to check on doctor's directives when coming on duty or going off at the end of her duty shift. Have they been carried out? Does the staff following her have full knowledge of what is expected of her in this regard?

It is thus clear that a doctor's round can be a very valuable teaching strategy if it is regarded and utilised as such. Students must be guided and taught to carry out ward rounds with doctors until they are completely confident and competent and are, in their turn, capable of teaching and guiding the newer recruits to nursing.

9.24 PEER GROUP TEACHING

A peer group is composed of members of one's own kind, a group in which relative equality exists. A peer is of equal standing. Thus, in the nursing care unit situation, student nurses form one 'peer' group and registered nurses another. It follows that 'peer group teaching' means teaching done by other members of one's own group, for example by fellow students.

Peer group teaching is one of the most important strategies in the nursing care practice situation. To deny its existence or importance shows complete lack of understanding of the unit learning-teaching situation in nursing. There can be very few nurses who have not at some stage or another been taught some aspect of nursing practice by one or more members of their peer group. True, the member doing the teaching may be more senior in nurse training, that is, she has passed further along the road to professional adulthood, but remembering the relative equality mentioned earlier, she is still a student and therefore a member of the 'peer group'.

Peer group teaching may be quite informal, making use of the 'teachable moment', or it may be quite formal. It may even be subconscious, such as a chance remark regarding an observation made during nursing care.

What must never be forgotten is that it must deliberately be employed by the unit head as part of her unit teaching strategy, for it lays the foundation for future teaching by the registered nurse in the area of nursing practice and it must be guided and stimulated from early on in learning the practice of nursing.

By using this method, students learn to pay particular attention to observation, they learn to assess and to exercise judgement. If they are compelled to present formal teaching sessions, they must be able to organise their thoughts regarding patient care into logical sequence, to master nursing care techniques and the underlying theory in order to be able to demonstrate intelligently. They must be able to establish priorities, to research cases, cause and effect and develop a skill in communicating their skills and knowledge to others. They learn to accept constructive criticism and to evaluate their own performance and that of others, so that they, in their turn, can give constructive criticism. The need for peer group approval, common to all, can motivate students to further reading, practice and ultimately to make themselves better practitioners of the art and science of nursing.

194

By planning and encouraging peer group teaching, the unit professional nurse helps students to develop greater and greater independence; the student learns thoroughness, pride in her work and a practical and realistic approach to the practice of nursing. In the beginning stages of formal peer group teaching, students are assigned fairly simple tasks to teach. The complexity of the nursing practice which she is required to present in formal peer group teaching is increased as the student progresses along the path to professional adulthood and independent practice. It makes teaching part of her nursing way of life and not a separate entity which must be undertaken by others.

The early inculcation of correct attitudes to teaching nursing practice, by making use of peer group teaching in the unit situation, stands the neophyte practitioner of nursing in very good stead. It develops her ability to teach and her appreciation of the fact that a nurse has a teaching function which is inherent in her practice.

Very important in guiding peer group teaching, is the attitude of the unit head or her deputy, or a teacher from the clinical teaching department towards the student engaged in teaching. It must be one of helpfulness, guidance, and constructive criticism. It must built up the confidence of the student and not break it down.

The student's lack of experience must be appreciated, and she must be helped to gain perspective, to understand the relative importance of various facets of the nursing actions used in the care of the patient. She thus becomes able to interpret nursing care and patient needs for the benefit of her own professional growth in nursing practice and for communication to others in the peer group.

9.25 WRITING, GIVING AND RECEIVING REPORTS AS TEACHING STRATEGIES

Writing and handing over ward reports may be considered management techniques whereby recording patient care given and instructions for the continuation of that care are conveyed to those responsible.

This is true, but there is such a large teaching/learning component in this process that it cannot be omitted from a discussion on teaching strategies. It can be used quite formally as a teaching technique, but it is also an informal teaching strategy par excellence, though its important contribution to unit teaching may not occur to those who use it daily. Thus the teaching-learning value inherent in this daily occurrence may be lost or dissipated. If every unit professional nurse and student or pupil realises its teaching and learning potential, it will be more fully utilised and the writing, giving and receiving of reports will be more than a chore which has to be carried out.

Handing over reports offer many teachable moments which should be grasped.

The following aspects of report writing and the giving and receiving of reports are of the utmost importance if maximum use is to be made of every opportunity:

(a) Clarity in writing and verbal description: A written report must be clear, concise and accurate. The unit professional nurse must guide the writing and insist on these points. Nevertheless, verbal amplification in response to queries or observations may be necessary.

(b) An open mind ready to enquire, to suggest and to look beyond the written word: A facial expression, a reaction to what is said should be observed and elucidation required. Giving and receiving reports should provide golden opportunities for eliciting comment and encouraging participation at all levels. A junior nurse may have valuable information which can contribute to better care and she should be free to mention anything she has heard or seen which has a bearing on the ultimate well-being of a patient or client.

(c) Comments which are relevant are important: The progress which the patients are making or the lack of it, as seen in the context of a report which is a legal document, presents valuable teaching opportunities which *must* be grasped. A relaxed, yet professional attitude to the whole matter of handing over reports must be cultivated.

(d) The use of carefully worded relevant questioning will help to stimulate thought and learning and assist in the correlation of theory and practice.

9.26 TEACHING THROUGH SUPERVISION

To supervise, according to *The Concise Oxford Dictionary*, is 'to direct or watch with authority the work or proceedings or progress of, oversee'. The key words would seem to be to direct, to watch with authority, to oversee, to which might be added 'to control', to *co-ordinate*.

What does supervision mean to nurses? The answer to this is probably very varied. Many will regard supervision as 'being spied upon', 'minding other people's business', and similar ideas. This is indeed a false premise. It should, in fact, be seen as a means by which an expert practitioner in the art and science of nursing guides and direct the work of someone who is less expert. The aim of this guidance is to help the one who is less expert to improve performance and obtain work satisfaction so that the ultimate purpose of maintaining quality patient care is achieved. Supervision has three important aspects:

• The preparation of the supervisor for her supervisory function

- The teaching function of the supervisor
- The creation of an environment conducive to good supervision.

9.26.1 The preparation of the supervisor for her supervisory function

Supervision occurs at many levels in the nursing hierarchy. In this work we are more concerned with the supervisory function of the unit head, or ward professional nurse.

A 'unit' or 'ward' professional nurse needs to be competent in supervision techniques and it is necessary that these be taught to her during her student days. Part of her function is administration or management of her unit. This administrative function is an enabling one in that it must enable patient care to be given – patient care of a high standard. Details of the type of supervision for which she will be responsible, will be discussed at some length.

Supervision as a teaching function is of interest here, and the need for students to acquire skills in supervision must begin early in their preparation for nursing practice. A competent professional practitioner must be able to supervise. A great deal will be learned by precept and example, but advice, positive guidance, assisting students in the practice of nursing so that faults – which are noticed in the process of 'overseeing', directing or watching with authority – are discussed and eliminated. The management function which must be taught to students includes:

- The use of control measures (record-keeping, checking, etc)
- The determination of *what* must be done in order to provide care and *what* is needed in the way of supplies and equipment for it to be done efficiently
- The determination of priorities *(when)*
- The allocation of staff so that tasks to be performed are assigned to competent personnel *(by whom)*
- The creation of a safe environment for patient care *(where)*
- Ensuring that students become competent at carrying out necessary procedures *(how)*
- Ensuring that care is given with knowledge and understanding, according to the needs of the situation.

The student of nursing must be taught all these aspects during her preparation for practice. The supervision teaching strategy ensures that the student is led to semi-independence in a given area as her competence and learning improve. This enables her to achieve complete functioning independence upon qualification. It has already been pointed out that all teaching of students is aimed at the production of a professional adult, and an adult is one who is capable of independent thought and action, and of assuming responsibility for her own actions.

A student can actually be supervised when she is supervising in order to teach her the technique. This can be achieved by allocating certain checking functions to a student, or asking her to watch and comment upon the performance of another.

In using supervision as a teaching strategy, the supervisor has to have criteria against which she can judge patient care. In preparing her for practice, the student is indeed provided with such standards. In preparation for her supervisory role, she must also be given the opportunity to use considered judgement, to be flexible according to the needs of the situation and to be able to eventually establish criteria, or to assist in the establishment of such criteria. Supervision always incorporates a measure of evaluation which will be discussed in a later paragraph.

9.26.2 The teaching function of the supervisor

Supervision is teaching. Therefore, all potential supervisors must be made aware of this and accept it. A supervisor must be able to build up mutual respect between herself and her students. She must, if she wishes to be respected, show respect for students. The supervisor must ensure that students assigned to her unit are aware of their duties and obligations. The students are there to learn and learning opportunities must be made for them, but they, in their turn, must make use of these opportunities.

A supervisor, as part of her teaching function, must always evince a fair and impartial attitude towards students who must be guided by her towards personal emotional control, patience and loyalty. A supervisor who loses her temper, becomes impatient and annoyed without cause and is disloyal to her colleagues, her employing authority or her profession, should not hold such a position.

Students will need to be corrected, even to be reprimanded, but the manner in which this is done – the student must gain and patient care must improve – is vital. Reprimands do not take place in front of other students, patients, clients, other members of the health team or other categories of workers. Good practices in supervision not only achieve more, but the attitudes displayed by the supervisor and her methods are transmitted to students, who will try to model themselves on the good role model presented by the good supervisor.

The supervisor, as part of her supervisory teaching function, insists on the maintenance of standards, and she makes sure that the students are taught such standards. All teaching strategies are interrelated, just as is all patient care. Supervision overlaps with teaching by means of ward rounds, precept and example, and other aspects which have already been discussed or which follow.

The supervisor or anyone using any of the other teaching strategies should always remember the value of praise where praise is due. Praise encourages the learner, it shows her that she is measuring up to the desired standards and that she is progressing and developing along the road she has chosen. The withholding of well-deserved praise can, on the contrary, be discouraging, even frustrating and does not engender a good learning situation in a unit.

9.26.3 The creation of an environment conducive to good supervision

The components necessary for this have already been mentioned. The main points will be summarised here.

(a) An atmosphere of mutual respect and trust in the unit so that *supervision is accepted* by all in a positive light
(b) Competence in her own practice so that she is truly known to be one who can 'watch with authority', who has the *right to supervise*
(c) Readiness to *help and guide during supervision* – not merely to offer carping criticism – so that the learner has an opportunity to learn
(d) Ability to adapt to the needs of the situation, so that the *type of supervision,* though not the quality, is changed when necessary
(e) Ability to motivate learning by showing *interest in the progress and ability of learners* as well as in the progress of those receiving care at their hands while *carrying out supervision of care*
(f) Proper employment of the *management function* required to enable nursing to be done, that is the provision of stores, equipment and personnel as and when required and *ensuring that these are correctly used*
(g) Noticing areas during the *process of supervision where improvement* is necessary, planning such improvement, teaching persons so that the plan can be implemented, and evaluating results
(h) *Acknowledgement of the value of other members of the staff as part of the supervision* of patient care and providing learning-teaching situations so that they in turn also become good supervisors
(i) Insistence on the absolute safety of the patient, his dignity, comfort and the confidentiality of his affairs as *part of the supervisory function.*

Thus supervision as a teaching strategy, though closely linked with others, can be seen to be one that is used – often unthinkingly – during every day of patient or client care. If the supervisor is prepared for this role during her training and if thought is given by the supervisor to the positive teaching component that is part of supervision, then it will play a vital role in the unit teaching and learning situation. It will form an even more useful strategy, to be employed by those interested in preparing nursing students for professional practice.

9.27 PROBLEM SOLVING IN THE UNIT

As with other teaching strategies in the unit situation, problem solving has both informal and formal aspects.

9.27.1 Informal

Problems in patient care, in staff allocation and many other areas are part of the everyday working world of the nurse. They are so much of daily occurrence, and are mostly solved on an *ad hoc* basis that they tend not to be seen as problems, but as routine. Nevertheless the manner in which these problems are tackled and solved, is part of the informal teaching which is carried out in a unit. It is part of teaching a student to manage problems herself. The problem-solving technique is really very basic, involving as it does:

- recognition of the problem
- collection of facts
- analysis of facts
- deciding on a course of action
- implementing that action
- evaluation of action – was the problem solved?

In the informal use of this technique, these phases are almost automatic and may follow one another very rapidly. An example may be quoted to illustrate this point:

Problem: A patient is uncomfortable in bed.
Facts: Age, sex, diagnosis, present treatment, position, temperature of room, symptoms of distention – excretion difficulties, post-operative pain, thirst, inability to turn or move – all these and more are looked for.
Analysis: Mrs Brown, 66, hemiplegic, slipped down in bed, positioning of limbs uncomfortable, cold, thirsty.
Action: Change position, supply more warmth, give warm drink.
Implementation: Delegate to persons capable of carrying out actions – supervise.
Evaluation: Mrs Brown, after action, looks more comfortable and is resting quietly.

This is simple to understand. Countless examples could be quoted.

9.27.2 Formal

Teaching in the clinical/learning situation which makes use of the problem-solving technique follows the same pattern of identifying problems and helping the students to do the same. Then the problem-solving technique is followed through to its logical conclusion. The problems will be diverse and may include those caused by

- the actual diagnosis and treatment of the patient;
- the progress or lack of it being maintained by the patient;
- the environment;
- interaction between patients/clients and their relatives and friends, health team workers and others;
- the social circumstances of patients/clients;
- a shortage of staff both in quantity and/or quality; and
- a shortage of equipment.

During the course of her learning the student must be guided towards the identification and solving of problems.

Even more formal teaching can occur in a unit revolving around problem solving if the person in charge, or someone delegated to do so, selects problems which have occurred in the nursing care of patients and organises problem-solving sessions around them. These should not be too far removed from the present time. In fact, they can be future oriented, for example, 'Tomorrow the operation slate is so and so'. 'How can we deal with the situation so that no one is neglected, all treatments are carried out and that the operating programme proceeds smoothly?' This gives students a chance to think and to plan, which is a vital part of learning for future practice. The competent ward professional nurse has her ward or unit running so smoothly that students who are not made aware of the problems give them no thought until confronted with them in the future.

If students are to be taught as part of their preparation for practice as registered nurses, then this formal problem-solving teaching technique is invaluable. It is also stimulating to the teachers who may tend to get into a rut. It is a method capable of infinite variation, depending on the imagination and resourcefulness of the unit professional nurse. It may be applied equally well in a ward, a specialised department or an outside clinic, but problem solving in a district, or in home nursing requires skills of a special nature.

9.28 THE NURSING PROCESS

(This is closely linked with the nursing care plan, just discussed.) A process may be defined as a series or sequence of actions, events or operations. The art and science of nursing entails a series of sequential actions, events and operations based on scientific knowledge and principles aimed at providing continuous personal care of a highly skilled nature to people and their families who are exposed to or are suffering from physical or mental ill-health.

Thus, the 'process of nursing' – the series of sequential actions that the nurse employs in carrying out her caring function – is the same as the 'nursing process'. It is not a new concept, although Yura and Walsh (1973) spelt it out very clearly.

The dimensions of the nursing process which they identify, are:

- Assessment
- Planning
- Implementation
- Evaluation.

To this, we in South Africa add the dimension of *record-keeping* which is seen as essential because the South African nurse is accountable for her own acts and omissions and must therefore provide proof of what care she has given the patient; record-keeping also safeguards the patient. This can be seen as a fifth step or as an integral or underlying part of all the other steps.

The five steps in the process of nursing will now be examined separately and the teaching component inherent in each part will be pointed out so that the use of such a mechanism for teaching can be clearly understood. Many of the teaching strategies already dealt with in this chapter will be used in the teaching component of the nursing process. It does, however, serve as a very good working model, not only for ensuring quality patient care, but also for the presentation of the total picture of teaching/learning in the unit situation. Therefore, if properly used, it helps to produce the proficient professional adult nurse capable of giving and supervising quality care, which is the aim of nursing education.

9.28.1 Assessment

The nurse must be able to make all the relevant observations of the patient or the client for whom she has to care, whether these be in the preventive, promotive, curative or rehabilitative field of her work. Moreover, these observations must be made with intelligent insight. This means that there must be a very good correlation of theory and practice. What she learns in the classroom must be related to what she experiences in the clinical field. Thus, the 'tutor' should also be involved in the nursing situation as part of the teaching programme, the 'clinical' teacher must stress underlying theory to help develop that intelligent insight into relevant observations. The unit professional nurse should act as the soldering mechanism where theory becomes blended with practice into one insoluble whole.

Having made relevant observations with intelligent insight, the nurse must be able to synthesise this information in order to carry out the next phase in the sequence. In order to learn to do this, the student will need guidance from the registered persons with whom she works and who are responsible for teaching her the practice of nursing. Observing how others use information obtained from *observation* is part of this, but teachers in the unit situation must make every effort to help students to understand the relevance of observation and point out to them how this is used in providing total nursing care to each individual patient. Total nursing care must be seen as an integral part of the overall patient or client care which includes medical care and that provided by other members of the health team.

The professional practising nurse must be able to diagnose the nursing needs which form part of her independent function, so that she can take appropriate action at all times. While the nurse in charge of a unit does this as part of her everyday work, she must use it as a teaching mechanism. This will enable those under her to develop their skills in this direction until they are competent to fulfil this part of their function, not because it is thrust upon them when qualified, but because it has, during the course of education for nursing practice, become second nature. Students who have been well educated, will also see it as part of their function to pass on such skills and understanding to neophytes.

The nurse must also be able to diagnose patient care needs which need referral to a medical practitioner or other members of the health team and know the proper means of instituting this referral. This should not occur by trial and error, but as a result of teaching and learning, by means of guidance, example and use of the teachable moment, supervision, handing over of reports and other appropriate teaching strategies.

Included in this assessment dimension, the professional practising nurse in the unit situation must also be able to diagnose the need for emergency action and be competent to carry out appropriate action. Again the teaching component of this section is obvious. If a nurse is to learn to recognise the need for emergency action and the appropriate steps to be taken, she not only has to learn the medical problems which may arise and the signs and symptoms thereof, but she must also be shown medico–legal hazards inherent in the environment and in the treatment programme, and must be taught their prevention as well as appropriate emergency treatment, should the patient suffer mishaps. This can be taught in theory, but reinforcement in the ward or unit situation is essential.

9.28.2 Planning

Having assessed the situation and determined the needs, the nurse must plan her course of action. This, as has already been pointed out, may necessitate immediate and swift emergency action, which cannot be carried out unless teaching and learning has preceded this need for emergency action. So again the teaching dimension of this phase of the nursing process is obvious.

Planning also entails the establishment of priorities, the decision as to what must be done without delay and what can and should in fact wait. Planning must be both short term and long term. In educating a student for the practice of professional nursing, the manner in which she must assume charge of a ward or unit where she will have to make the plans should not be left to chance. Students must be taught to make nursing care plans, to allocate or delegate duties, to order equipment, stores, dietary requisites, linen, cleaning material and other essentials, and to make out duty rosters or 'off-duties' so that patient care can proceed smoothly. A great deal of this is learned in the course of working in a unit. It should, however, be part of the teaching objectives of every person in charge of a unit. It should form an integral part of her teaching plan, based on her assessment of student needs.

9.28.3 Implementation

Having assessed the situation, established needs and planned the course of action, the nurse has to see that the plan is implemented, either by carrying out the action herself or by breaking it down into units and delegating the units to those working with her. Perhaps the most readily understood teaching component lies in this implementation dimension of the nursing process, for 'doing' requires many skills which have to be taught. These are usually well understood by the person in charge of a unit, even if they are not clearly identified as teaching by the ward professional nurse.

A student could, no doubt – given time, a well-illustrated guide, and the necessary apparatus – eventually learn to give an injection, but no one would dream of employing such an unwieldly, time-consuming learning technique, fraught, as it would be, with many potential dangers. It must, however, be remembered that 'showing how' is not the full story of getting a plan implemented. The intelligent understanding which is necessary must be based on theory, on the application of knowledge and scientific principles to the course of action. Thus teaching in order to promote learning is vital to implementing the plan, which must also be flexible enough to allow change, should the need arise. This again is a teaching opportunity, that is, how and why the plan must be amended in the light of changed circumstances.

9.28.4 Evaluation

This vital phase of the process of nursing entails deciding whether the action or actions planned and implemented are having the desired effect, in other words whether the client, the patient or the community is reacting as anticipated to the planned nursing action. If not, then re-assessment, re-planning, re-implementation and re-evaluation become necessary. If re-implementation is not possible, then evaluation will show where mistakes could be avoided in the future.

This dimension again presents many teaching opportunities. Some would be quite informal, but others would be deliberately planned. The nursing process can be used on an organised basis to provide patient care, if some form or record system requiring completion is devised, based on the various dimensions of the process. It would be similar to a nursing care plan, but would be put together in a slightly different manner and would incorporate the whole process including implementation, evaluation and record-keeping. A form of this sort, properly devised and used, would also present endless teaching opportunities.

All four phases which have so far been discussed, namely assessment, planning, implementation and evaluation in the nursing process, apply to the carrying out of nursing actions and are those duties which fall within the practice of nursing. They require not only practical skills which can be taught, but also a trained mind which is kept acutely aware of patient care needs and of the ever-increasing changes which occur in nursing and medical treatment. It is part of the teaching function of the professional nurse in charge of a unit to guide students so that they develop such a trained mind. They must be stimulated to think, learn and act. Planned, thoughtful use of the nursing process would be invaluable to this end.

9.28.5 Record-keeping

This step in the process of nursing is considered essential in South Africa. The professional practising nurse in South Africa is a registered person, accountable for her own acts and omissions in the care she gives to her patients and clients. Record-keeping, besides showing the progress of a patient towards or away from recovery, is a means by which proof can be presented of the care which has been given. Omission to record presents a picture of omission to give care. Thus, the importance of record-keeping must be stressed throughout the nurse's education for practice and insistence on accurate, clear record-keeping is one of the hallmarks of good unit administration.

The practising nurse must also safeguard herself against possible accusations that she was overstepping her nursing role, and practising as a medical practitioner. Record-keeping in all its dimensions provides a means of doing this.

The fact that a person in this country, under common law, is entitled to the safety of his person, his name and his property must also be remembered. Record-keeping assists in this aspect. It also provides a means of bringing home to nurses this important part of their caring function; in other words 'teaching' them.

In order to fulfil the requirements spelt out above, the accurate recording of the four steps in the process of nursing is essential, this thus constituting a fifth phase in the process.

Record-keeping – apart from being a valuable teaching mechanism in itself, enabling the 'why' underlying such humdrum 'routine' procedures as the charting of temperature, pulse and respiratory rates to be taught – produces documents which are ideal visual aids upon which to build teaching sessions. If they are used in this way, concurrently with care being given in the unit, then the live situation will serve to engender greater interest than if they were to be used retrospectively, that is after discharge of the patient, although such records could then still be valuable teaching aids.

The process of nursing is continuous, with all its phases leading into one another. In a busy unit, various phases of the process applied to various patients will be occurring simultaneously. It is not only part of the giving of patient care, but it is also part of the teaching 'how' that care should be given. To summarise, teaching can and should occur through the following:

(a) *Assessment of the needs* of patients or clients and of the total situation in which care is sought and/or given
(b) *Planning to meet these needs* on a short-term or a long-term basis. The reality principle must not be forgotten in planning so that the next step is possible
(c) *Implementation of the planned course of action* be it preventive, promotive, curative or rehabilitative in accordance with the total care needs of patients or clients
(d) *Evaluation of the effects* of actions taken, which in turn leads to re-assessment, re-planning, re-implementation and re-evaluation until the objective is achieved
(e) *Accurate record-keeping* which also forms the basis for re-assessment, re-planning, re-implementation and re-evaluation for the present and the future.

The nursing process as a teaching mechanism is invaluable, for it serves to place nursing care in perspective. It is during her work with patients and clients that the student of nursing should develop her understanding of the theory which she has been taught as it relates to the practical situation which makes up a large part of her nursing life. During the process of nursing, if use is made of the teaching opportunities inherent in its considered, planned application, the student correlates theory with practice and begins to recognise the problems inherent in nursing practice. By developing an enquiring mind capable of considered judgement, the nursing process serves to produce a confident, competent practitioner who obtains job satisfaction in the practice of her profession. The logical sequence of events and the safeguards built into each phase as it moves on to the following in a circular continuum, provide guide-lines for practice which will stand her in good stead throughout her professional life.

A word of warning: The system of nursing process used must be practical and allied to reality. A method that entails a great deal of writing takes too much time and will, in actuality, not be used. A danger also exists that the patient may be overlooked as the nurse may look past him in concentrating on the form, which defeats its own object. The nurse may be nursing paper instead of people.

9.29 WORKSHOPS

The workshop as a teaching form is probably limited in its application to basic forms of nursing education, although it can be used in the more senior levels, in in-service education and for post-registration courses.

It is a term that is unfortunately applied somewhat indiscriminately, and its meaning has been diluted and applied to many educational forms, including seminars.

In its essential form, the workshop is considered by many to be one of the most effective methods ever devised for group learning. The workshop begins by assembling a group with some common interest. In the case of nursing a workshop could be arranged, for instance, for tutors, or nurse-educators having a common interest in the implementation of the syllabus and directive for general training.

A workshop group can be arranged for groups of any size between 40 and 200. The time allowed for an effective workshop should be a minimum of one week, depending on the scope of the subject (shorter times for a very limited subject are possible, but students should have ample time for group interaction).

Three weeks is considered to be a reasonable and desirable time allocation, but truly difficult subjects can be tackled over a much longer period. It might even be possible to employ the workshop technique dealing with a particular subject throughout the year. Workshops are often residential in nature, but this is not essential.

When structuring a workshop, the general plan must be worked out and the participants divided into small groups, each group being assigned a specific aspect of the central theme to study.

There must be a steering group to co-ordinate the group work, to act as resource persons, to ensure that a programme is drawn up, that facilities required are available, that participants know what is required and that the whole organisation runs smoothly. Members of this steering group should circulate among the working groups, joining in, guiding, suggesting ways of dealing with problems that may have arisen, or simply listening and encouraging.

A typical programme would include a general assembly session where the workshop co-ordinator welcomes participants, explains the general format and modus operandi, and identifies the steering group and staff members. A general layout of the area, the locales to be used and the time scheduling are explained. A handout to each participant giving these details is also helpful. The overall topic is given and then the assembly could be asked to identify aspects which require attention. The steering group will already have considered this question, so that aspects which are not identified could be brought to their attention, and a general scheme of tackling the subject worked out. The number of groups necessary is then decided upon, and the total participants are divided into groups. Although participants can be allowed a certain amount of choice, groups must be more or less evenly constituted numberwise, otherwise difficulties may be encountered when groups are too large or too small. A technique which is sometimes employed is to have some type of schedule drawn up. The name of the topic heads the list and numbered spaces are set out below. Participants are then given the opportunity to fill in their names under the topic of their choice. If the list of his first choice is full, the participant must make a second choice. This can be scheduled to take place during a fairly lengthy tea break.

Time blocks are allocated so that the workshop participants have time for

- workshop group sessions;
- daily general assembly sessions with a brief report-back from each group;
- time for research which may be necessary, library work, consultation with experts, etc;
- time for meals, relaxation and some social activity;
- special assembly sessions for the showing of any relevant films, etc.

Groups could also arrange combined sessions of two or three groups to discuss aspects of the general subject which their specific allocated topics have in common.

Once the individual work groups are formed, each group meets separately and chooses from amongst its members a group leader who has to keep the group work flowing, and a rapporteur responsible for the reporting back at interim of general assembly sessions, and the final report. Groups may further decide to form small subcommittees to research certain points relevant to their discussions. These committees can meet or pursue their individual research activities during the time allocated for this.

In organising a workshop, meticulous planning is necessary, which allows sufficient flexibility to cope with the unexpected, where the participants are oriented to the purpose and methodology of the workshop, and where provision is made for communication of some sort between groups, apart from verbal report-back. If the workshop lasts for any length of time, a roneoed bulletin of progress should be circulated among groups.

The workshop provides an opportunity for students to learn what they are most interested in learning instead of what others think they should learn. The field of andragogy is particularly suitable in this respect. It also forces the student to do research in her own area of interest. All this occurs in a climate conducive to learning with group support from the participants for her endeavours.

9.30 TEAM TEACHING

This form of teaching involves the organisation of the student learning experience by a group of nurse-educators.

Together they assess the needs of the students for the particular section of the course for which they will be responsible. This assessment of needs will be built upon a knowledge of what the student has learnt up to that stage.

They then plan the course for which they will be responsible, allocating different segments, such as paediatric nursing, orthopaedic nursing and nursing of diseases of the various systems. In other words, the work is divided up into modules and course objectives are set for each module. By working together as a team in this planning phase, unnecessary duplication of subject-matter can be avoided, and the students will benefit from having a variety of teachers with different talents, methods or teaching techniques, and the best use can be made of the teachers' special expertise in the clinical field.

The plan is then implemented, the team having worked out a time schedule which does not overload the student, and which gives each teacher sufficient time to fulfil her part of the teaching programme.

During this implementation phase, team teachers should meet frequently to discuss progress and to iron out any difficulties. When the particular programme has been completed, the team also meets to evaluate the results, the learning achievements of students and to replan the next programme for the next group.

The schedule of activities for all members of the team as well as for students must be drawn up. Many different teaching strategies can be scheduled, including laboratory work, seminars, projects, group discussions, clinical teaching sessions as well as the more formal lecture sessions. Individual tutorial sessions can also be scheduled.

Team teaching also allows for planning independent study sessions, which can be guided by one or more members of a team. The success of such a method will be dependent on the teachers' truly forming a 'team' with good interpersonal interaction. It is a method that can be exciting and stimulating for teachers and students alike, and although a good deal of time needs to be devoted to the planning phase, it is well worth trying.

Too often a tutor is expected to teach everything, to be an expert on all aspects of the syllabus, and ends up by being inadequate in everything, because no one can be an expert at everything. It is so much more interesting for the student to be presented with subject-matter by a member of the team who knows the subject well, and therefore presents it in a lively, exciting way which awakens interest, so that learning is facilitated.

In this chapter an attempt has been made to explain many of the strategies which can be used to teach the practice of nursing. None will be sufficient by itself. A carefully thought out combination of teaching strategies to meet the students' needs, the course requirements, the talents of individual teachers, and the circumstances in the live situation where live nursing practice occurs, is essential.

Time available, teaching material available and personnel available will all influence the use of various strategies. Whatever the strategies used, they have only one aim, namely *to teach effectively the practice of excellent nursing care* for the benefit of all those who receive it, both now and in the future.

9.31 COMPUTER-ASSISTED INSTRUCTION (contributed by Hilla Brink)

Computer-assisted instruction is a teaching strategy which has been used with considerable success in several schools of nursing in the United States of America, and is now gradually being introduced into some of the nursing colleges in South Africa.

Computer-assisted instruction is an example of an indirect educator/learner relationship. The student is positioned at a computer or if the time-sharing system is used, at a computer terminal, and responds by means of a keyboard to information displayed by the computer on a television-type screen. The information is presented by a computer instead of the tutor or a textbook.

Micro-computers and mini-computers, which are now widely advertised at affordable prices and can even be bought at some supermarkets, are extremely well-equipped for such instruction. A typical micro-computer is composed of several components referred to as hardware, such as a keyboard, the central processing units (made up of micro-chips); the monitor, which looks like a television screen; a disk-drive, which is a device on which information is stored, and which reads it from a plastic disk, similar to a 45 rpm record, or a cassette tape recorder; another device for storing information; and the printer, which prints information on paper. All micro-computers possess capabilities for receiving, processing and transmitting information. In computer-assisted instruction the computer can present material, ask questions, receive and evaluate learner responses, and make decisions based on the evaluation. If the computer detects the need for review of certain material, the computer programme will automatically guide the student through an appropriate review. The computer can also function as a tool that aids students and teachers to perform calculations, analyse data, keep records and write papers.

The value of any computer-assisted instruction will of course depend on the quality of the programme used. Programmes, also referred to as software, are used to give directions to the computer. Programmes are acquired in a variety of ways, such as
- tutors writing their own programmes
- purchasing commercial software
- contracting a professional programmer.

Several computer manufacturers have developed very useful computer programmes that assist the teaching process. An example is the Plato system. This system can provide animated displays, and tie in to both audiocassettes and 35 mm slide presentations. It includes programmes that teach about drugs, teach the student the fundamentals of the foetal circulatory system and test the student's knowledge of the working of the human heart. By means of other available programmes, students can become involved with a hypothetical patient, identify nursing problems, test solutions and find out the results of their interventions, without involving real patients.

Advantages of computer-assisted instruction

(a) *Self-pacing:* The programmes are designed to proceed at the pace of the student. The fast worker can work through the lesson rapidly and progress to the next, without having to wait for class-mates, while the student experiencing difficulty can work at a slower pace, reviewing (revising) troublesome sections and requesting additional practice until he has mastered the work. This type of instruction can thus be geared to the specific needs and progress of individual learners.

(b) *Drill and practice:* The computer can present drill as long as the student likes. Practice problems appropriate to the learner's performance may be provided in different amounts, based on needs. Drill and practice programmes are probably the easiest programmes for tutors themselves to write.

211

(c) *Personalised feedback and instruction:* Like programmed instruction, computer-assisted instruction is designed to elicit active responses from students. Once a response has been given, immediate feedback can be presented, indicating whether it was correct or incorrect. In addition, the computer allows the responses, along with other pertinent information to be stored and used to generate personalised messages and prescriptions. For example, a pretest of a module could be designed so that if a student has more than three errors out of ten questions, she is directed to another programme and told to complete a certain number of exercises. In addition, the programme can be arranged in such a way that, based on the success or otherwise of early examples, the difficulty level and/or number of further examples is increased or decreased accordingly.

(d) *Multisensory presentations:* Computers can utilise a variety of presentation modes, including test illustrations, movement and sound, and thereby provide alternatives for students who may experience difficulty in learning from a particular mode.

(e) *Simulation:* The computer can be programmed to represent a corresponding set of events in reality. A complex clinical situation could be presented and the students required to analyse the situation and solve a problem. Considerable latitude for students' responses can be built into such a programme, and feedback can be provided to students on their progress.

(f) *Motivation:* Friendly, low-pressure competition seems to be a good motivator of learning and can be built into computer programmes. In problem solving for example, the student could be kept informed of her performance relative to some standard.

(g) *Providing and storing information:* The computer is known for its ability to provide and store immense quantities of information.

Disadvantages or limitations of computer-assisted instruction

(a) As it is only a machine, the computer does not have the human ability to provide meaningful support and encouragement.

(b) It lacks flexibility, and is not well adapted for instruction requiring extensive reading.

(c) Its effectiveness depends on the available software and the tutor's skill in selecting or writing appropriate programmes.

(d) The computer is expensive to install.

In the light of these limitations, it should be clear that computer-assisted instruction is a teaching strategy/resource for assisting tutors/educators, and not a means of replacing them.

Research evidence is generally supportive of computer-assisted instruction, indicating small but significant contributions to course achievements, considerable savings in course completion time and more favourable attitudes towards instruction.

9.32 VALUES CLARIFICATION (contributed by Hilla Brink)

Values clarification is a relatively recently adopted teaching strategy within nursing education. It is especially recommended for the teaching of ethics and decision making.

The values clarification approach attempts to make one consciously aware of the values and underlying motivations that guide one's actions. It provides opportunities for learners to clarify and defend their values through the 'valuing process'. The valuing process includes the steps of:

(a) Choosing from alternatives after thoughtful consideration of the consequences of each alternative
(b) Prizing or cherishing and publicly affirming the choice made
(c) Acting on or doing something with the choice made.

Whenever possible, values clarification should be carried out in group sessions. A group process allows additional opportunities to clarify one's values. The individual members of the group will probably hold differing values. The individual becomes aware of the values of others as well as learning about self with help of group members.

Climate setting is important when a group strategy is selected so that respect for all group members is assured. Values cannot be strengthened when an atmosphere of fear and mistrust prevails. The nurse-educator must ensure that

- the atmosphere is relaxed
- nobody is made to feel uncomfortable and threatened
- the values of each person are respected
- negative feedback is discouraged
- she, as educator, responds to ideas expressed by learners.

A values clarification session could proceed as follows:

- Start off by setting the tone or providing a warming-up session.
- Next, explain the purpose and ground rules of the session.
  The *purpose* of this session is for students to
  - learn ways of valuing – not a particular set of values
  - discover their standpoint on issues they may be facing.

213

- A ground rule for this session is that students who do not wish to discuss their standpoints need not do so.
- The nurse-educator explains her own understanding of values and valuing and illustrates with examples.
- The theoretical framework of values clarification is introduced.
- Proceed to some values clarification exercises in which the steps of the valuing process are used.
- Clarify with the group what congruence they can identify between their personal values and the professional values they have observed so far in their experience.

Examples of values clarification exercises are:

(a) Students could be asked to list five values which guide their daily interaction and then rank these according to their priority. Students could then be paired and each pair could compare and discuss each of the values they listed, giving reasons why these guide their interactions.

(b) Students could be given alternatives and asked to rank the alternatives and write the value that emerges in response to their first choice. For example:

What would be the most difficult for you?
counsel a dying child
counsel a dying adult
counsel a parent whose child has committed suicide.

The values inherent in the first choice are then identified. Such exercises require students to identify values, choose from alternatives, state or affirm their choice and explain their position – all of which form part of the valuing process.

(c) Students could be presented with a problem with several alternatives from which to choose, such as being given a profile of six patients waiting to be seen in casualty, and then asked to indicate the order in which they think the patients should be examined, the basis for their decision, the values that influenced their decision and the values they consider most important. Having completed this, students should compare their rankings with those of their class-mates and discuss the similarities and differences in values that affected their decision.

(d) Finally, students can be assigned a clause from the international code of ethics and asked to compare the values expressed in it with the personal values which they had affirmed earlier.

The size of the group, the time and resources available together with the personal preferences and the level of their own group will determine which of the strategies will be used.

Values clarification is a strategy for:

- making nurse-practitioners more humanistic (aware of human needs)
- assisting in promoting personal growth
- establishing values which are consistent
- fostering the art of professional practice.

9.33 STUDENT PLANNED LEARNING

This is a method which can be used with success in senior groups and post-registration courses. Within the parameters of the course which they are following, the person in charge of the course/class asks students to identify particular topics that they want covered. Depending on the size of the group a student may be asked to present from two to ten points/subjects which she feels are particularly relevant and on which she would like information.

All the points are then collated, duplication eliminated and the group requirements discussed with them.

Although the lecturer supervising the course has to check that vital points in the syllabus are not omitted, it will generally be found that the topics presented cover the prescribed ground adequately.

Once the topics have been identified, students, in a group discussion session, can organise these into some form of order so that a working format is obtained. Students may also identify teaching methodology which they prefer for different sections.

It will be found that students become more motivated when they are part of the planning process.

This teaching strategy makes use of the andragogic principles of 'active participation in the learning experience' and 'assumption of responsibility for learning'.

Those who employ this method find it very stimulating and rewarding, although it may take more time and effort than some other methods.

9.34 THE CASE STUDY METHOD (contributed by Hilla Brink)

The case study method as a nursing teaching strategy can be used in both the clinical situation and the class-room. It is usually directed toward a real or a theoretical situation, a community group or institution or an individual, and requires in-depth analysis of the area of concern followed by judgemental decision making to solve the problem.

When used as a clinical teaching strategy the case study is usually based on a health-care consumer, for whom the student is responsible for providing care, or is derived from a clinical situation in which the student has been previously involved. The subjects available for case studies are limitless. Case studies in class-room teaching present problems, dilemmas and ethical questions, or areas that concern social or organisational relationships.

Examples of problem areas used as case studies in teaching nursing are:

(a) Miss Green is the only registered nurse on duty on Sunday in a ward with 40 acutely ill patients. In dividing the work she struggles to decide whether the patients should be divided equally among the three assistant nurses and she herself be available briefly to all patients, or whether she should give direct care to the most seriously ill patients, and have the assistant nurses care for the other patients with little or no supervision.

(b) Mr X is faced with the decision of whether or not to have a high risk, but life-extending major operation. You are his private nurse. Discuss how you would handle the situation.

(c) Miss Z, a tutor, is faced with a low-achieving student with an IQ of 140. Discuss how she should manage the situation.

(d) Mrs Y, a professional nurse in charge of a paediatric ward, is faced with an irritable mother who claims that her child is being treated inappropriately. Give her response and explain why she should answer/act in this way.

(e) Elaine is a premature infant with severe congenital abnormalities. The parents show increasingly less interest in Elaine and her progress. They visit, and when you tell them about Elaine's progress, the father blurts out, 'I wish you people would stop trying; what are you trying to prove by keeping a thing like that alive?' Discuss how you might react in this situation.

Students are required to examine all dimensions of the given problem and then make judgemental decisions and justify their choices.

As can be seen from these examples a case study offers only a small piece of reality. It has no real beginning or ending. It is never possible to supply all the facts. This is also true of reality. Decision makers rarely have all the information they would like to have.

Procedure for the case study method

The case study method involves four independent stages.

Stage 1   Students read independently and consider the case.
           While reading the case in preparation for a discussion, the student may be asked to identify major and subsidiary issues/problems, and formulate a tentative analysis of the case.

Stage 2   Students analyse and discuss the case study with each other.
           Each student helps and learns from the group. During this process they may gain new insights into their own beliefs and those of others, as they have to explore all aspects of the issue objectively.

Stage 3	Students compare their own independent analyses of the case study with those of the group.
Stage 4	Students apply current experiences to related and/or new ones.

The tutor should act as a facilitator throughout and assume the role of a learning resource person. She should therefore be knowledgeable about the subject, informed about group dynamics, an astute observer of human behaviour, and familiar with the decision-making process.

Advantages of the case study method

- It allows risk-taking without the fear of harming clients.
- It generates creative and innovative approaches to finding solutions to problems and helps students to realise that there are no magical solutions.
- It provides opportunities for students to present a supportive rationale for the solutions to problems; to examine the interrelationships of multiple phenomena in the clinical situation; to acquire skill in problem solving; to organise ideas logically in written form; to practise higher levels of cognitive learning as they make inferences, apply theory, analyse and synthesise knowledge relevant to a specific hypothetical situation, and evaluate the product.
- It increases the retention and transfer of learning.

Limitations of the case study method

Limitation are related to how the case study method is used. For example

- the tutor may have difficulty in writing or developing good case study material
- students may lack sufficient experience to assess the case study adequately
- study material may be so complex that students do not have the necessary knowledge and/or experience to analyse the problem adequately.

217

10 *Aids to teaching*

In all the teaching strategies described in chapter 9, some form of aid for the teacher was suggested: a chart, a chalkboard, an overhead projector etc. Even the most formal lecture is supplemented by the use of visual aids, and lecture notes as such are also a form of teaching aid. This chapter will look in more detail at various teaching aids and suggest means for their effective use.

10.1 THE CHALKBOARD

The chalkboard is one of the oldest and best known teaching aids and mastery of its use is essential for all nurse-educators. Effective use of a chalkboard does not come by accident; it has to be planned and the basic techniques must be practised.

Chalkboards are not simply enlarged 'scribbling pads'. Although they may be used informally for the elucidation of a problem or for a quick calculation so that the whole class can see what is going on, they can be put to much better use.

Before the start of a class, a whole scheme can be set out on a chalkboard – sketches can be made or simply outlined. If there are sliding chalkboards one can be prepared and left behind the other, and then slid into place at the appropriate moment. The same can be done with folding boards which can be opened out as the class proceeds. A chalkboard provides the educator with an inexpensive and adaptable visual aid which lasts indefinitely. All that is required for its continuous use is a ready supply of white and coloured chalk.

10.1.1 Uses of the chalkboard

The uses of a chalkboard are the following:
(a) On the board a framework of the lecture may be set out, which can then be filled in during the class. Sections can be rubbed out and the framework used for revision, with the students supplying the missing parts.
(b) It provides a means of progressing from simple to complex ideas, and developing each explanation point by point.
(c) Diagrams, symbols, charts and even more complicated drawings can be added at the appropriate time to bring life and meaning to a subject.

218

(d) Questions or problems to be discussed can be listed on the board. New or difficult words can be spelt out so that students can copy them or become familiar with them. Statistics can be put up to illustrate a point.

(e) A space is provided for the lecturer to record suggestions from the students as the class proceeds.

(f) Tests can be written on the board.

(g) It provides a space upon which students can be asked to illustrate explanations so that the entire class can participate in what is being said.

(h) A few, sometimes evocative words which serve as 'mind grabbers' and rivet attention can be written on the board.

10.1.2 Effective chalkboard utilisation

Some hints on effective chalkboard utilisation are the following:

(a) Plan ahead as to how it will be used in a class. Lecture notes could include reminders of what to put on the chalkboard, when, and how.

(b) Writing and drawing should be sufficiently large, clear and visible to all.

(c) The whole surface of the chalkboard must be visible to all.

(d) The work to be covered should be organised into sections with appropriate headings. The writing of one section should not run into another.

(e) Erase work as soon as its usefulness for the lesson has been expended.

(f) Where possible put summaries, words, sentences, figures or diagrams on the board as they develop in the lesson. If an elaborate drawing or diagram has been prepared beforehand, label each part clearly as the subject unfolds.

(g) Boards should be kept clean with felt or sponge erasers as is appropriate. On some very modern varieties of the chalkboard, use is made of felt-tipped pens, and then special erasers are necessary. Felt erasers should also be kept clean.

(h) Lighting should be such as to prevent glare.

(i) All students should be able to see the board at all times.

(j) Lecturers should take care to speak to the class, and not to the board.

10.1.3 Effective writing and drawing on the chalkboard

(a) Write so that all lines are horizontal. Use a liner if your handwriting tends to slope. Light lines can be drawn on the board beforehand, or a few dots to help keep writing straight. Practice usually corrects this tendency.

(b) Stand sideways to the board when writing, so that your back is not turned completely to the class. The chalkboard user should turn frequently to look at the class to establish eye contact.

(c) The chalk should be held between the thumb and forefinger with about 2,5 cm projecting upwards towards the board. An angle of approximately 30° to the board should be aimed at. This helps to prevent the chalk from squeaking.

(d) Chalkboard lettering should receive special attention. Legibility depends largely on the size and the style of the letters used, bold block letters being the most appropriate. Letters should be used in a uniform way, with capital letters at the beginning of phrases or sentences, or the whole heading. Mixing up capital and small letters without thought, and changing style in mid-sentence spoil the appearance of chalkboard work and diminish its effectiveness. For comfortable viewing in a ten metre room, letters should be at least five to six centimetres high and the lines about one centimetre wide. In smaller class-rooms of course, smaller lettering may be used.

(e) The lighting must be sufficient for students to see the writing on the board.

(f) The choice of chalk depends on the colour of the chalkboard. Coloured chalk can be used very effectively to point out contrasts and is indispensable in, for example anatomical diagrams.

(g) Neither writing nor drawings on the chalkboard should be too detailed. Matchstick men, in contrast to full-bodied figures, are often more effective.

(h) Attention should be paid to proportion. For example, the head of a human being should not be bigger than the trunk. Outlines of buildings should not be smaller than a person in front of them. A car is bigger than a dog. A syringe is smaller than a trolley.

(i) Spacing between letters and words should be consistent. Letters should not run into one another.

(j) If it is necessary to show overlapping, use contrasting chalk.

Chalkboards may sometimes have a magnetic backing which enables lettering, sketches, arrows and other symbols, pictures or photographs, that are mounted on cardboard with magnets taped onto their backs to be used to supplement chalkboard work.

10.2 CLOTH BOARDS

These are also an old form of teaching aid, and are still very popular. They are often called by the name of the material used in the construction of the board, such as flannel, felt, velvet or velcro.

A cloth board consists of a piece of board covered by the chosen material. Cut-outs are then made of pictures, diagrams, signs and symbols, lettering or any other form that can be depicted. Commercial advertising pictures, for instance, provide good material for cut-outs to illustrate a lecture on nutrition.

The back of the cut-out can consist of any rough material which will stick to the material on the board. Flannel sticks very well to flannel, and sand paper as well as other rough surfaces can be used effectively. Heavy material or objects cannot be used with success, nor where the board is likely to be subjected to movement as the attachment is minimal.

However, a cloth board covered with sturdy nylon material called velcro which is available in many colours and sizes, is very suitable and provides a firm base attachment. A piece of a roll or strip of velcro companion material is attached to the back of the visual material and when the two types of velcro material are pressed firmly together, the surfaces adhere securely. A fairly small patch of the loop or companion material can support quite a heavy weight, which gives the opportunity for three-dimensional display. (This material is actually used to replace zip fasteners on clothing and may be familiar to many as it is often used for attaching the cuff of a baumanometer.)

Guide-lines for the use of cloth boards:

- Boards must be visible to all students.
- Materials used must be clearly recognisable.
- Visuals should be kept simple, and boards should not be too cluttered.
- Any lettering or symbols must be large enough to be clearly visible.
- Make sure that the presentation is lively and provokes interest.

Visuals can be preserved for use in future lectures. They should be packed in labelled envelopes or in cellophane packets, and grouped appropriately. If the containers are stored in files or boxes, these should be clearly marked for easy access when needed. A list of prepared materials should be kept with the number or filing code next to each item.

The cloth board is particularly useful in health education programmes.

10.3 THE OVERHEAD PROJECTOR

This is a simple and effective teaching device which can be used in almost every class-room under normal lighting conditions. It requires some form of projection screen, and while an ordinary one will serve the purpose, the projected picture will be somewhat distorted. An angled white board gives a straight image.

10.3.1 Advantages

- The educator is in full control of the material at all times. He chooses what to show, when, how and why. The timing can be suited to the progress of the class.

- The educator never turns his back on the class, thus visual contact is never lost.
- Transparencies can be prepared in advance, presented as required, and quickly removed when they have served their purpose.
- Projectors are simple to operate.
- Projectors are relatively inexpensive.
- By using suitable pens, the screen itself can be used as a chalkboard, and wiped clean immediately.
- A stock of excellent teaching material can be built up and easily stored for future use.
- An out-of-date transparency can be extracted and replaced without disturbing the whole package of learning material.
- Control of the visual part is possible by simply using a piece of paper to cover all or part of the transparency, and moving it down as required.
- The lecturer can see what is being shown above his head on the screen in front of him.
- Transparencies can be prepared with overlays, each of which can be placed on the first and subsequent transparencies, to build up a composite whole with labels, symbols or additional lines. If these overlays are taped to the basic transparency frame and numbered, the operator (lecturer) can manipulate them very easily as required, and they will remain in the correct position.
- Materials can be produced easily and effectively with very little inconvenience by most teachers. If the assistance of those who draw well can be obtained, so much the better, but simple tracing is often enough. Use can be made of commercially produced lettering, which will add a very professional touch.
- Real objects such as bones can be used quite effectively for projection.

10.3.2 Methods of producing transparencies

Commercially produced transparencies on a variety of subjects are available and can be very useful. These are mounted in frames and can be hinged for overlays. However, it is possible for teachers to produce their own with the expenditure of a little time and effort and not much else.

In order to produce transparencies for viewing, the following materials are necessary:

- Transparency film, a thin sheet of clear acetate: This can be obtained in different colours which are useful for overlays.

- Felt-tipped pens and pencils: These may be water-based so that markings can be removed with a moist cloth or piece of cotton, or they may contain permanent ink which can only be removed by special solvents. Care must be taken to use pens or pencils which show up in colour on the screen. Those that are opaque or light only give a black image.
- Cardboard frames, if the transparencies are to be kept for future use: By punching holes in the sides they can be stored in sequence in leverarch or ringback files.
- Material such as masking tape for making hinges.
- A special transparent film for use in ordinary copying machines can also be used to prepare transparencies from drawings, etc.
- Commercially produced lettering if desired.
- The material to be copied, traced or an outline of the lettering required: It is possible to produce really elaborate pictures, but this usually requires the services of an artist and the use of special machines.

Some overhead projectors have an attachment for slides, so that it is possible to show one or two slides, say of diseased tissue or some skin condition, during the course of presenting the bulk of the visual material in the form of simple transparencies on the projector.

When using an overhead projector it is important to switch it off when the image is not actually relevant to the discussion, as the image or the light being presented continuously can distract the students.

10.3.3 Filing and storing transparencies for overhead projection

Because many transparencies can and will be used many times, it is worth arranging them in some system which will facilitate easy storage and quick retrieval.

Transparencies used frequently should be mounted on cardboard frames, each of which should be clearly marked. They should then be classified under appropriate subject headings, titles of units or modules, or specific topics for lectures.

The method of storage must then be decided upon. There are several possibilities:

- Filing cabinets
- Boxes of approximately the same size
- Ringback or leverarch files accommodated in bookshelves.

There are some important points to be remembered about every method:

(a) The box, file or filing cabinet must be clearly labelled and immediately visible.

(b) Boxes should not stand one on top of the other, but side by side. It is a great inconvenience if the box containing the desired transparencies is at the bottom of the pile or if the files are lying on top of one another.

(c) Detailed lists of the numbered transparencies contained in the box or file should be pasted inside the box or file. In the case of filing cabinets, files containing transparencies should be numbered, and a card index file kept for detailed cross-reference.

(d) Transparencies should be reviewed from time to time to check whether the information they contain is still relevant.

It must be remembered that in teaching the practice of nursing, suitable transparencies can be prepared and kept in wards and departments. They can quite easily be shown against an X-ray viewing box for the benefit of small groups.

The only requirement when operating an overhead projector is to focus it before starting and to be able to place transparencies on the screen and operate the on/off switch.

10.4 FILMS, FILM SLIDES, FILM STRIPS, VIDEO-CASSETTES

Any material captured on film can give a very realistic view of the real thing. Today, with colour films, this aid to teaching is absolutely invaluable.

10.4.1 Motion pictures

These are so much part of the everyday life of students that they need no introduction. Modern film projectors are relatively simple to operate, and many excellent educational films are available on loan from provincial libraries, commercial firms, libraries of state departments and other sources. Many films suitable for nursing courses can be purchased and used again and again. It is even possible, though somewhat expensive, to script and produce one's own films.

In order to ensure successful use of films, the following should be done:

• Decide what film is suitable for which group.
• Order films in good time.
• A preview is necessary before showing them to a class to assess their suitability for the level of the students or relevance to the course.
• Return them immediately after use. Also films must not be kept unused for any length of time.
• Keep an evaluation list of all films shown for future reference.
• Report immediately, in writing, any damage to films.

- If films are purchased, ensure their safe storage, easy retrieval and quick repair if they become torn or damaged.
- Prepare the students for what they are to see – point out specific points to be observed.
- Introduce any strange words to the class before the film is shown.
- Hold a general discussion immediately after the film and re-show sections or the whole film if necessary.
- Prepare a list of questions or a post-film test.
- Ensure that the projector is in good working order.
- Assign reading matter to supplement what has been shown in the film.

Motion pictures have many uses. They are as follows:

- They allow many people (students) to see all aspects of, for example, water purification works which groups cannot see clearly on visits. Commentary points out important aspects as the camera zooms in on the section of the plant being shown.
- They can help to facilitate understanding of concepts or terms such as 'electricity' by means of viewing a sound film which would otherwise be incomprehensible in the written text.
- Micro-photography can make visible what cannot be seen by the naked eye.
- Films can be slowed down, stopped or 'frozen', or even reversed and re-played to enable students to see some point they have missed.
- Open-ended films can paint a picture and pose questions which can initiate fruitful debate.
- Films recreate real or imagined events, actions or processes that have occurred, that may possibly occur in the future, or that can only be depicted in animated form. Bodily functions, particularly of internal organs, fall into the latter category, although modern photographic techniques have made things visible which were thought impossible not long ago.
- Processes which normally take months, such as the development of the foetus, can be condensed into a short time. The birth of a baby can be shown in half an hour, instead of the hours it would normally take.

The possibilities are endless.

10.4.2 Film slides

Film slides are valuable teaching aids. They can be prepared at little cost either by the teacher or in special audio-visual departments, or ready-made slides can be purchased.

Advantages of slides as instructional aids

- They are fairly cheap.
- They can be stored easily.
- They can be used to illustrate various medical pathologies or microscopic structures photographed by special cameras. Many rare conditions which may otherwise be difficult for students to see can be illustrated by slides.
- Excellent colour projection is possible.
- The attention of students can be focused on salient points in a lecture.
- Slides can be shown sequentially and thus present a picture of various stages of development.
- It is possible to point to specific aspects on a projection slide by means of a pointer or a special torch-type indicator.
- A sound-track tape which synchronises with the slides can be produced so that student self-study programmes can be produced.
- Slides are a very flexible type of visual aid – they can be removed or added at will.
- Slide projectors are relatively cheap and can be operated with very little trouble.

For the successful use of film slides as a teaching aid, the following points should be borne in mind:

- Slides to be shown should be carefully chosen to illustrate a specific point.
- Slides should be of good quality.
- Slides to be shown should be previewed and put into the correct sequence for showing.
- Lecture notes should be marked so that the appropriate slide is shown at the correct time. With remote control switches, it is quite simple for the lecturer to operate the slide projector herself.
- The projector should be set up, tested and focused before the lecture starts. Re-focusing may be necessary, but this can also be done by a standard remote control switch.
- The number of slides shown should be limited. Too many spoil the impact.
- Proper storage facilities should be available. Hanging slide holders that fit in ordinary filing cabinets are valuable, as are containers which fit the projector.
- Slides should be labelled, listed and numbered individually.
- Slides should be mounted in proper frames, and should be checked frequently in case the frame has been damaged, or the film has slipped.

10.4.3 Film strips

These are a related sequence of slides printed in logical order on a short strip of 35 mm film. A special camera is required for their production as is a special projector.

Some advantages of film strips

- They are an economical means of presenting information.
- They can be used for independent, small group or medium group study.
- They are convenient and flexible to use.
- They can provide a framework of the work to be studied.
- They can be projected forwards or backwards, making it possible to re-view material.
- Film strips can be accompanied by some form of recording device, which enhances their use for self-study.
- It is possible to return to a previous frame if a question arises later during the showing.

For successful production and operation of film strips, the following points should be remembered:

- Plan the filming operation carefully, as the pictures to be shown must be shot sequentially.
- It is essential that the lecturer prepares for using the film strip.
- Film strips must be carefully selected, and relevant to the course.
- Students must be prepared for viewing by means of scene setting, talk or questions.
- Students should be encouraged to participate during the showing; to ask questions, jot down notes, etc. Thinking should be stimulated – comment can be invited.
- Follow-up activities after the showing enhance its use:
  - Questions and answers
  - Discussion
  - Asking students to write down main points
  - Assignment of additional research on the subject
  - Re-showing if necessary.

10.4.4 Video-cassettes (video-tapes)

Video-tapes or video-cassettes for viewing on a television screen are also useful teaching aids. They are more expensive to produce, the hardware is expensive, the component parts are fragile, and maintenance costs are high. Scripts must be written, and the technique of producing video-cassettes needs mastery. When used to give students immediate feedback on performance in practice procedures, role playing or simulated situations, it can be invaluable, and is particularly useful in the training of teachers. Video-tapes used for this type of machine can be 'wiped' clean and re-used on many occasions.

Video-tapes can be prepared to demonstrate procedures in the live situation, as for example operation procedures or specially complicated procedures such as strict isolation nursing to prevent infection, using all the modern equipment available. It is possible to video-tape actual TV shows to show to a class at a future date. Many uses can be envisaged and, as cameras and equipment become easier to operate and less expensive, the use made of this teaching aid will increase. More and more commercially produced material will also become available, which if carefully reviewed and selected, should make the use of this medium more prevalent.

10.5 CHARTS, FLIP-CHARTS, DIAGRAMS

10.5.1 Charts

These are probably one of the best-known teaching aids. The charts produced commercially to illustrate anatomical structures are familar to everyone who has done a course in nursing. The clarity of the sketches combined with the necessary captions are invaluable. They can be used to illustrate many other aspects of nursing, such as injection sites, common sites of fractures, reasons for complications in injuries, and many more. Commercially prepared charts which illustrate subjects such as sanitation, water collection and purification, the growth and development of the foetus, anatomy, and many more are available.

Charts may be pictorial only or may include graphs, diagrams and symbols. A diagram is a schematic presentation of a subject without the detail given in the true-to-life picture of the subject.

Charts can be rolled up and stored for immediate use in a wall frame, or duly labelled and kept in an easily accessible container. In that case a suitable hook or stand must be available in order to hang the chart when it is required. Charts may also be fixed to the wall, and remain in view for varying lengths of time. Care must be taken in the class situation that such hangings do not become too distracting. Charts to be used for teaching can be covered with sheets of plain paper. These are then removed when the particular point to be illustrated occurs in the lecture. A complete sequence can thus be built up by the use of single or strip charts.

Pointers should always be used to focus attention on particular areas. Care should be taken to position oneself to one side, so as to avoid obstructing the view of the students. If the chart is positioned to the side of the dias at the front of the class-room or on a stage, the presenter should not stand towards the centre of the 'teaching area', but should place herself nearer to the side wall. In this way the students' vision will not be obstructed. Very effective charts can be prepared to illustrate a lecture or to supplement a demonstration. A little ingenuity is required in the design and preparation of such charts. Bold outline drawings or cut-outs from magazines can be useful. Labelling should be clear and concise. The use of commercially produced lettering or stencils makes for a professional finish and renders the self-produced chart more acceptable. Various forms of material are available, for example poster cardboard. Charts can be given a longer life if they are prepared on a suitable form of paper, and then glued to a piece of material. Thin rods which are easily available can then be fixed at each end to keep the whole chart stable, and also to facilitate rolling. A cord for hanging can also be fixed to the chart.

Many freely available materials can be used in producing home-made charts. These include sticks of various shapes and sizes pasted on coloured paper; felt-tip pens in various thicknesses and colours; a variety of letter, number, and figure stencils; and commercially produced lettering, usually available in black, white and gold.

10.5.2 Flip charts

These are aimed at presenting a sequence of information which would be difficult to show on a single sheet. They can be used, for example, to illustrate the different steps to be followed in carrying out a procedure.

Flip charts should be prepared on reasonably durable material, with a material backing as described above or on particularly durable cardboard. They can then be fixed together sequentially in several ways, one being by punching two or more holes in the top of the chart, strengthening the holes to prevent tearing and fitting rings through the holes. These are then slipped over a rod which can be fixed to a stand. One stand can of course be used for several flip charts, which are removed and stored when not in use.

Another method is to fix the charts, again arranged sequentially, together with thin metal or wooden strips at the top. One strip should be in the front and one at the back. A cord running through the rings would then allow the whole chart to be fixed to an easel. In both these cases the charts can then be flipped over as the lecture proceeds.

10.5.3 Diagrams

A diagram is either a figure made of lines, a sketch showing the essential features of an object, or a symbolic representation of a subject. Diagrams are widely used to illustrate texts, and are equally useful for chalkboard work or for charts. They can be used to illustrate the sequence of events in a physio-logical process; the life cycle of disease-bearing parasites; the flow of work in nursing administration; the responsibility of various categories and the work relationships; and the basic structure of the heart.

All these chart forms, in order to be successful teaching aids, should meet certain requirements. These are the following:

- They should emphasise one principal point.
- Only *correct* information should be presented.
- Correct grammar and spelling are to be used.
- They should be legible.
- Capital letters should be printed and about three to five centimetres high, while lower case letters should be at least two to two and a half centi-metres high.
- Letters should be formed with great care.
- The diagrams should be uncluttered.
- Words and terms used should be suitable to the level of the student being taught.
- The diagrams should be able to attract and hold attention.

10.6 POSTERS

These are large notices, designed to convey information in such a manner that they attract attention. Posters should be vivid, attractive to look at and convey the message clearly.

In the field of nursing education, they can be used to announce courses, ad-vertise films, displays and exhibitions, even the availability and costs of new textbooks.

To achieve their objectives posters must be

- directed towards *one* specific aim;
- clear – not ambiguous in any way;
- accurate;
- able to furnish all necessary information, or to direct viewers to another source for more details;
- colourful;
- large enough to be seen *and* understood at a glance;
- balanced in design; and
- bold in execution.

The making of posters for a specific purpose can be used as a teaching/learning activity for a group of students. The finished poster can serve as an instruction instrument on its own, but the potential for learning which is presented when students construct posters themselves, is unlimited. The challenge to students to play, design, write, draw, paint and display offers them an opportunity to learn a great deal more about the subject in the process, to pick out salient points and develop creativity. The use of poster production as a teaching/learning technique can add an effective dimension to the learning event.

Commercially made posters advertising various commodities can be used as cut-outs, or irrelevant or inappropriate advertising matter could be edited out for the purpose of the class.

10.7 BULLETIN BOARDS AND TEACHING DISPLAYS

Bulletin or 'notice boards' which may be extended into teaching displays and even exhibitions are inexpensive teaching resources, and with a little forethought can serve as a very useful teaching/learning technique.

Most modern class-rooms are equipped with bulletin boards, otherwise a board is often to be found outside. The material from which the board is constructed must be of a kind onto which paper could easily be pinned, and as easily removed.

In education, bulletin boards can be used for the following purposes:

- *Current events:* On this board (or section of the board), the lecturer or students affix paper clippings, articles and notices which are relevant to either a particular subject being studied or nursing as a whole. These must really be kept *up to date.* Once they are no longer newsworthy, they should be removed, and may then be pasted in a scrapbook; a series of items on a subject might thus show developments or changes brought about, to serve to remind people of particularly interesting events
- *Display of particularly good work* done by students
- *Announcements* (or notices) of importance to students
- *Indication of progress* of a project
- *Requests for assistance,* information, ideas or contributions to a common goal
- *Facilitation of class study of material* of which there is *only one copy* available
- *Stimulation of student interest;*
- *Saving of time;*
- *Provision of a review* of general class activities
- *Presentation of individual or group reports* in a summarised form.

By extending the bulletin board into larger display boards which can be used for exhibitions, teaching opportunities are also extended. In this way it will

- encourage student participation;
- assist students to communicate by means of visual presentation;
- making class-rooms dynamic, relevant, attractive and interest-provoking;
- stimulate interest by encouraging students to research a subject thoroughly in order to present an exhibition or display;
- act as a showcase for the work done in a certain department.

In order to present an exhibition, the following points should be remembered:

- Start planning early.
- Decide on a theme.
- Get a responsible group together to estimate time needed, resources needed,; finance available and needed; to determine for whom the exhibition is intended; and to consider means of advertising and the space required.
- Detailed planning is then required. *Who* is to be responsible for *what, when, where, how,* with the *why* underlying all planning. This will include making of sketches, space allocation, collection and use of materials, use of outside people for visualisation and other purposes, safekeeping of material exhibited, etc.
- A file should be compiled and added to at each exhibition, which gives details of sources and display material, resource persons and any relevant matter.
- Use of colour, grouping in the room, incorporation of audio-visual programmes, real objects, models, and many more need to be considered. Glass exhibit cases may be required. Handouts should be given attention.

All the activities required to present an exhibition, or a smaller exhibit, have learning potential.

To round off an exhibition, the following must be done:

- Return borrowed items.
- Thank those who assisted, *in writing*.
- Salvage label and file or store materials that have long-term uses.
- Dispose of other materials.
- Evaluate the success or otherwise of the exhibit, and file a report.

10.8 REAL OBJECTS

No form of visual aid, picture, film, simulation, model or anything else can produce exactly the same effect on the learner as that of the real object. In teaching and learning the practice of nursing, there is no substitute for practice with real objects or of nursing the real patient.

232

Many objects which are in use can be readily obtained, such as syringes, needles, scissors, forceps, tubes, medicine glasses, cradles, equipment for making beds, thermometers, baumanometers, catheters, suturing material and needles, drip stands, respirators, bandages, and dressings to name but a few. All can be obtained and used for the purpose of practice. What is often not available, is the actual stitch to remove, the drain to shorten, the wound to irrigate, the patient who needs catheterisation, or the person needing the assistance of the respirator. Here films, simulated wounds and other models must be employed in order that a technique can be practised. Often too, real objects such as syringes can be used with some fluid, even water, and an injection given to an 'unreal' thing, such as an orange. This ensures dexterity without subjecting a patient to unnecessary anxiety at the hands of the non-expert. True, the time will arrive when the student who has practised a manual skill in a simulated situation has to transfer this skill to a real-life situation. Her previous practice with the 'real' object will have given her a certain amount of skill, and thus confidence.

Real objects are three-dimensional, and *are* the real thing. Thus the use of such materials is always realistic in part. The senses of sight, feeling, touch and even smell or hearing in some instances, are all involved.

Real objects are costly and must be handled with care. They may involve some danger in the handling, but that can be a positive teaching point, as ways of avoiding injury and medico-legal hazards can be emphasised.

There are three types of real objects which can be used in teaching the practice of nursing:

(a) *Unmodified* real things such as syringes, needles, instruments, even monitors: Various scopes are another example. They can be handled, felt, tested, taken apart in some instances and re-assembled.

(b) *Modified* real things such as skulls, the whole skeleton or human bones: These may have been disarticulated, sawn through to show the medullary cavity or the base of the skull. In other words, elements of the real object are separated and rearranged to clarify relationships and structures. Bones, for instance, can be painted to mark muscle attachments, or sections can be cut out to permit viewing of the internal structure.

(c) *Specimens:* Teachers or students of anatomy will know what valuable teaching aids these can be. They are taken surgically from a human body or from a body after death. They are real objects, but except for frozen sections for immediate laboratory investigation, have to be preserved in some way. This will alter the texture of the specimen, as those who have dissected cadavers will know very well. Removal of thin sections, which enable microscopic study, is also possible. Many specimens are preserved in bottles, jars or other containers which permit direct observation and study.

Specimens are of course also used in zoology, biology and other sciences.

Pathological specimens which are removed surgically or post-mortem, are also valuable teaching aids.

Fresh animal specimens, such as eyes, lungs and liver or kidneys are useful in teaching, and muscle meat can be used to practise stitching, or the performance of episiotomies.

10.9 MODELS

Models are reproductions of real objects which may be too costly, too delicate, or impractical to obtain. They are also three-dimensional.

Some models are smaller than the real object, some are life-size and many are larger. They are usually constructed in such a way that they can be taken apart to permit easy study of internal structures and relationships. All nurses should be familiar with the model of the human body complete with eyes, heart, ears, kidneys and other structures. As long as these are related to reality, they serve as excellent teaching aids.

It would also be possible to construct model sewerage disposal works, water purification works, and monitors or respirators. The model upon which cardio-pulmonary resuscitation is practised, is also well known. So also are the life-size, but not very life-like, 'dolls'. It is possible that one day life-like dolls with properly articulated joints and a more realistic body and orifices will be produced. Many children's dolls have already progressed along this line, while dolls approximately human in terms of weight, flexibility, etc, are used extensively for testing safety devices in vehicles. Perhaps an almost real 'Mr Brown' to be studied in nursing will also appear before too long.

10.10 AUDITORY MATERIALS

It is so easy to record sound nowadays that ever-increasing use of auditory material in teaching the practice of nursing can be foreseen. The sound of normal and abnormal breathing, lung sounds, the sounds made by persons with various speech difficulties or with deformities leading to speech defects, are obvious examples of the use of tapes or other forms of recording.

A lecture on the heart beat, with a tape-recording of the various normal and abnormal rhythms to illustrate each type, would have more impact, and thus effect more learning than does the tapping out of rhythms that are even today the most frequent method employed in this teaching section of the syllabus. Teaching physical assessment skills without such aids is very difficult indeed. Tape recorders are relatively simple to operate, are not expensive, and good quality tapes can be re-used time and again.

There are so many ways in which sound can be used in nursing education, that it is difficult to mention them all. Films have sound tracks, and tapes can be synchronised with slides. Sound can be used as part of a self-instructional package, and lectures can be taped and played back by students themselves.

The voices of well-known personalities can be taped and used in future history lectures; short excerpts of actual taped speeches can be used to excellent effect to illustrate a specific point.

Sound tracks as part of a video-tape presentation is of great use in teaching the practice of nursing. It forms part of micro-teaching, which is an excellent technique.

Tape recorders can be of great use to student-tutors in practising 'crit' lectures. By playing back to yourself what you want to say, you can learn a great deal about yourself, your voice and your speech habits. All problems can then be ironed out.

It is as well to remember that listening to sound is not the only means of teaching and learning. Students retain surprisingly little of what they hear. It is said that only 20 to 33% of the lecture is retained by the young adult, while even mature persons will retain only 50%, no matter how hard they try. It has also been shown that two months later they will be unable to recall even half of that. Thus if 20% of what is heard is retained with no reinforcement, only 10% will be retained in the longer term: a sobering thought.

Nevertheless the judicious use of auditory materials as illustrations of reality, does have impact and is valuable.

10.11 PRINTED TEXTS

Printed texts may be in the form of textbooks, magazines, booklets or pamphlets. Every form of teaching will require the use of supplementary literature, beyond that which is presented in a formal class-room or lecture setting.

10.11.1 Textbooks

These are books which contain basic texts around which whole courses can be structured, or serve as reference books for particular aspects of the course, or to provide more detailed information. They can also be used for background reading or simply for the enrichment of the student. They are of course portable and can be consulted at will, the use of the index being particularly helpful in this regard. They can be skimmed through to give an overall picture before proceeding to a more detailed study of certain sections (wholes before parts). They are reasonably easy to store, and require little maintenance. They are often very well illustrated, which makes study more interesting as well as elucidating pertinent points as they occur in the text.

Advantages

(a) *Individualisation of teaching:* All students read at their own rate. They can go over and over the printed text until they have mastered it. They can study in more detail any aspect which particularly interests them. Students have the opportunity to select what they think is relevant to their own needs, or the needs of the study they are undertaking.

(b) *Economy:* Textbooks can be used and re-used. Although the costs of textbooks have escalated, they are still far cheaper than similar information contained in charts, slides, films and other visual aids, which are not readily available in any case.

(c) *Organisation of subject-matter:* Any well-planned, well-written textbook works to a design so that students are guided to an orderly study of the subject-matter. A logical sequence is followed.

(d) *Stimulation of thought:* By posing special questions in the text or at the end of chapters or simply in the written word, a well-prepared textbook can stimulate thought.

(e) *Alternative source of information:* When students experience difficulty understanding class instruction, they can devote more time to the points which particularly puzzle them, without holding up the whole class.

(f) *A foundation upon which to build a course:* A textbook cannot constitute the complete course, but may form a basis upon which to build the whole teaching strategy.

(g) *Supportive of lecturer's statements:* If the student retains only 20% of what he hears, the supportive reading will help to reinforce what he has heard, will make for better retention and will confirm what he has heard in cases where he may doubt the information given by the lecturer (who *must*, of course ensure that his facts are correct).

Disadvantages

(a) Many books especially in the scientific field, become outdated very quickly. Teachers must be on guard against this. A physiology text, for instance, printed ten years ago, will contain inaccuracies in the light of recent research findings.

(b) Prescribed texts may become the be-all and end-all of student study. Therefore it is essential that students are given other references, as well as reading assignments that necessitate their use.

(c) Badly written books, with language that mystifies rather than clarifies, do not contribute to learning.

It is clear that the evaluation and selection of textbooks which are suitable for the course and the level of student knowledge at various stages of the course, should be an ongoing activity for every tutor. Of course she will not be able to read and evaluate all new textbooks, but it should be possible for her to study those relevant to her subject, and most publishers are willing to supply review copies for this purpose.

Schools of nursing could also have a committee which deals with the evaluation of textbooks and their selection for general use, or for purchase by the library. They will also reject texts which are totally unsuitable for their purpose.

A few criteria for textbook evaluation might be the following:

- *Content:* Is it related to the course and up to date?
- *Depth:* Is subject-matter dealt with in sufficient depth?
- *Appropriateness* to the level of student learning for which it is being considered.
- *Language:* Is the language used clear, readily understood and easy to read? Long, complicated sentences or ambiguity should be avoided.
- *Size of type:* Is the textbook easy to read in that the print is large enough and sufficiently spaced out? Are pages uncrowded?
- *Binding:* Is the book sufficiently reinforced and bound?
- *Paper:* Is this of reasonable weight and durability?
- *Index and glossary:* Is there a clear and accurate index, as well as a glossary, if appropriate, of difficult words?
- *Summaries:* Are well-organised summaries included at the beginning or end of each chapter?
- *Diagrams, pictures:* Are these clear, of good quality, properly labelled and integrated into the text?
- *Bibliography:* Does this contain recent texts from which more information can be obtained? Is it comprehensive?

Textbooks as teaching aids can be of great value to students. The teacher must use them according to her planned teaching programme. They must not be seen as a substitute for teaching, but should supplement it. Carefully chosen textbooks which are used with skill and discrimination can improve student study and learning.

10.11.2 Journals

These are the life-blood of any scientific discipline. Professional journals publish the results of recent research long before it reaches textbooks. New technology is explained and thought-provoking or informative articles dealing with many subjects are stimulating to students and lecturers alike.

A representative supply of journals should be available at all nursing colleges and universities, as well as at the hospitals where practica are undertaken.

Students should be encouraged to make full use of such journals. Photostat facilities which enable students and others to make a photocopy of any article of particular interest or relevance to them, should be available.

Copies of professional journals should be bound and kept for reference in libraries. They should also be accessible to students and tutors. As teaching aids, journals cannot be bettered. They help to keep teaching personnel up to date, and the habit acquired as a student of consulting them regularly stands the erstwhile student in good stead for the rest of her nursing career.

10.11.3 Pamphlets and booklets

They are often a valuable source of specific information, and can be used as handouts to supplement instruction. Many useful pamphlets are prepared as advertisements, or as a special information service by persons concerned with health education. Such material can also be used to great advantage when exhibitions are planned.

10.12 MOCK-UPS

A mock-up is in fact a simplified version of the real thing. It is constructed in such a way that it highlights the essential part of a subject or its functions, and eliminates unnecessary detail. Some may be smaller than in real life and some larger. Size must however be proportionate so that relationships are clearly seen.

A mock-up of a ward can be made inside any building, with chalk lines on the floor to demonstrate walls, or a scale model can be made. It is then possible for students to 'see' a ward which appears on a plan. It is a means of bringing reality to the reading of plans. Many other examples could be given.

A mock-up is really something between a model and a simulation, and is a form of teaching aid which would bear further investigation.

10.13 SCRAPBOOKS

In teaching the practice of nursing, small groups of students or individuals could be asked to compile scrapbooks on a specific subject. The material inserted in the scrapbook could include paper clippings, photographs, pictures, photostat articles, pieces of material – the list is endless. Any relevant material flat enough to be stuck in a book and which does not deteriorate or disintegrate in storage, can be used. The materials should be carefully displayed and linked together by labels (written or typed) and dated. A collection of such scrapbooks over the years can become a valuable supplement to learning.

The exercise of compiling such books is a teaching aid in itself. The compiled books, stored and accessible to future groups, add another dimension to available instructional material.

10.14 LEARNING RESOURCE CENTRES

Learning resource centres are places which supply the resources so that learning can occur. Although many teaching aids are available, and in fact form the core of the learning resource centre, it is more than a collection of such aids or a storage place.

In order to make it a true learning resource centre, teaching and learning materials must not only be collected and stored, but students and staff must be able to retrieve and use such materials.

A true learning resource centre should comply with the following requirements:

- It should be readily accessible to those wishing to use it.
- It should be open for at least 14 hours per day.
- Learning packages, including necessary tapes, slides and other materials must be made available and accessible in the same way as library books are issued.
- The necessary equipment such as viewing boxes or screens, projectors and tape machines must be available as needed.
- Resource staff must be available for students to consult for the full period that the centre is open. This is difficult when staff shortages are the order of the day. It is nevertheless essential if the learning resource centre is to serve its purpose.
- There must be sufficient, separate carrels/work stations/booths at which students can work independently.
- The centre should have certain specialised work stations, such as practical practice areas and equipment which students will share with others.
- There must be preparation room where materials can be gathered, and study guides and learning packages prepared.
- At least one small assembly room for tutorial sessions, progress assessment and other such activities must be available.
- Have one larger assembly room capable of holding all the students engaged in any one course at one time.
- Lighting must be good at all times.
- It must be well ventilated at all times.
- It must be equipped with a bulletin board.
- Vending machines for coffee, tea, or cold drinks should form part of the equipment, so that students can take a break without leaving the area.
- Electrical outlets must be sufficient.

- A technician must be available to deal with equipment if it should break down.
- It must have a large supply of reference books; a library is basically a learning resource centre.

The following is an example of how a learning resource centre should work/function:

The student, on entering the centre, collects the appropriate study guide and equipment for the unit of work which she has to cover. The course or section which is being covered by independent study has already been divided into units, and the appropriate learning package prepared. She signs for it, and the unit she has taken is marked off on her individual chart or her section of a composite chart.

The student now takes the package to a carrel where other resource material is set out. Any equipment that is needed is now set out, such as cassettes into the tape recorder, a slide container into the viewing box or projector, and anything else, including reference books required.

The student settles down in the carrel, studies the course objectives, and then starts the tape which will guide her through a variety of learning experiences and activities. She may be referred to a film, her textbook, other reference books, a microscope or other appropriate materials, specimens, a diagram or chart or to models or real objects. There are times when she may be required to work out a problem or to answer questions on a blank space provided in the study guide.

The tape is not a substitute for a lecture. It is part of a form of programming a student through learning experiences. Teaching staff must be available at all times to assist students who are experiencing problems or difficulties with their learning programme. The student should be at liberty to call a member of the teaching personnel at all times, in case of need.

Students following a specific course are called together for *general assembly sessions* at the end of each week. This session is used to show a film, present an outside lecturer, for major tests or examinations, etc. Smaller assembly sessions where about eight students meet the instructor, are held each week, usually at the end. This session takes the form of a tutorial or quiz session where the instructor can assess student progress, clarify certain points, and ask one student to tell the group what she has learnt about a specific item or unit of work during the week.

Students can thus work through a whole course or sections of a course in a learning resource centre when it is used as a centre for individualised or independent learning systems.

On a simpler scale it can be an extension of library facilities, or smaller learning resource centres can be organised, attached to specialised depart-

240

ments such as intensive care, midwifery, paediatric units, and others. However, this will necessarily entail duplication of equipment, which would add to the expense.

Learning resource centres are expensive to create, equip and maintain. If they are to justify such outlay in monetary terms, as well as in terms of personnel, they must serve a purpose. *They must be used.*

Before embarking on such an exercise, careful *planning* is essential. A committee which consults regularly with all the teaching personnel as well as with a representative section of other personnel, should be established. This committee should determine the following:

- The *philosophy* underlying the establishment of such a centre. Something of this nature might meet the needs: 'It is believed that learning can be facilitated when individuals work through guided programmes or do independent study, which relate to their current needs, and at the same time achieve defined educational goals'
- *The aim of the learning resource centre* – again the following might be appropriate: 'To provide educational material which is conveniently situated and easily accessible, and which will encourage and facilitate independent self-paced learning'
- *Definition of users,* for example students, registered nurses, etc, and estimated numbers of each category
- *Determination of physical resources necessary,* which include:
  - Space required
  - Equipment required including carrels, educational hardware and software
  - Books
  - Storage space, and type of storage

- *Personnel required* to run the centre
- *Control measures*
- *Existing resources*
- *Classification and indexing system*
- *Student access*
- *Sections of courses* or complete courses to be put into learning packages
- *Topics* for which resource material is to be provided on a reference basis
- *Staff required for* preparatory work
- *Time required for* preparatory work
- *Estimated original cost*
- *Annual estimated budget.*

A well-planned, well-run learning resource centre is a tremendous asset to all teaching programmes and combines many teaching aids in one unified concept.

Teaching aids must always be seen as a means to an end, and must never become the end itself. Time taken to produce visual aids must be part of an overall teaching plan. It cannot be the only effort put into teaching preparation.

11 Clinical teaching

The word 'clinical' comes from the Greek *klinikos*, meaning a bed. Basically therefore it originated from *bedside*, the patient receiving clinical care being 'in the bed'. Nursing has moved away from *bedside* care to *patient*-side care, as patients and those for whom nurses give health care are not always confined to bed. However, bedside care must not be forgotten as it is still very much part of patient care, but has expanded, changed and moved away from the bedside only. Clinical nursing care too, is given to everybody requiring nursing care, and thus clinical teaching is not confined to teaching nursing skills in caring for bedridden people. It is this aspect of modern nursing that often causes the greatest misunderstanding amongst those who still see all nursing as the care given by nurses to *patients in bed*.

Clinical teaching is necessary to ensure that the recipient, be he in bed or out, is given the nursing care to which he is entitled. It may be preventive, promotive, rehabilitative, maintenance or terminal nursing care. Clinical teaching is the means by which the student nurse learns to apply the theory of nursing so that an integration of theoretical knowledge and practical skills in the clinical situation becomes the art and science of nursing.

Teaching the theory of nursing in the class-room situation enables the student to learn, assimilate and store knowledge for future use, and to apply the nursing care which is given to patients and clients. A nurse who is a theoretician only, is no nurse. Academic achievement without the ability to translate it into practice is useless.

Physical skills, such as caring for a patient's tracheostomy, performing a bladder catheterisation or removing sutures, must be allied to arts and skills such as observation, the making of skilled, educated judgements, interpersonal relationship skills and effective communication.

A nurse must be able to put into practice what she has learnt in theory, and apply the knowledge she has obtained in the class-room to exercise educated judgement, and to making skilled observation throughout the giving of patient care.

This correlation of theory and practice and the building up of meaningful experience, must take place in the field of clinical practice, be it the hospital ward, special department, casualty department, out-patient department, day hospital, clinic, old-age home, or the home of a patient or client. It is only in

243

the clinical situation that nursing care becomes a reality, and the nurse can also observe the responses of patients/clients to illness, to nursing and medical care and treatment. It is in the clinical situation that nurses encounter the people for whom they are caring, as people. It is there that the human side of nursing is in evidence. The nurse comes into contact not only with the client or patient in the clinical situation, but also with his relatives and friends. The nurse learns to interact skilfully with these people and with other members of the health team. Nursing is one profession which cannot be practised in isolation.

The following should be borne in mind about clinical teaching:

- It occurs in the *real-life* situation; it translates theory into reality.
- The student is an *active* participant.
- It is a *small* group activity. Physical limitations make the number of students who can be involved very small. It may even occur on the basis of one patient, one teacher and one student only. This naturally limits its utilisation.
- The student is enabled to develop *self-confidence* by performing under expert guidance.
- It affords the student opportunities for *observation* and *decision making*.
- It allows assessment of the degree to which educational objectives have been attained.
- It centres around *patient care*.
- The real-life situation needs careful handling to prevent both patient and student from being placed in a difficult position.
- It is an invasion of the privacy of patients and can therefore only be carried out with the consent of the patient.

11.1 THE AIM OF CLINICAL TEACHING

Clinical teaching is aimed at producing a competent registered nurse, capable of giving expert nursing care which is based on sound knowledge and practised skill. The care given must be an interaction between two or more human beings, the recipient of care and his family on one side, and the nurse or nurses on the other.

In order to achieve this aim, clinical teaching must be based on theory, and applied to practice. It must include teaching such skills as leadership and administration. It must include teaching and organisation and control of staff, the determination of work methods and procedures, the economical use of equipment and materials, the drawing up of appropriate nursing care plans and supervision, and control of the unit as a whole.

Clinical teaching must include teaching the practical side of methods of clinical teaching so that the student can become proficient in peer group teaching and will later be ready to take her place as the teacher of students and pupils in the clinical field.

11.2 WHO IS RESPONSIBLE FOR CLINICAL TEACHING?

A great deal of clinical instruction, formal and informal, lies in the hands of the unit professional nurse. She has been the traditional teacher in the clinical field. The passing on of the expertise which has been developed over years of thoughtful and observant practice, is of inestimable value to the student. This fundamental aspect of the work of the professional nurse in charge of the ward has never been taken away from her, and nor should it ever be. The professional nurse in charge of the ward needs acknowledgement and support, even assistance, but it is a responsibility which she cannot sidestep.

11.2.1 Teaching as an integral part of giving patient care – the unit professional nurse

The main function of every registered nurse is to ensure that the patient or client entrusted to her care obtains the best possible health care. In order to achieve such quality care in the unit, the registered nurse has to ensure that those to whose care she entrusts her patient, that is the students and/or pupils, are capable of providing it. If they are unable to do so, it will be her duty to teach them. This is another responsibility which cannot be side-stepped.

The teaching given by the unit professional nurse may be either quite informal, for she is in the best position to make use of the 'teachable' moment, or it may be more structured and formal, such as the demonstration of a nursing technique supported by theory. The unit professional nurse is responsible for enabling the student who has been assigned to her unit for experience in the specific area of nursing, to encounter and cope with such situations, which will enable growth and development into a component, independent practitioner.

The student is *not* assigned to a ward primarily as a 'pair of hands', but to learn the practice of nursing. The unit professional nurse is accountable not only for patient care, but also for teaching students and/or pupils to give that care.

The unit professional nurse acts as a role model for the student nurse who learns a great deal, often unconsciously, by imitation. As the person always present and in charge, the unit professional nurse has a great responsibility to teach, by example, such intangible matters as attitudes as well as ward administration.

The task of teaching specialised skills may often be allocated to a unit professional nurse. This is very often done in a haphazard manner, instead of being planned and allocated so that each one is aware of her special tasks. Each unit should be allocated a list of, say, six procedures which are commonly found in the ward (depending on its category), which the professional nurse in charge of a ward or her deputy *must* demonstrate each month. She must also be expected to have the theoretical background to make her demonstration meaningful.

It is necessary that the professional nurse in charge of a ward be fully aware of the practical progress of each student allocated to her unit. When it is evident that a student is already proficient in a procedure, she may ask the student in question to demonstrate the technique to others. This will encourage peer group teaching and prepare the student for a future teaching role.

The professional nurse in charge of a ward must be very well aware of the need to do incidental or situational teaching by seizing every teachable moment which presents itself. She must also be aware of her role in the continuous assessment of the nursing proficiency of the students in her unit. Her work in the abstract field of teaching attitudes, communications, interpersonal relationships, the making of sound professional judgements, and the maintenance of professional standards and ethical behaviours, and in the day-to-day counselling of students must also not be forgotten.

11.2.2 The clinical instructor or the clinical teacher

The clinical instructor should be seen as supplementary to the teaching role of the professional nurse in charge of a ward, and should not be seen as the only provider of instruction in the clinical area.

Ideally the clinical instructor should be allocated to units or wards with about 60 beds in her area. A specialised 'clinical teaching department' can be used, but the personnel operating from such a department tend to be seen as separate from the main stream of nursing practice, and as such are less likely to have good liaison with the professional nurses in charge of a ward.

11.2.2.1 Clinical instructors allocated to units

These professional nurses come to know the areas they serve, the particular likes and dislikes of doctors serving the area, and are able to build up a close working relationship with those in charge of the units. Of course it will mean a fairly large number of clinical instructors, but the resultant benefit to training and thus to patient care, makes it a worthwhile system.

The instructor, in this case with 60 to 80 beds as her field of clinical practice, will have 12 to 18 students under her tutelage for at least a month at a time. With such a number she will have

- several students at the same level of training;
- an opportunity to know each student and her learning needs;
- knowledge of the day-to-day happenings in each ward, the patient needs

and the practical training opportunities;

- the opportunity for working closely with each student almost every day;
- the chance to plan her teaching programme to meet the unit, patient and student needs, and arrange the timing of her teaching activities to meet the unit timetable and to be of assistance in carrying out nursing care rather than being 'in the way';
- the opportunity to establish good interpersonal relationships and mutual trust with professional nurses; and
- ample time to assess student progress.

11.2.2.2 A clinical teaching department

This is a specialised department set up for the purpose of co-ordinating and organising clinical teaching throughout the hospital. A well-organised department can be of great advantage, but may also have many disadvantages. It can become remote and out of touch with reality in the day-to-day ward situation.

Because the personnel are not closely in touch with the wards, the patients and the professional nurses in charge of wards, many opportunities for close contact with students in the working environment and appreciation of their needs and problems are missed. The work of the department then tends to become procedure oriented and not patient-care oriented.

Because the clinical instructors work in isolation, their acceptance by the unit professional nurses is less likely than those who are working under the first-mentioned system. Ward professional nurses are less likely to consult the clinical instructor from a remote department about problem nursing situations, problems with students and general changes which may occur in the prescribed treatment.

If the clinical teaching department is so organised that its personnel are allocated two wards each, under overall jurisdiction of the department, and that reliefs are supplied from the general pool in times of leave and sickness, it would have a better chance of success.

A certain measure of standardisation is also possible – whichever method is used, regular consultations with unit professional nurses must be standard practice. Each section must know what the other is doing, and must have the opportunity to consult one another on a regular basis.

11.2.3 Appointing the clinical instructor

A clinical instructor should be chosen very carefully and should have the following characteristics: she should
- be a skilled practitioner of nursing;
- have an up-to-date theoretical background which she maintains by read-

ing, enquiry, attending up-dating lectures, courses, symposia, etc;

- be able to instil confidence into those she is guiding;
- have a flexible attitude so that changes which could possibly improve nursing care can be evaluated and adopted, adapted or rejected according to the merits of each;
- have high professional standards, honesty, integrity and objectivity, and an ability to interpret the norms and values of her profession and make them part of her lifestyle;
- have an even temperament and balanced judgement spiced with a sense of humour;
- be resourceful, so that unforeseen occurrences are dealt with calmly and constructively;
- possess a knowledge of the resources available, both in the hospital and in the community, which could be of use in drawing up a meaningful programme;
- have excellent interpersonal relationships, so that resentment among ward professional nurses is avoided and willing co-operation is obtained;
- be able to manage her time and organise that of others to the maximum benefit of all;
- have a realistic approach to all that she undertakes. This does not imply a lowering of standards, but a sensible application of the basic principles to any given situation;
- have the ability to impart knowledge and skills in a clear, understandable manner so that those she is teaching gain maximum benefit from the time spent with her;
- be approachable so that students will feel free to go to her for assistance, not only in connection with the practical work problems, but also when they experience emotional difficulties, such as when patients die, are permanently physically handicapped, or terminally ill;
- accept that it is a fundamental part of her responsibility to prepare future professional nurses for their role and function;
- possess a sense of responsibility and accountability;
- display leadership qualities;
- exhibit thought and the ability to use innovative ideas; and
- place a high value on human life and dignity.

11.3 WHY IS CLINICAL TEACHING UNDERTAKEN?

Clinical teaching is necessary to ensure that students learn the practice of nursing, that standards of patient care are maintained and improved, that competent practitioners of the art and science of nursing are produced and in so doing, that quality patient care is practised from one generation of nurses to the next.

Nursing techniques must be taught and practised, technical skills must be acquired. Nursing judgement based on knowledge and skilled observation must become part of the armamentarium of every would-be nursing practitioner. Nurses' patient-nurse relationship attitudes need clarifying and reinforcing.

The ability to run a unit or department, to control and organise personnel and to co-ordinate the health care of the patient must be mastered. A full professional who will be an asset to her patients, her medical colleagues, her employer, the community and her profession must be developed. This person never ceases to learn and grow in professional expertise and has the ability to render humane, compassionate, skilled attention to those in need of nursing care, be it preventive, promotive, rehabilitative, maintenance or terminal.

11.4 WHAT IS TAUGHT IN CLINICAL TEACHING?

The first thing that comes to mind in answer to this question is nursing care, which is rather oversimplified. Perhaps the following list will give some idea of what clinical teaching should encompass:

(a) Guidance towards *professional adulthood*, which will enable the nurse to practise her independent functions in the knowledge that she, and she alone, is responsible for her actions.
(b) *Technical skills,* based on knowledge.
(c) *Observation skills* upon which her nursing care is planned.
(d) *Critical judgement* in all health-care situations.
(e) *Responsibility* for the care of her clients or patients, for the teaching of the students or pupils and *accountability* to patients, colleagues, the employing authority, the public as a whole, and to herself for her acts and omissions.
(f) *Attitudes, norms and values* which are appropriate for the subsystem which is nursing, and which identify and meet patient attitudinal requirements.
(g) *Appreciation* for the points of view and needs of others, and for the fundamental differences in human beings, their culture and backgrounds and their varying needs.
(h) *Appropriate behaviour* in a wide variety of situations, from crisis conditions to mundane, routine events.

11.5 WHEN IS CLINICAL TEACHING DONE?

Again this question is simple to answer. *All the time,* whenever clinical nursing occurs. It can be a formally organised occasion with due warning, it can be by precept (do as I say), or example (do as I do), or by situational teaching when the teachable moment occurs.

As the opportunity for clinical teaching is always available, the whole organisation of the programme can be very widely based. Certain procedures may be more difficult to demonstrate because of the rarity with which the condition necessitating such treatment occurs, but because nursing care is given 24 hours a day the *when* will, on the whole, depend on those responsible for patient care and for clinical instruction, and the availability of the student at that time, and on little else.

11.6 WHERE DOES CLINICAL TEACHING OCCUR?

Wherever nursing care is given. It may be

- at a bedside;
- in a clinic;
- in casualty;
- in an operating theatre;
- at the side of a patient or client who is not in bed;
- at a health centre;
- in an old-age home;
- in a private home;
- at a first aid post;
- at a primary health care centre;
- in a doctor's consulting rooms, etc.

The list is endless. The main point is that clinical teaching occurs mainly in the *real-life situation*.

11.7 HOW IS CLINICAL TEACHING DONE?

Many of the methods already discussed in chapter 9 are particularly relevant to clinical teaching. A few of those strategies which are particularly appropriate are listed here.

- The demonstration, which is particularly useful for teaching techniques: If it is properly applied with pre-teaching as well as follow-up work, and the patient is seen as a person and not a case, this will be particularly useful.
- Precept and example: Precept consists of telling someone what to do, while example is showing them what to do. This is often the setting of an example by one's actions in the nursing-care situation, which is then imitated by students. A good role model will have a *positive* teaching effect, whereas a poor role model can have a negative effect.
- Use of the teachable moment.
- Ward rounds, including doctors' and nursing rounds.

250

- Drawing up of nursing care plans.
- Case discussions.
- The use of problem-oriented nursing records.
- Case studies, if discussed in the clinical setting.
- The use of workbooks to direct attention to clinical care.
- Peer-group teaching.
- The writing and giving of reports.
- Problem solving in the unit.
- Simulation techniques.

The use of media such as real objects, transparencies, slides, films, closed-circuit television and video-tapes, models, specimens, charts, and text-books, can all be included in clinical teaching.

11.8 GENERAL ASPECTS OF CLINICAL TEACHING

Clinical teaching, if it is to serve its purpose, should be available in a training hospital for 24 hours a day. Students work in units and clinical teaching should thus be conducted at the same time.

Clinical instructors should work the same shifts as the students, including night and weekend duties. The number of instructors required for certain shifts and for night duty could be reduced, but rosters should be worked out carefully so that students have the opportunity to receive guidance from their instructors when they need it. When inexperienced students have to assume night-duty responsibilities far beyond what they should normally be expected to undertake, they could gain support and grow in confidence if they were able to call on instructors for assistance. This task should not devolve upon the skeleton trained staff on night duty, who are in any case over-burdened with keeping the hospital running and are dealing with acute cases. Special 'night-duty' clinical instructors, with clearly spelt out job descriptions should fulfil this task. Then night-duty experience would indeed become a learning experience and not simply a working situation, fraught with anxiety and danger.

All this sounds as though a large team of clinical instructors is needed, for relief will have to be supplied for off-duty days and nights, for shift work and for leave. This is indeed the case, but if the student nurse is to be treated as a student, and if the time spent in clinical practice is divided up a follows:

Total	36	months (a three-year training course)
Less	3	months leave
Less	10	months block
	23	

then these 23 months *should* have more teachers than the class-room period of ten months. Some of this teaching will be done by ward professional nurses, of course, but a good case can nevertheless be made out for more, well-selected clinical instructors. This can be adapted to any length of course.

Clinical instruction should go far beyond ensuring proficiency in technical skills. It should also embrace the following:

- Developing skills in making independent judgements regarding nursing needs and care
- Developing the interpersonal skills necessary to deal with patients, relatives, visitors, other members of the health team, and personnel from ancillary services
- Developing communication skills
- Developing skills of giving emotional support to those with special needs
- Developing teaching skills
- Developing the ability to manage units and personnel with skill and discrimination
- Internalising professional ethics, standards and behavioural patterns so that the student becomes a mature professional adult, with the ability to present a good role model to the neophytes in the profession.

The clinical instructor is a teacher and not an examiner. Although a small part of her time could be occupied in assessing student proficiency, her main concern should be directed towards *teaching the practice of nursing in the clinical area, and correlating theory and practice*. The teaching should be patient-care oriented and *not* procedure oriented.

11.9 THE PROGRAMME

In order to make clinical instruction or clinical teaching effective, it is essential that a plan or programme be drawn up, according to which the whole process will occur.

Drawing up such a programme will require the following:

- A knowledge of the curriculum
- An ability to organise material to be covered in clinical teaching according to the educational needs of students at different levels
- An ability to plan systematically and to be realistic at the same time
- A decision regarding the method to be followed
- Co-operation from personnel in the clinical areas and the opportunity to consult them about their needs, convenient times and assistance that can be given to them

- Planning to ensure that each student knows what is expected of her, and when
- Clear definition of general as well as specific objectives
- Division of available time and allocation of personnel so that all students have an equal opportunity to benefit
- Setting aside specific times when students are released from the wards for certain formal activities, such as demonstrations. These times must be known to ward personnel, who should have a say in the choice of suitable times, and students alike
- Incorporation of ward personnel with special expertise in a formal programme
- Flexibility in planning to meet unforeseen eventualities
- A system of record-keeping so that it is possible to see at a glance if all students have the opportunity to benefit from the programme and if they, in their turn, fulfil their obligations with regard to maximising clinical practica experience
- Standardisation of nursing and other procedures to facilitate nursing care and teaching
- Evaluation procedures
- Every registered participant in the programme, that is unit professional nurses as well as clinical instructors, must be provided with an outline of the programme and the specific contribution she is expected to make. General and specific objectives must be spelt out, as well as a list drawn up of suggested teaching strategies. It may be necessary to organise programmes of continuing in-service education to keep personnel aware of their responsibilities and of teaching techniques and evaluation methods
- Medical and paramedical personnel must be consulted and involved in providing a contribution to the clinical training of students who are being prepared for service to patients. Health services rely so heavily on nurses for provision of care that other members of the health team should be made aware of their responsibilities. Without nurses, patient care on an organised basis would grind to a halt.

11.10 EVALUATION IN CLINICAL TEACHING

As a complete chapter is devoted to evaluation in nursing education, evaluation in clinical teaching will only be touched upon here for the sake of completeness.

Evaluation of the results of clinical teaching include:

- the quality of care which patients receive
- the progress made by individual students
- the effectiveness of the teaching programme

- the integration of theory and practice.

Evaluation in the clinical situation is the responsibility of many people, including:

- the unit professional nurse in charge
- the clinical nursing service manager
- the specially assigned clinical instructor
- the tutor
- other registered nurses
- those who make use of the services of nurses.

The evaluation process has several important aspects, and could include:

- student progress reports, usually on a monthly basis
- continuous evaluation of work in the unit, which should be noted and reported
- special proficiency evaluation
- completed workbooks which are assessed
- reports on positive as well as negative aspects.

The person doing the evaluation:

- must be proficient herself
- must be able to assess objectively
- must have an appreciation for what can reasonably be expected from the student being assessed
- must have criteria against which to measure performance
- must have the ability to get the best out of students
- must be unbiased in her judgements.

The aim of evaluation in clinical teaching is to improve student performance. The assessment, report or whatever form the evaluation takes, is part of the evaluation of nursing education as a whole.

Clinical teaching, as was stated in section 11.1, aims at producing a competent registered nurse, capable of giving expert nursing care which is based on sound knowledge and practised skill. Evaluation of her proficiency in the physical, cognitive and emotional supportive dimension is thus of the utmost importance.

12 *Curriculum development*

Before discussing curriculum development, it would be as well to identify what is meant by the word curriculum. *The Concise Oxford Dictionary* defines it as a 'course (of study)', while *Chambers Twentieth Century Dictionary* says that it is 'a course, esp. the course of study at a university'. It is derived from the Latin *curriculum*, from *currere* = to run.

Carol Clark (1978: 46) says that 'a curriculum is an educational programme designed to meet specific goals', while Allan Waldren (1974) states:

> A curriculum is many things to different people. Generally it is regarded as a programme of instruction for an educational institution. To students, curriculum is usually an array of required or elective courses that must be taken in order to graduate. To teachers, curriculum may be a sequence of 'packages of knowledge' to be 'taught' in certain ways at certain times by subject specialists. To administrators, curriculum is a way of organising and departmentalising a school into manageable administrative units. To society, curriculum often represents a time continuum of 'school activities' that have been designed to prepare students for future roles in the community. Additionally, curriculum can be thought of as the content for instruction; the standards for student learning; a programme for processing students; a tradition for the school to follow; a set of guidelines to serve society's needs; or a primary vehicle for change in education.

This somewhat lengthy quotation points out clearly that there are many facets to curriculum development. In the nursing context it is as well to be aware that people have different ideas that need clarifying before the actual development of curricula is tackled.

If one looks at the origin of the word *currere*, to run, the idea of a course that has to be run emerges. But what course? The object of teaching the practice of nursing is to produce trained nurses from students. Therefore the course to 'be run' or at least followed, is *a course in the art and science of nursing*. This leads us to the assumption that it is a *planned educational programme* for student nurses (or if preparing for the roll, pupil nurses) to enable them to achieve a *specific goal*, namely that of becoming a registered (or enrolled) nurse. There are various forms of curricula planning which will subsequently be discussed.

255

12.1 OUTLINE CURRICULA

This curriculum serves as a *broad outline* for the course, stating principles only, and is laid down by the examining and/or registering body. In the RSA these curricula for basic as well as post-basic courses are drawn up by the South African Nursing Council.

Although curricula are constantly under review, changes cannot be made too frequently as all regulations made by the Council have to be promulgated in the *Government Gazette* by the Minister of Health, Welfare and Population Development, and frequent changes would be impracticable. It is for this reason that the curricula prescribed in the regulations are stated in broad principle and outline only.

The Council then draws up directives which can be changed according to changing needs, without promulgation in the *Government Gazette*. These directives supply minimum requirements and give guide-lines as to how the curriculum should be interpreted.

In designing broad outline curricula, various factors have to be taken into account. These include the following:

(a) *Design* to meet the needs of all groups training in nursing education programmes and not the specific needs of one group only
(b) *Delineation* to meet the health needs of all population *groups* and all strata of society without deviating from the broad principles
(c) *Allowance* for the incorporation of any advances in the medical, nursing and technological fields within the limits of the curriculum
(d) *Flexibility* of the curriculum, which would be sufficient to accommodate social changes which affect health
(e) *Incorporation* of education in promotive, preventive, curative, rehabilitative, maintenance and terminal care in institutions, as well as in the community
(f) *Realism*, so that excessive cost is avoided in the establishment and maintenance of training establishments
(g) Educational *requirements*, in line with the ability of the average student who leaves school with at least a senior certificate, which must be met
(h) A reasonable *ratio of practica* to theory and practica that are designed to lead to competent nursing practitioners at the end of the course
(i) Maintenance of *standards* which will ensure good, safe patient care
(j) The possibility for defined *objectives* to be met.

12.2 DETAILED CURRICULA

These are designed by the nursing school to flesh out the skeleton provided by the Council. The setting out of more detailed curricula or courses, which

256

follow the broad principles of the South African Nursing Council can then be undertaken at various levels. These include overall planning by those responsible for the provision of nursing education, such as the provincial authorities, and planning done by the schools themselves. This is also subdivided as Clark puts it, by 'organising and departmentalising a school into manageable administrative units' and then into special curriculum planning segments for different courses, where details are worked out by the tutor and which are also available to students to guide their learning.

12.2.1 General aspects

Organisation must follow a process of assessing needs and facilities and planning to meet these needs within the framework of requirements of the registering body and the employing authority and of the facilities available, implementing the plan and evaluating its success.

12.2.1.1 Regional or overall curriculum planning

When the training school forms part of a larger provincial authority as is general practice, then the authority responsible for the provision of nursing education should appoint a working committee at regional level, with representatives from the respective schools. This committee should plan policy with regard to the overall implementation of training regulations and determine how much control or latitude is to be allowed to individual schools. Finance, time allowed for block periods and student utilisation in wards, hours of work, etc, form part of their terms of reference. Some of the planning will be dependent on South African Nursing Council examinations and deadlines to be met, but a uniform policy regarding the implementation of the curriculum should be determined, so that students who may have to transfer from one school to another within the same province, will not be penalised by variations in different schools.

Regional or overall planning should also contain a clear statement of

- the *learning* needs of students, particularly in the practical situation;
- *duties of registered staff* relating to student training;
- policy regarding *night duty*, including *clinical teaching* responsibilities on night duty;
- policy regarding personnel responsible for *non-nursing*, domestic or 'hotel' duties;
- *educational needs* of students at each level of training; and
- the *student's* role as a *student*. Although a member of the team, students must be seen as individual students.

257

12.2.1.2 Training school: curriculum

Armed with a clear policy statement from the authorities responsible for implementing nursing education programmes, which they as members of the committee have helped to draw up, it is then necessary for the individual school to plan more detailed curriculum development.

The guiding curriculum planning will have stated the following:

- Hours of duty
- Block periods
- Guide-lines for broad division of subjects in each block
- Student requirements regarding testing, promotion to subsequent blocks and procedure to be followed regarding failures, number of attempts allowed within a plan flexible enough to accommodate the student who tries but is slower than average, remedial teaching and illness
- Responsibilities regarding allocation of students for practica
- Student roles
- Registered staff responsibilities.

It is now up to the training school to get down to detailed planning. The overall plan will be flexible enough to allow for individual differences, such as the use of various teaching strategies, the internal testing programme, allocation of teaching personnel according to their special interests and abilities, and the allocation of students, according to their learning needs, to wards and departments. Far too often this part of curriculum planning is left to persons who see it as a duty which is concerned only with service needs and not as part of the 'educational programme to meet specified objectives'. In training-school curriculum planning the unit professional nurse, the clinical teachers, and the persons responsible for student allocation *must be part of the planning committee.*

The student comes to a nursing training school for a specific purpose, namely to learn the art and science of nursing, and her overall educational programme is what must concern those dealing with her in college, as well as in the unit. In times of staff shortage this can cause problems, but if the ward staff were seen in a different light and more use were made of part-time registered or enrolled nurses who are often prepared to work 'peculiar' hours, better education of the student could be planned, and at least some student wastage could be avoided. Before employing part-time workers, special shifts could be worked out and workers could then be asked to apply for such shifts, and be appointed for those times only. Howerver, a long discussion on this subject is out of place here. It is only included to indicate that curriculum planning entails planning the course of *nursing education* which the student must follow, and *not* a course to be run haphazardly, which eventually may meet requirements only in the number of hours spent by students in various units, and not any real *educational* requirements.

Training-school planning must be designed in such a way that those responsible for carrying it out are accountable to the South African Nursing Council, to the educational authority, usually the province, to the *student* who is the core around which nursing education centres, to the *patient* she is being educated to serve, and to the *taxpayer* at whose expense her education takes place.

Part of the responsibility of the training-school curriculum committee would be to do the following:

- Undertake detailed task analyses before tackling curriculum design.
- Assess what is already done, what needs to be done, and who is available to do what, for only then can successful curriculum planning occur. Redesignation of functions, re-allocation of tasks, scrapping of redundant tasks, and the introduction of new ones must be based on facts and not assumptions. Rationalisation and reduction of tasks, rather than constant addition, is the crux of the matter.
- Ensure that there is no overlapping in teaching. If an integrated course is followed, then each responsible teacher must know for which section of the work she is responsible.
- Constantly review planning in the light of achieved objectives and changing needs.
- Provide for administrative back-up to ensure smooth running of the programme.
- Gear timetable planning to curriculum planning.
- Ensure that each person responsible for teaching is given a clear outline of her specific function.
- Draw up a clear programme of activities, which is made available to all.
- Ensure that 'new material' is not simply added to existing curricula without a careful assessment of what is already taught, what is relevant and what is not essential. Curriculum planning must be *planning* based on *investigation* of *reality* and designed to achieve *order*.

12.2.1.3 Individual curriculum planning

This type of curriculum planning is done by the individual tutor or clinical teacher.

Here the real flesh, perhaps even a bit of padding, is given to the broad outline laid down by the registering and examining body, by the allocation of a particular course or section of a course to the individual and the availability of teaching facilities for use in her individual planning.

In chapter 9 a good deal of emphasis was placed on the planning of lectures and individual classes. Various strategies were discussed. It is now necessary to go a stage futher in course planning. A curriculum must be drawn up so that the course content can be covered during the period allocated, and that it is possible for the average student to follow it successfully and to achieve the set objective. In the short term, this is the successful completion of the specific course, and in the long term, the achievement of state registration (or enrolment) and the competence to practise with confidence, safety and efficiency, as a registered or enrolled nurse.

In dividing the work allocated to her, in planning how it is to be covered, and rate at which she will present the work, and the activity itself (including self-activity which the student must complete), the tutor or clinical teacher must make certain decisions.

She will have to

- define objectives;
- divide the work to be covered into meaningful units;
- draw up guide-lines for each unit;
- draw up work activities for students;
- plan regular evaluation; and
- provide students with outline guides to each section, set deadlines for self-activity and testing, and stick to them.

12.3 CURRICULUM DEVELOPMENT: SOME UNIVERSAL ASPECTS

Curriculum development is not a new concept in education. The influence of the *Greeks* on education is well known. In ancient Greece a planned programme was followed which included the study of such subjects as music, reading, writing and arithmetic. This education programme commenced at the age of seven, for boys only, while geography, literature, grammar and rhetoric, mathematics, and citizenship were included later. Some of the brighter students later studied science, psychology and philosophy. It would appear that their curriculum was divided not only into subjects, but also into a form or primary, secondary and tertiary education.

Roman education was somewhat different. Their curriculum had to meet the needs of their particular form of society as does ours today. Reading, writing and oratory, including the art of debate, were important. The curriculum of the Middle Ages was also geared to meet the needs and knowledge of the times and included rhetoric, grammar, music, astronomy, arithmetic and geometry.

Universal education, that is education for all the people, is a relatively modern concept. In 1870 a bill aimed at bringing elementary education within the reach of every child in England was brought before the English Parliament. This made *elementary* education possible, but it only became *compulsory* for all children in 1880, just over a century ago. And even then this was *elementary* or primary education. Secondary education followed in 1902. Education for girls was slower to get off the ground.

12.3.1 Setting objectives: curricula objectives

An objective is aimed towards bringing about a change in student behaviour, through learning. Curricula objectives are the changes or results which, it is intended, will be brought about by teaching and learning. In the nursing context, the objectives to be defined must specify what the student should be able to do after having completed a particular aspect of the curriculum. It naturally includes cognitive as well as psychomotor skills.

In drawing up curriculum objectives in nursing education, evaluation of student progress, both in technical as well as theoretical areas, must be planned. These must be designed to measure what it is intended to achieve, and requires clear thinking.

Basic principles in curriculum planning include the following:

(a) Assessment of the needs of society both for the nation as a whole and for local needs. Nursing needs are not constant throughout the country. Urban and rural differences, population density, cultural practices, degree of industrialisation, coastal areas or inland areas all affect health and health-care services.

(b) Consultation could also occur on the level of patient needs, learner needs, service needs, and needs of medical men for skilled observation and nursing care on the part of the nursing staff whose patients are also the patients of the doctors.

(c) An arrangement of needs according to Bloom's taxonomy of educational objectives. He distinguishes: (a) *the cognitive domain,* which consists of knowledge to be acquired, comprehension of what has been learnt, application to the 'real-life' or practical situation, educated analysis of effects of action, discrimination, synthesis of all the foregoing so as to plan, re-organise, review, revise and reimplement as necessary, evaluation of outcomes for future action; (b) *the affective domain,* where the nursing student must be able to *receive* the message, signal or communication, to *respond* by taking intelligent action, *supporting* the person in need emotionally as well as physically, making thoughtful assessment and evaluation, reporting with insight and developing an appropriate system of values for the nursing subculture. It includes the solution of problems; and (c) *the psychomotor domain,* which pertains to the demonstration of motor skills, but interrelated with cognitive and affective aspects.

12.3.2 Required knowledge

Basic curricula based on broad objectives will have been laid down. In individual planning certain decisions will have to be made. These entail:

- Content of courses
- Depth of knowledge required
- Textbooks to be used
- Method of making courses relevant to the subject of man, his health needs and his human needs, so that all subjects have meaning for the student of nursing as part of the study of nursing
- Planned evaluation techniques
- Consultation and co-ordination with others in order that the knowledge required from students is clearly defined.

12.3.3 What curriculum planning should achieve

(a) A plan for a basic nursing education programme which provides a broad, solid but realistic foundation upon which the effective practice of nursing can be based, and which acts as a cornerstone for continuing post-registration, or advanced nursing education.
(b) An environment for learning and opportunity for student growth towards professional adulthood.
(c) The opportunity for students to achieve their maximum potential in the practice of the art and science of nursing.
(d) Stimulation and encouragement for the student to learn and grow in technical skills, sound nursing judgement and interpersonal relationships.
(e) An opportunity to acquire sufficient knowledge in
  - the natural and biological sciences, so that she can apply scientific principles to patient care;
  - the social sciences so that the patient is seen as a person with human needs, that he is recognised as a person coming from a family, from a specific strata of society and work environment, to which he will return. This will also help her to make personal social adjustments with others, and be able to build up good interpersonal relationships as well as communication skills.
(f) The chance to learn and become expert in skilled technical practices, applied with judgement and humanity.
(g) The development by the student of the ability to work as a competent nurse practitioner, with assurance and with due regard to the independent functions which are her responsibility.
(h) An integration of theory and practice into a unified whole.

There are many books available on curriculum planning. All that has been attempted here is to place it in perspective, and give guide-lines to those who have to undertake such an exercise for the first time.

12.4 EXPERIMENTAL COURSES

Experimental courses are those which are tried out on a group of students in order to find out whether they will work, whether they are an improvement on existing courses or whether they are worse than those already in practice.

There are a few important aspects which must not be forgotten:

(a) Students following the experimental course must in no way be penalised. They must be registered or licensed in exactly the same manner as are other students on successful completion of the course.

(b) The course must have official approval from the registering body.

(c) It must be carefully planned and implemented under strictly controlled conditions, with clearly defined regulations, curricula, criteria for admission, examinations, practica requirements and any other conditions.

(d) It must be planned for a specific purpose. A proliferation of experimental courses could lead to chaos.

Experimental courses have been planned and implemented in the United Kingdom with variable results. Some have led to basic changes in existing courses, others have not.

The closest South Africa has come to conducting experimental courses has been to introduce courses at provincial level, which were later taken over by the South African Nursing Council. A case in point was the introduction of a course for nursing auxiliaries for which provincial curricula, examinations and certificates were issued. These certificates were later recognised by the South African Nursing Council, which enrolled the holders as enrolled auxiliary nurses (later enrolled nurses) and controlled the training, examination and enrolment.

A similar situation has arisen with the short course for occupational health nurses which was run under the auspices of the South African Nursing Association. The South African Nursing Council has now promulgated regulations for this 'short course'.

Although the South African Nursing Council has changed its regulations pertaining to various courses quite drastically over the years, it has never to date actually run an experimental course of its own. There is nothing, however, that prevents it from doing so, should the members so decide. Britain, for example, has run shortened courses leading to registration. This has never been attempted here.

The purpose of including a short note on experimental courses in this chapter is simply to emphasise that no course can be run without some form or structure, and also require curriculum development. Thus rules and regulations have to be made and a *curriculum* has to be drawn up. That *planned programme of instruction* and *set of guide-lines* has to be there or the *course to be run* will have no validity.

Curriculum design is a difficult process, requiring experience and insight. The new tutor will need guide-lines and help even at the level of preparing her own work and dividing it into units, planning the methodology to be used, and directing her students through their learning experiences. Her colleagues and the head of her college should assist here.

Curriculum planning in clinical teaching is so new a concept that a great deal of assistance might be necessary in the early stages if effective curricula for clinical teaching were to be drawn up.

A curriculum is much more than a list of procedures to be carried out, or subjects to be covered. It needs thought, practice and skill. Detailed programming and clear explanation, including pilot studies, revision, the co-operation of all concerned, and making the programme known to all students involved, are essential.

Curriculum planning at higher levels demands experience, practice, insight, time and patience. Senior staff members need to develop these skills or they will fail in their task of providing effective nursing education, a task which, to say the least, is unenviable, but very necessary in order to keep the standard and the relevance of nursing care at the highest possible level.

13 *In-service education and continuing education*

As this book is directed at teaching the practice of nursing, and as such at the neophyte nurse-tutor, the subject will be dealt with mainly from that point of view. As Mellish's doctoral thesis dealt with in-service education, this chapter will be based largely on that work.

13.1 DEFINITION OF IN-SERVICE EDUCATION

- In-service education is education given to people while they are employed.
- In-service education is deliberately planned.
- In-service education is designed to meet specific needs, to fill gaps in learning or to remedy deficiencies in knowledge and skills of employees.
- In-service education aims at more efficient functioning on the part of the employee.
- In-service education aims at better functioning of the organisation.
- In-service education usually follows on a period of pre-service education.
- In-service education is only part of continuing education (Mellish 1978: 12).

Before discussing the value of in-service education for those preparing to teach the practice of nursing, the last concept, namely 'in-service education in only part of continuing education' demands more attention.

Continuing education in nursing, as in any other field, has a much wider meaning than does in-service education. Continuing education is an ongoing process which is not necessarily given to or followed by persons who are employed. Even though nurses are sent to undertake post-registration courses on a full-time basis and receive salaries if they are away for a period of time longer than that normally occupied by their annual leave, they are no longer in a 'working' situation, and therefore the course they take is continuing education, *not* in-service education.

There are many nurses working in fields outside nursing or for that matter not, at that stage, working at all, who do a great deal of professional reading, attend seminars, symposia, and the like. They are also engaged in continuing, but *not* in-service education.

13.2 WHO NEEDS IN-SERVICE EDUCATION?

The obvious answer is *everyone*, but let us not be too simplistic, and list those in nursing who require specific in-service education.

13.2.1 'Returning' nurses

Many nurses complete their formal education, work for a short time in their chosen field, and then marry. Some continue to nurse until the arrival of their first child, when they leave the profession. When the youngest child starts to attend school, many feel the need or desire to return to work. Some do so from financial necessity while others feel time hanging on their hands. These women would often like to return to their chosen profession, but are afraid of what they might find upon their return or of becoming obsolete and having lost their skill or competence.

A large amount of money goes into the preparation of the registered nurse. If these nurses do not return to nursing, but take up employment in other fields, then those resources are being squandered. Registered nurses, seeking employment after a break in their nursing career, fall into this category. They are often not utilised in spheres of work commensurate with their education.

No country can afford to waste its potential trained manpower in this way. The need for this category of workers to receive in-service education which would restore their original peak performance and confidence as rapidly as possible, is self-evident.

Other categories of nurses, apart from those who left to bring up families, such as divorcées, widows, or those who interrupted their careers to devote time to the care of for example a parent who subsequently died, are all potential 'returners'. In these days of shortages, properly planned, organised and advertised programmes for updating prospective 'returners' could help to alleviate some of the staff problems, and the 'returner' would quickly regain her competence and confidence.

13.2.2 Nurse-educators

Trained nurse-tutors should be better equipped than many other nurses to keep themselves up to date. In fact, they owe it to their students to do so. Nevertheless, the sheer pressure of coping with ever-changing classes in the 'block' system may leave them little time for personal reading and research. They need encouragement in the form of arranged in-service courses, and other in-service activities to stimulate their self-learning activities.

It is unfortunately true that professional nurse-tutors are to be found who all too frequently have used the same methods and presented the same material in the same manner for the past ten to 15 years. These professional nurse-tutors often stifle the enthusiasm and readiness for change that tutor training courses attempt to engender in their students. Recently qualified nurse-educators become disheartened and in their turn, stagnate.

Nurse-educators are not the only category of teacher that falls prey to this type of teaching practice, or rather, lack of activity. Teachers who should be at the vanguard initiating change are, all too often, those applying the brake on others who are trying to prepare the up-and-coming neophytes to deal with and prevent 'future shock'.

13.2.3 Nurses moving from one institution to another, or one field of nursing activity to another

These groups need orientation to their new spheres of activity. True, many will learn by 'experience', but again, can the country afford to use expensively trained and often highly paid personnel so uneconomically? Surely the sooner they are prepared to function to maximum capacity in the new work environment, the less the expense to the consumer, who in this case is the general public in need of health services. Why should people have to flounder around in their new work situation, trying to find out such things as what methods are employed to obtain supplies, how and by whom patients are transported to other departments, or what the lines of communication are in the hospital or agency, to quote but a few? An up-to-date manual and two or three days in an orientation programme would obviate all uncertainty and have them performing their nursing duties in the new situation quickly, efficiently and with confidence. This must lead to more efficient patient or client care, which is the aim of all health-care institutions and health-care personnel. It is also the desire of the consumer, that is the patient or potential patient, of the future.

The frequency of such programmes and their content would vary, but they should be ongoing programmes which are properly planned and co-ordinated.

13.2.4 Nurses who show signs of obsolescence or are in need of remedial training

These groups may be the most difficult to convince that they are in need of in-service education. It is often true that one is the last to recognise one's own inadequacies. These people will seldom seek in-service education of their own accord. Their needs will have to be recognised or elicited by other personnel, and programmes designed for them will need special planning and presentation. When persons who have been forced into such programmes come back 'asking for more', the in-service education programme has really taken off.

Other gauges of success will obviously be the increased efficiency in the performance of nursing duties, increased interest in new ideas and more smoothly flowing work with better interpersonal relationships, especially amongst and with the young and still enthusiastic students.

In classifying nurses into this category, it must be taken into account that many nurses are reluctant to break away from the established routine of 'having always done it like this' because of fear of failure, lack of confidence in their ability to tackle something new, a tendency to prejudge, self-satisfaction with their present performance, the inability to realise that improvements are necessary or even possible, and an inflexible attitude to life in general.

Special efforts will have to be made to reach these nurses, that is those who are obviously obsolescent or in need of remedial training because of a lower standard of performance, to attract them to in-service training, and to motivate them so that they are able to derive benefit from such programmes.

13.2.5 Special groups

These groups are in need of special courses to teach new techniques, to prepare for special assignments, or to fill in gaps in training. This type of in-service education is an absolute necessity if it is desired that the employee should function to maximum capacity.

In order to get a special job done, or to introduce new, and in these days always expensive equipment, or new sophisticated techniques, in-service training not only ensures optimum performance in a minimum time span, but also makes certain that the job is done properly, the expensive equipment used efficiently, or the sophisticated technique carried out competently. This not only leads to job satisfaction and gives confidence to workers because they feel adequate to deal with the new situation, but it prevents damage to equipment because of mishandling and obviates the breakdown in sophisticated techniques, such as reverse isolation or modern isolation techniques because of inadequate knowledge.

The groups identified above can, of course, be subdivided. Additions can no doubt be made. It must be emphasised that all nurses, at various times in the course of their nursing practice, from the recently qualified sister to the chief nursing officer, need in-service education of some sort. Many will realise their own needs and ensure that these needs are met, others will need pushing, prodding and forcing.

13.3 THE NURSE-EDUCATOR'S RESPONSIBILITY IN IN-SERVICE EDUCATION

Nurse-educators are so busy with basic nursing education that they have little time to consider in-service education as a separate entity. It is my premise that they have a threefold responsibility with regard to in-service education, which they cannot escape.

That is:

- Responsibility towards themselves and their students
- Responsibility towards those they have trained
- Responsibility towards the profession as a whole.

If one considers that the aim of nursing education is to prepare competent nursing practitioners to care for patients or clients efficiently and humanely, that underlying responsibility must not be forgotten.

13.3.1 Responsibility towards themselves and their students

No tutor who has completed a nursing education course and commences teaching can labour under the impression that she 'knows it all' and will never again have to study. She will be only too well aware that she has only scratched the surface.

The first difficult hurdle will be for her to assess what she has to teach her students. Many new tutors make the fatal mistake of thinking that students following basic courses must be given all the information which they themselves were given.

Once this has been resolved, tutors can become complacent and feel that much of what they had learned was wasted and they consequently lapse into a 'learning stagnation', which is equally wrong. For the benefit of themselves and their students, they must read constantly and keep abreast of new developments, or they may find themselves teaching material which, although at one time accepted as fact, has since been proved wrong, and new, more up-to-date, presently valid material is necessary.

How can tutors keep up to date, and keep their material relevant? Here are a few suggestions:

- By reading professional literature, especially professional journals, regularly and thoroughly
- By discussions with other tutors
- By frequent visits to the clinical areas and by discussions on new techniques with the unit professional nurses and the resident medical personnel
- By attending any medical lectures whether they are aimed at the general public or not
- By gaining access to medical meetings and discussion sessions
- By attending symposia whenever possible. These should include not only those on medical subjects, but on related social issues and on teaching techniques
- By being given at least a month a year to spend on self-study activity away from the class-room situation.

All this may sound ideal and impractical in the light of staff shortages, but if some sort of policy which will serve as a guide for the future is not laid down, we will never emerge from the crisis situation. Too many tutors become frustrated and move away from tutoring, and too many potential tutors who see the conditions under which our present tutors work, are lost to the ranks because they cannot see themselves functioning under such conditions.

The idea that a tutor must be in front of a class from eight to four, or that she must be on the college premises for eight hours a day, unless granted special permission for absence, else she is not 'working', is antiquated. The odd shirker will be quickly detected, and the freedom to work where and when you like, for preparation, marking and such activities, provided one is available for special periods for student consultation, makes for greater job satisfaction and often increased performance.

Financial provision for tutors to attend 'away' symposia should also be part of employment policy.

If a tutor keeps herself up to date and is encouraged to do so, then she meets her responsibilities towards herself and her students.

13.3.2 Responsibility towards those they have trained

It is very often the case that a course is completed, a lamp-lighting ceremony is held, speeches are made, and congratulations are the order of the day. Students then enter the ranks of registered nurses and the tutors, beyond a cursory glance at photographs on the wall, forget all about them.

Should it not be the stated policy of the school and of the tutors who were responsible for the education of the students, as well as the clinical teachers, to immediately follow up with an organised programme of continuing education on an in-service basis, so that student interest and enthusiasm are not lost after they have finished 'training', and that there is still some forum where problems can be discussed?

At this stage it is suggested that an in-service period be put aside for newly qualified professional nurses only, during working time, where discussions can take place with the people who trained them, where special points can be clarified, requests for special talks complied with, and where the 'new professional nurse' is given the opportunity to feel that she has not been deserted by those who trained her, and yet is given a chance to spread her wings.

It is not suggested that this be a formal teaching situation for giving students what should have been part of their basic course in any case, or a grouse and grumble session. It should provide security, continuity and a stimulus for new professional nurses to continue their education.

In this way too, tutors could become aware of the needs of students which should have been met, but for some reason were omitted; in this way future courses could be improved. Many new ideas could be discussed which could only improve training. A session of this sort could be held on a weekly or fortnightly basis for a period of six months, and be *compulsory* for all new diplomates, even from other hospitals. New diplomates would join as they complete their courses, so that it would be an ongoing programme. In this way the responsibility which those who teach have towards their students, could be met.

13.3.3 Responsibility towards the profession as a whole

While advocating that every hospital should have an in-service education department to meet the specific needs of its personnel and its service, it is suggested that the nursing colleges should play a far greater role in in-service education programmes. This is to be done not only by the participation of individual personnel, but also by the arranging of symposia, workshops and other techniques of presenting programmes on at least a yearly basis. This should stimulate interest and give practising nurses, at least from the hospitals they serve, an opportunity to attend short courses, symposia of particular interest and workshops. This is a responsibility that those with the know-how of organising programmes, with contacts with knowledgeable speakers, and with the opportunities for determining specific needs, have towards the nurses of the country.

Two or three universities have started such departments of continuing education, and are very active in the field, and some branches of the South African Nursing Association have at various times organised such programmes. Nursing colleges as such have done little.

Again, it is well known that there is a shortage of tutors, and that these programmes would seem to place an added burden on them, but the enthusiasm that can be generated and the benefit that all can derive from participation might result in tutors remaining in teaching and encourage others to join the ranks.

It is the responsibility of the employer to

- provide in-service programmes to meet the needs of employees;
- make it possible for employees to attend courses at their own institutions as well as those offered by others;
- set up in-service education departments in the health-care institutions;
- support part-time programmes so that the personnel can benefit and be given consideration in terms of time off to attend regular short courses (or even in the wider field of continuing education courses leading to the acquisition of additional qualifications).

Thus they may meet their obligations to provide quality patient care by in-

271

vesting time, money and personnel in keeping employees up to date, competent in all new fields of medical care, and capable of giving modern, efficient health care to all persons in need of such care.

13.4 BROAD BASIS FOR IN-SERVICE EDUCATION

Any form of in-service education should be based on the following:

- Determination of learning needs
- Planning of learning experiences to meet the assessed needs
- Division of learning experiences into units
- Setting objectives to be met
- Survey of available resources
- Provision of facilities including a budget for courses
- Choice of participants
- Selection of personnel to provide programmes
- Methodology to be employed
- Detailed planning of individual course
- Announcement/advertising course
- Record-keeping
- Evaluation.

Much has already been written on in-service education. The student tutor with a special interest in the subject is referred to such literature for further study.

At present it is, unfortunately, approached on a haphazard basis. Perhaps the 'new tutors' of the future and nurse-administrators in general will soon realise its importance, and get down to tackling it in an organised manner. Proper in-service education could do much to improve job satisfaction and keep in the profession many who might otherwise be lost.

14 Administration and control of nursing colleges and schools: Aspects of inspection

14.1 ADMINISTRATION

Basic principles of administration

In order to understand and to be able to apply the basic principles of administration in the college or nursing school situation, it is necessary to define administration and clarify some of the concepts involved. Before studying the administration of a nursing school in detail, therefore, the fundamental principles of administration will be discussed.

Administration is derived from the Latin *ad* = to and *ministrare* = to serve. Thus administration 'provides service to'. It is a process which in the case of nursing school administration enables *nursing education to be undertaken*. In this particular context, it is the service rendered to students (or pupils), to colleagues, and to employing authorities to enable students (or pupils) to be educated and prepared for professional practice.

Nursing college administration can also be seen as a collection of activities which are carried out when two or more people work together, in order that the service of providing nursing education may be achieved, which will eventually produce efficient nurse practitioners, capable of managing their independent functions in a responsible and humanitarian manner (the objective).

14.1.1 Principles, processes and effects

Henri Fayol, one of the early writers on administration, defined three principles of administration, each of which had a *process* (that which had to be done), and an *effect* (the end result).

A principle may be seen as a fundamental or primary element – a starting point, something from which a start can be made, in some cases also described as a fundamental truth. A process is a sequence of events or actions, that is what is done, and an action is the effect of the sequence of events or the action taken.

In order to understand these so that they can be applied to the administration of a nursing college or school, each principle, its process and effect will be dealt with separately.

PRINCIPLE (primary element)	PROCESS (what occurs)	EFFECT (end result)
Investigation	Forecasting (prediction)	Planning
Reality	Organisation	Co-ordination
Order	Command	Control

14.1.1.1 The principle of investigation

This is the basis upon which all administration rests. To 'investigate', to 'examine' or 'enquire' into, is derived from the Latin *in* = into and *vestigare* = to track. Therefore research is also investigation, or enquiry into, and is not something outside medical or nursing administration.

The need to apply the principle of investigation before any action is taken is important to any form of administration and nursing school administration is no exception.

Decision making, which forms a major part of the work of those to whom the administration of a training school is entrusted, must be made on a sound basis and not on 'intuition', 'feeling', or other emotional grounds. Sometimes the *process* of forecasting or predicting which follows on the investigation may, because of the nature of the work and the urgency of the situation, be very rapid indeed, but at other times it may involve long and careful enquiry into all the circumstances before planning can be done to solve the problem or to institute a new method of work, to reorganise the teaching methodology, or to initiate another system.

A quick *investigation* in a nursing college may be undertaken simply to find out why class members arrived late, the result of which may show that a meal was not served on time, and the matter can then be dealt with and plans made to prevent its re-occurrence. Nevertheless all the steps following on the *investigation* have been taken. An investigation into staff grievances, student wastage, failure rates, reasons for staff resignations and failure of nurses to come forward to train as tutors, may take many weeks before forecasting and planning can follow.

Having decided that the principle of investigation on which all good administration rests, must be applied, the *sequence of events* or process is followed, so that the end effect, which is planning to deal with the case, can occur.

Let us consider the sequence of events. A problem must be *investigated*. This need not necessarily be a problem in the sense of an unpleasant or unfortunate occurrence, but can be something in the nature of the establishment of a new nursing school, or the introduction of a new course at an existing school.

Forecasting must be done as to the reason for the occurrence of the problem or the argument for or against a new school. *Planning* must then occur to meet the needs identified or to arrive at a solution to the problem. In order to follow this logical sequence, *facts* must be sought. A very useful aid to the investigation or the procuring of facts in a daily administrative situation is the use of Rudyard Kipling's 'Six honest serving men':

> I kept six honest serving men
> They taught me all I know
> Their names are WHAT and WHY and WHEN
> and WHO and WHERE and HOW.

The use of these six 'gentlemen' as part of the process of investigation can be easily understood if illustrated by the following example in the nursing school context.

Problem: Examination results have shown a distinct decline during the past year.

The following questions arise:

WHAT results?
To WHAT extent have results declined?
WHAT staff changes have occurred?
WHAT is the academic standard, that is matriculation symbols and subjects?
WHAT correlation is there between examination results, college examination results and practica reports?
WHY has the decline occurred? Is it a result of, for example:

- Less study time?
- New methods of teaching?
- Student dissatisfaction?
- Too large classes?
- Excessive work pressure?

WHEN did the decline commence:

- After staff changes?
- After shortages in teaching and ward personnel?
- After student unrest?
- After changes in teaching strategies?
- After changes in the examination system?

WHO is failing, or performing poorly – is it those with poor potential anyway?

WHO is doing the teaching? For example, if a student's examination results decline despite his being taught by tutors who normally have good results, the probable cause might well be elsewhere.

WHERE did the decline occur?

- In all groups
- In groups at specific times of the year
- In specific subjects only.

HOW?

- By outright failure
- By failure in some subjects
- By fewer distinctions.

HOW many times did the same students fail?

(This is simply a brief outline of how facts can be assembled in an orderly manner.)

Having assembled all the facts they must now be studied, analysed and decisions made to deal with the situation. Immediate plans must be made as well as those which will prevent future problems. The administrator must be able to *think*, to *learn* and to *plan*. It should be fundamental to all administrative practice that *investigation of all facets* of a situation be undertaken before decisions are made. The decisions must not be hasty, but based on carefully assembled and analysed facts.

14.1.1.2 The reality principle

If investigation is the foundation of good administration, then the *principle of reality* forms the bricks and mortar with which it is built.

In administration it is absolutely essential to be *realistic*. No amount of idealistic planning can be implemented, no matter how desirable it may be, if the means of putting it into practice do not exist. If investigation is properly undertaken, all factors such as human and material resources including available finance, would have been identified and thus planning would be based on realism. Nevertheless, identified needs may have so overwhelmed the forecasters that planning may not have been realistic, and therefore the next principle of Fayol, namely that of reality, puts things into perspective. This does not mean that more and better resources should not be sought for the future or that long-term planning should be neglected, but simply that plans for the present must be tempered by what is available, and that long-term planning must be continued. A building selected for use as a college may not be ideal, but adaptations could be made and a school started, while future planning for new buildings and equipment proceeds. It is amazing what can be achieved with the resources available, and a new school which has just been started and which proves its reason for existence, can look forward to the provision of more resources and facilities as time and realistic planning permit.

If approached from the angle of reality, the process of *organisation* can make the best use of the available facilities, so that the effect of *co-ordination* of available resources could be achieved.

If the training or education of nurses it to be continued so that patient care can also be given on a continuous basis, then action must be taken. Sitting back with folded hands because there is too little money, too few staff or too little equipment, achieves nothing but frustration. Nurses should be resourceful people who will make the best of any situation, while constantly planning for improvement. Ill-health will increase and not decrease if the population as a whole suffers from financial difficulties. A community can only have the health services it can afford. If lack of finance makes it difficult for trained manpower to be produced, the health of the community will only deteriorate.

Lack of trained nurse–power demands *realistic* planning, even though this will limit the services which can be provided. Reality also dictates that training opportunities be *organised* to make optimum use of what is available. *Co-ordination* must take place, so that resources are pooled and the nurse–power situation improved. Reality also dictates that enough nurses of the various categories be trained to meet the existing needs and that the *organisation* of their training be founded on *investigation*. Is it economical to have a multiplicity of small training schools, even when the student nurses attend the same college, or would it better meet the needs of the community to train *more* enrolled nurses locally at the smaller schools, and concentrate on training for registration at larger centres? Does not the reality principle also suggest that small classes of one language group be accommodated in larger groups, and that not every college always strive to keep both language media going, which is certainly not a realistic use of nurse–tutor power?

14.1.1.3 The principle of order

Order must be obtained and maintained among both human and material resources, or nothing will come of the preceding principles, their processes and effects.

In order to maintain an orderly sequence of events, authority is needed. Thus in the process of achieving order, authority is used, not only in the sense of giving orders to personnel, but also in that there must be an authoritative body in *control*, the ultimate effect in the administrative process being control. This is easy enough to understand in the administration of a nursing school.

The overriding authority which is legally responsible for nursing education in South Africa is the South African Nursing Council. It is a statutory body and lays down regulations, prescribes curricula, training regulations, fees to be paid, examinations, practica and requirements for admission to the courses and those for registration or enrolment. It prescribes the conditions for recognition of training schools. With the new comprehensive course, it recognises training schools and nursing colleges in association with universities, and approves curricula and examinations held by these institutions, while having the right of inspection. It also has disciplinary powers. In fact, it governs the practice of nursing.

The next authority to be considered is that providing the facilities for nursing education to be carried out. This is in the main still in the hands of the provincial authorities, who provide colleges or schools, personnel, facilities, training posts for students, practical experience and the finance needed. The legal aspects of this financial provision were discussed in chapter 4, and will not be repeated here. Suffice it to say that the provinces are chiefly responsible at an overall level for the provision of nursing education. Private institutions are becoming involved in nurse education and, of course, many organisations are involved in the training of nursing assistants.

The process whereby they exercise *order* is through a system of *command,* a form of power delegated to officials at the nurse-training establishments, and a comprehensive system of control in the form of record-keeping, report back and inspection.

The third principle of order is implemented by appointing persons to positions of *command,* in other words creating posts for the purpose of running colleges and schools, with clearly defined methods of control, so that the work actually done can be checked and the required record-keeping used not only as a control measure at local or even provincial level, but also for future *investigation,* forecasting, planning based on reality with its organisation and co-ordination aspects, and leading to order through command and control.

14.1.2 Generic processes

Administration can also be discussed in terms of six generic processes (generic = characteristic of, and process = sequence of events or actions).

Thus, the six aspects or characteristics of a sequence of events or actions, which is administration, may be identified as follows:
(a) The process of *policy making,* which leads to planning and programming
(b) The process of *financing* in order to obtain money to pay for resources and actions required by policy

(c) The process of *organisation* to provide those who are to carry out the action which was planned under policy making, with what is required to attain the stated objectives

(d) The process of *providing and utilising personnel* so that institutions or organisations charged with carrying out the policy are provided with enough suitably qualified staff, who then perform the actions needed in order to attain the objective

(e) The process of *determining work procedures* so that members of the team charged with policy implementation can work together in an orderly, constructive manner

(f) The process of *control*: All work must be controlled so that it can be ascertained whether pre-determined goals have been attained. Control has two dimensions, namely that of checking to see that work is performed safely within the specifications of the policy, and that of rendering account of what has been performed.

These six generic processes will be discussed in some detail in their relation to the administration of the nursing college or school situation.

14.1.2.1 Policy making

As has already been said, a great deal of policy making in nursing education is done by:

- The South African Nursing Council
- The authority in charge of the provision of nursing education
- The local body providing the education.

14.1.2.1.1 *The South African Nursing Council*

The Council is comprised of 30 persons of whom 17 *must* be registered nurses, while seven more *may* be registered nurses. It is furthermore laid down that the president and vice-president shall be nurses. Thus the basic policy making, at the Council level, is in the hands of nurses.

The executive committee of the Council consists of the president, and the vice-president (both nurses); the treasurer; one member who is an officer of the Department of Health, Welfare and Population Development, who is a medical practioner *or* registered nurse; one member who is a lay person; and the director of hospital services of the province concerned, or a person in the employ of the province, who is a medical practitioner *or* a registered nurse; and other members as the Council may determine. This means that there must be two nurses on the executive committee, while there could be at least five. This could present problems, except that the executive committee has no power to set aside or amend any decision of the Council. Any act performed by, or decision taken by the executive committee shall be in effect and in force *unless it is set aside* or amended by the Council at its next ensuing meeting.

As far as the policy-making powers of the Council are concerned, it is empowered by the Nursing Act, 1978 (Act 50 of 1978) to

- keep registers and rolls according to the criteria established by it;
- register or remove persons from the register or rolls according to its prescriptions;
- draw up and promulgate training regulations;
- inspect training schools;
- approve training schools;
- conduct examinations;
- register additional qualifications;
- draw up regulations regarding the scope or practice of registered or enrolled nurses, and the conditions under which they may carry on their profession for promulgation. The Minister may promulgate the control which shall be exercised by specified officers of the Department of Health, Welfare and Population Development or local authorities over the practice of enrolled nurses, and the inspections which shall be carried out in connection with enrolled midwives.

The powers of the South African Nursing Council are therefore quite extensive, but are subject to the approval of the Minister and must be carried out in accordance with the Act.

14.1.2.1.2 *The authority in charge of the provision of nursing education*

The provinces which, at present provide the bulk of nursing education, have to function within their powers and in accordance with their ordinances. They are nevertheless responsible for the following types of policy making:

- Siting of training schools
- Decision on types of training to be offered
- Facilities and resources, both human and material, to be supplied, and budgeting
- Inspection of their own training schools
- General standardised form of overall record-keeping
- Periodic feedback from training schools
- Training of teaching personnel
- Criteria for the selection of post-basic students; recruitment and motivation
- In-service opportunities and programmes to be provided for personnel

- Policy regarding language media to be used
- Recruitment of students for all schools.

14.1.2.1.3 The local body actually providing the education

Here we get down to the nitty gritty of running the training school. Policy making, although much has been done and imposed by higher authorities, can still be altered if enough time, thought, and motivation are given to aspects laid down by the higher authority which do not appear to meet local needs or which cannot be complied with in the local situation.

Apart from this policy making by higher authorities, every local situation needs policy decisions which are peculiar to it. These pertain to (a) block periods, or other systems of nursing education; and (b) time allocated for block periods, study days, etc. The following aspects will receive attention in this respect:

- *Who* teaches *what*, *when* and *how* – in other words a policy regarding team teaching, subject teaching, the whole syllabus for a block system of teaching, the use of outside lecturers and their availability. Hours allocated to study periods, self-activity, projects and the like
- Compulsory study periods
- The use of notes instead of textbooks
- Policy regarding the use of films
- Safekeeping of audio-visual apparatus and materials
- Making and storing of slide collections, etc.
- Timetables, and who is responsible for their compilation
- Availability of library facilities and other learning aids; times open, etc; control measures
- Learning resource centres and their staffing
- Duration of lecture periods/formal teaching sessions
- System of record-keeping, such as lecture records, class attendance, etc.
- Breaks during the day
- Recreation facilities and encouragement to use them
- Projects, assignments, workbooks.

All these and more are part of local policy making which require attention. They are also interwoven with organisation.

14.1.2.2 Finance

Nursing education is financed by the taxpayer via provincial and state budgets. Beyond supplying motivation for specific needs and application to the relevant authorities, there is little that can be done at local level to provide for a large capital outlay.

Nevertheless, each school of nursing should draw up its own budget to meet its own needs. This should not be the exclusive task of the administrative officer, but should also involve the principal of the college, or the person in charge of the training school, and at lower levels the tutors, who may desperately need new equipment or facilities, but who are seldom consulted. It should be policy that each tutor keep a list, during the year, of *urgent requirements* or replacements for equipment which she has been unable to obtain. Date, time, reason for request and disadvantages of not having received them should also be specified. When the time for drawing up the budget draws near, the principal of the college then collects and collates this information, and uses it to good effect in budgeting expenses for the next year.

Another aspect of finance which must receive attention, is that it is the responsibility of every staff member of a college to use materials and equipment effectively but economically. A tutor is just as accountable to the public for wasting its money by negligence and extravagance as is anyone else. Expensive equipment that is never used is also a waste of public monies for which one can be held accountable.

A third aspect of finance, which often escapes the tutor's attention (although in these days of shortages it is difficult to imagine), is that it is a part of the professional responsibility of every registered nurse, tutor or otherwise, to ensure that she herself renders a full day's work for a full day's pay, and *that her students do the same*. It is all very well to continually cry out for better salaries (which, in the case of students is actually a *training* allowance), but these must be earned. As said previously, a student spends only 23 out of 36 months in actual clinical practice. If she is to *earn that training allowance, the block time or study time must be fully utilised for study*. She is receiving and hopefully earning full 'pay' for the 23 months spent in the ward. Thus 64% of her salary can be regarded as pay for services rendered, but the ten months study time (or 28% of the time not used constructively for learning), is *not earned*.

The 8% left over is payment for leave due. Students who did not study enough and failed because of lack of application would not appreciate it if 28% of their training allowance were to be subtracted because of poor performance. This would of course penalise the hard worker who is a slow learner, and its practicality is therefore doubtful. The time has come for all students to pay towards their training. Perhaps then the squandering of taxpayers' money, which some students make a practice of doing, would be limited. Wasting one's own money is more acceptable than wasting that of others.

14.1.2.3 Organisation

The process of organisation is perhaps the most readily understood of the generic processes. Policy has been laid down, funds have been allocated, and now the work of running the college has to proceed within the limits imposed by policy and the budget. In order to achieve this level of organisation, *this giving of orderly structure to or making arrangements for the undertaking of an operation,* it is necessary to identify the component but interdependent parts of various tasks which need to be performed in a college or nursing school, in order for nursing education to proceed smoothly. In the analysis of the nursing college activities as such, sight must not be lost of the part of nursing education that takes place in the clinical field. In the initial planning and analysis stage, all those concerned with the education of the nurse must be fully involved, for nursing education cannot be planned in compartments but must be planned in its totality, and consultation must be continuous.

Organisation in the college itself will have to be planned. Not only must the work of educating the nurse be organised, but the available physical and material resources must be stored and controlled in an orderly manner so that they are easily accessible when and where needed.

Division of labour is part of organisation, as is delegation, co-ordination and communication. Organisation of all the multiplicity of activities that occur in a nursing college is essential to the effective functioning of the college.

The college principal is the co-ordinator of all the activities, but teamwork, an understanding of requirements, and communication amongst personnel, both nursing and non-nursing, are vital. Organisation is not merely the compilation of neat charts and diagrams showing *who* should do *what,* although this is part of it. It entails ensuring that *who* does *what* and also at least *how* and *when.* A nursing school will only function as effectively as its organisation allows.

In planning the organisation of a nursing college or school, the following aspects are essential:

- Courses offered, and their organisation
- Numbers of students to be catered for
- Regulations regarding courses
- System of nursing education used
- Curriculum
- Teaching methodology
- Outside educational facilities for fieldwork, etc.
- Facilities available

  - Personnel, nursing (tutors) and clerical
  - Class-rooms and other study accommodation
  - Office and teaching space as well as for clerical staff
  - Library
  - Other resources

- Record-keeping system including those required by registering authorities
- Evaluation procedures
- Timetables
- A chart showing lines of communication, delegation of work and authority. Responsibility and authority given to each member of the teaching staff, etc.
- System of running the residence
- Housekeeping and other 'hotel' services, staff and their responsibilities.

All this organisation will have to conform to the policy laid down by the overall or employing authority.

14.1.2.4 Provision and utilisation of personnel

Personnel for the teaching of students is again provided for by higher authority. The posts are there, but unfortunately they are not always filled. The reason for shortages and for resignations by tutors is important, but will not be discussed here. Availability of posts is one thing but filling and keeping them filled by utilising personnel so that they obtain job satisfaction is another. Many tutors are driven from teaching by unsatisfactory work conditions, by unsympathetic and even 'dictatorial' attitudes of seniors, by being forced to teach subjects in which they have little interest, not because there is no one else willing to do this, but by sheer lack of effective personnel management.

Effective personnel management, excellent interpersonal relationships maintained by those at the head of institutions, guidance and encouragement for new and inexperienced tutors and the creation of an atmosphere of trust, are essential. Delegation of responsibility must be coupled with appropriate authority. Fairness and impartiality coupled with praise when it is due, and correction of faults with sympathy and an attitude of helpfulness rather than condemnation, are required. A principal must have the intellectual honesty to recognise her own limitations, and the capacity to remedy shortcomings. She must also have the ability to encourage teamwork and motivate personnel to give of their best at all times.

In personnel management the following aspects need to be considered:

- The qualifications of teaching personnel, for example, post-registration qualifications apart from those of tutors
- The special teaching interests of teaching personnel
- The special abilities or talents of teaching personnel
- The workload of various members of teaching, administrative, counselling, and preparing staff

- Personnel policies pertaining to leave, sick leave, study leave, leave to attend 'study days', etc
- The type of schedule planned – does it provide for late sessions or even evening classes?
- Opportunities for further study
- Encouragement for further study
- In-service education for teaching personnel
- Clerical help available and use to be made of them by teaching staff
- Non-nursing personnel available for non-teaching tasks, such as maintenance of the library, supervision of student residence, health care of students
- Provision of opportunity for student counselling
- Encouragement to try out new teaching methods.

Careful attention to all the factors, which have only been outlined here, can make the utilisation of personnel far more effective. Choose the most qualified person for the job that needs to be done.

If there is a shortage of posts, then the usual procedure of appealing to the higher authority and presenting convincing, well-researched data is the method of choice.

14.1.2.5 Determination of work procedures

This generic process is less easy to apply in the administration of the teaching section of a nursing school, for many teachers find that methods which suit one person, are completely useless to them. Individuals differ, and so do groups of students, but in the administration of a nursing college as such, certain work procedures will have to be laid down and followed.

These include the following:

- Compliance with South African Nursing Council regulations
- Effective record-keeping
- Methods of ordering, obtaining and safekeeping equipment and using stock
- Budgeting and remaining within the budget
- Maintenance of buildings, grounds, etc.
- Providing accommodation
- Supervision
- Methods of dealing with complaints.

Planning must be such that any work procedure, such as the standardisation of a technical procedure in the clinical field, can be worked out, made known and included in the teaching programme.

14.1.2.6 Control

This process of administration is readily understood by nurses. It is part of their accepted work to supervise others, to check prescriptions, treatments, the administration and control of drugs, to control work schedules and chart treatments, and make controlled observation on a continuous basis, so that the matter of transferring this exercise of control to nursing education, and to the administration of a nursing school, is quite straightforward.

Nursing is a profession that demands control of or by others as well as self-control. Nursing education and the administration of a nursing college, where students are prepared to take responsibility for the lives of others, demand far more control than does a profession in the liberal arts. As nursing is concerned with the care of man, *control in nursing education* is and must be *compulsory*.

All student tutors should compile a file which includes copies of regulations relating to:

- The Nursing Act
- The election of the South African Nursing Council
- Distinguishing devices
- Conduct of registered nurses and midwives and all enrolled persons
- Registration of students and enrolment of pupils
- All types of training, basic and post-basic and relevant directives
- Inspections
- Enquiries
- Nursing agencies.

14.2 SPECIFIC DUTIES

14.2.1 The principal in charge of the college

Her responsibilities include the following:

(a) Organisation of her department and co-operation with those who are in charge of the services at her disposal such as stores, maintenance, engineering, cleansing, linen, pharmaceutical and dietary departments
(b) Student welfare especially while attending college
(c) Recruitment in co-operation with the nursing service managers of hospitals
(d) Student allocation in co-operation with the service departments to ensure that educational and service needs are correlated as much as possible and that blocks/study days are jointly planned

(e) Planning of the entire educational programme of the students, again in co-operation with the service department to ensure that the requirements of the South African Nursing Council are met with regard to lecture periods and subjects, presentation of curriculum, as well as aspects such as practica, internal examining, entrance to examinations and registration as students within the prescribed time

(f) Optimum use must be made of the available physical facilities

(g) Allocation of teaching personnel, making optimum use of special talents

(h) For maintenance of equipment and for prevention of loss by the introduction of reasonable control measures

(i) Drawing up job descriptions for each category of worker that falls under her jurisdiction, and introducing sufficient flexibility in the form of a duty schedule so that one person (eg tutor) could help another who is overloaded with work, or falls ill. The danger of overly rigid job descriptions is that people may tend to stick only to what is written, and regard other work as 'not my job'.

Housekeeping and clerical staff must not be forgotten. Refusal or unwillingness to undertake a task because it is not included in the job description must be prevented at all costs

(j) Ensuring that the service department is kept up to date with the curriculum followed in the school, and that any changes are immediately discussed and made known. All unit professional nurses should have, at all times, a short summary of what students are taught in each study unit

(k) Record-keeping: The principal must ensure that each student's record is kept completely up to date at all times, and that copies are kept in different places in case of fire, etc. The records must supply all the information required for completion of South African Nursing Council training forms, as well as be able to supply confidential reports when requested to do so

(l) Timetable planning: Although this can be entrusted to others, the final responsibility is hers

(m) Appointment of part-time lecturers in accordance with employing authority practice

(n) Arrangement of internal examinations as required

(o) Ensuring that students are prepared for external examinations in good time

(p) Guidance to tutors, teaching professional nurses and students

(q) Reporting to service departments regarding student progress

(r) Keeping educational objectives of the college constantly in mind

(s) Promoting the image of the college and training school at all times.

14.2.2 The individual tutor

Her responsibilities include:
(a) Keeping up to date by reading, paying frequent visits to wards and units, post-basic part-time study, etc
(b) Counselling students, especially those with learning problems
(c) Counselling students with personal problems
(d) Preparation of lectures, etc
(e) Being creative in her teaching presentation
(f) Keeping lecture records
(g) Ensuring that the material presented is at least sufficient for the average student to be able to pass her examinations
(h) Reporting on student progress to the principal, etc
(i) Maintaining discipline with justice and understanding in class
(j) Setting and marking tests and examinations as required
(k) Maintaining good interpersonal relationships
(l) Participation in group activities, such as timetable planning, course planning, project work, workshops, etc.

14.2.3 The nurse-administrator responsible for clinical practica

Her responsibilities include:

(a) Close liaison with the college to be able to correlate theory with practica in so far as this is possible
(b) Allocation of students to units keeping in mind the students' *educational needs* and not sacrificing these to service needs
(c) Allocation of non-nursing duties to other categories of workers and ensuring that this policy is carried out
(d) Planning a clinical teaching programme in consultation with the college and making maximum use of registered personnel in the wards
(e) Training clinical teachers for their functions
(f) Arranging a system of interviews, consultation hours, or other appropriate ways in which close liaison can be kept with students and clinical personnel
(g) Compliance with South African Nursing Council regulations regarding student practica
(h) Ensuring awareness of nursing personnel of South African Nursing Council instructions regarding the *purpose of the course,* and the *guide to each course,* so that all registered nurses realise their professional responsibility regarding student education, as well as to their own practice
(i) Ensuring proper record-keeping.

14.3 THE ESTABLISHMENT OF A NEW NURSING SCHOOL

Before a new school can be established and administered, there are certain processes which must be worked through. 'Let us build a hospital' is often the cry in smaller areas where the establishment of such an undertaking carries a great deal of prestige. Yet another frequent cry is 'let us start a training school'. It is therefore necessary that the whole exercise be approached and measured against well–thought–out criteria, which have stood the test of time. These are:

(a) The size of the community.

(b) The distance from other hospitals: With helicopter transport available to-day, distances have shrunk. Thus the building of a new hospital, let alone the planning of a training school is in many cases neither feasible nor necessary.

(c) The health needs of a community: A rapidly growing industrial area will have greater need of a hospital than a small rural community which is more or less static, and the idea of a training school would be viable as well as necessary in such an expanding community.

(d) The health service personnel available in the community: A hospital without trained nursing, medical and paramedical staff cannot offer training. Training for enrolled nurses may be possible if there are enough registered nurses of the right calibre to provide this training, but that is all. If there is no hospital, then training is out of the question, and the siting of such a new hospital might be quite impractical for other reasons as well.

(e) The availability of existing training schools in the vicinity: To be effective, training should surely be concentrated in areas where facilities are already established and tutors at least, exist, rather than dissipating resources unnecessarily by starting new schools.

(f) Sufficient young people with the required educational background from whom to draw potential students.

(g) Finance available: Training schools, especially their registration, are costly.

(h) Social and cultural factors, such as whether it is culturally acceptable for young women to leave home and be educated for an independent professional existence. Do cultural differences prevent different ethnic groups from working and studying together harmoniously?

(i) The effect that beliefs, customs and traditional health practices may have on potential students. These last two may appear strange to many, but we live in a multinational society where many Western health practices are not acceptable to large numbers of people, which can cause problems when trying to establish a new training school.

(j) Are sciences and mathematics which are basic to nursing study, offered by schools in the area, and do enough schools exist which will provide girls with the high school education necessary to undertake diploma courses?

It is suggested that those who are interested in more detailed aspects of nursing school planning, especially in the rural areas and in neighbouring states, consult Lyman (1961). It will give those who are concerned with any form of nursing school planning, beyond that in sophisticated Western areas, much food for thought and will also be of value to other student tutors.

14.4 ASPECTS OF INSPECTION

It has been stated that various bodies or persons are responsible for the inspection of schools of nursing, but how, when, why, what and by whom must inspections be done?

Inspection (according to *The Concise Oxford Dictionary*) means to 'look closely into', to 'examine officially'. Thus in undertaking an inspection, the salient aspects are *close scrutiny* that is *official*.

Nursing school inspection can be done at three levels:

(a) The national level when it is carried out by the South African Nursing Council
(b) The regional level when it is carried out by the authority responsible for the education of the nurse, that is the province or state health department (the financing authority)
(c) The local level where the principal of the college and/or the person in charge of the training school carries out periodic inspection of the department/s concerned.

How is the training school inspection to be undertaken?

14.4.1 At national level

(a) The South African Nursing Council has a policy of inspecting training schools at three-yearly intervals.
(b) The planned inspection tour is designed some time beforehand, and the schools to be inspected are notified in good time.
(c) A member of the Council or in rare cases, someone designated by the Council for the purpose, usually accompanied by a member of the registrar's staff or even the registrar himself, carries out the physical inspection.

290

(d) A detailed form requesting information regarding the training school is sent out some months before an inspection, and is returned to the South African Nursing Council. Details required include:

- Teaching staff and qualifications
- Organisation of the department concerned, including liaison with those in charge of clinical practica and other departments
- Courses and numbers of students following courses
- Subjects offered
- Class-room facilities
- Daily occupied beds in various specified departments
- Operations
- Out-patient attendance
- Casualty attendance
- Number of approved posts
- Number of posts filled
- Number of registered nurses who participate in the training and supervision of students
- Midwifery beds
- Number of deliveries (in midwifery schools)
- Psychiatric clinical facilities (specified in categories) (if applicable)
- Number of registered psychiatric nurses who participate in the teaching and supervision of students.

The following will also be subject to inspection:

(a) *Preventive and promotive health practica*
  - Facilities
  - Who supervises this practica?
  - Number of hours of practica

(b) *Clinical instruction*
  - Arrangements for teaching and supervision in clinical and other practical areas
  - Do final-year students get an opportunity to take charge of a ward?

(c) *Policy with regard to night duty*

(d) *Policy in respect of leave*
  - Sick leave
  - Vacation leave

(e) *System of promotion*

(f) *System of record-keeping*
  - Detailed breakdown of subjects

- Number of lectures and the qualifications of those presenting the subject
- Total hours of lecture and clinical instruction
- Distribution of clinical practia

(g) Where are *post-registration courses* offered?

Similar details are required for each course. The financing authority is always notified of impending inspections and they can delegate someone to accompany the Council inspectors, should they so wish.

It must be remembered that the inspection of training schools is to ensure that the regulations regarding the various courses offered are being met and to inspect *nursing education,* and not the administration of the hospital as such, except where it affects training.

Any deficiencies in training are pointed out to the hospital/training school being inspected, and a detailed report of the inspection of each school is sent to the Council. These reports are circulated to Council members and all matters requiring attention or arising from the report can be dealt with at meetings of the executive committee or of the Council itself.

Serious deficiencies are pointed out in writing and the school has to report on steps taken to remedy the deficiency within a specified period of time. In some cases, the Council can re-inspect the school if it appears to be necessary.

It must be pointed out that the South African Nursing Council has no legal jurisdiction over the running of training schools, beyond approving recognition of training. In very serious cases approval of training can be withdrawn. However, the Council only does this when there is no alternative.

Council inspections cover:

- Inspection of teaching facilities
- Inspection of clinical facilities both in the hospital and in the community
- The organisation of the system of education, that is block or study periods, timetables, day and night duty
- Record-keeping
- Assessment strategies
- Student allocation
- Leadership roles
- Qualifications of teaching personnel
- In-service education
- Availability of clerical and other personnel to avoid the use of nurses for non-nursing duties
- Implementation of teaching programmes in accordance with the South African Nursing Council regulations, guides and directives.

292

14.4.2 At regional level

Inspectresses are appointed by the financing authority to carry out inspections of their own training schools to ensure that training is being done according to the regulations. This is, however, a more personal approach. Regional inspections should be carried out at least yearly, according to a planned programme. Because more time is, or should be available, the programmes can be examined in more detail and deficiencies attended to on the spot or taken up at head office for urgent attention.

Inspection, that is examining closely and officially, must not be seen as a 'spying' activity, but as a teaching/learning situation where a good deal of counselling can take place.

As national and regional inspections have so much in common, a list of important points to be *looked at closely* could be given. A form or checklist could be drawn up so that no factor needing attention is forgotten. These forms will vary from one organisation to the next. Their compilation should be undertaken by a committee although it is hoped that the result will be something better than the muddle or 'hotch-potch' that a camel symbolises! Regular meetings, pilot studies and the application of the basic principle of *reality* should make it possible to draw up a satisfactory form which will ensure that all important factors are looked at but which will be simple to complete and will not require constant rewriting or hours of extra work. Frequent review to see whether the form is serving its purpose, which is to identify problem areas quickly so that remedial action can be taken as well as to ensure thorough inspection, is also necessary. The form must make provision for the following important information:

- Name of centre
- Date visited
- Length of visit
- Daily bed occupancy
- Does clinical material meet the educational needs of students and programmes?
- Number of operations and types
- Theatre record-keeping with its special needs and hazards
- Number of deliveries (in midwifery schools)
- Approved posts of various categories
- Filled posts and by what categories: training could suffer if there are insufficient trained staff
- Methods used for assessing workloads and motiviation for more staff
- Training records – average period of time spent by students in wards – method of allocation.

In *ward inspection* relating to training, the following aspects are investigated:

- Duty rosters
- Night-duty programming
- Trained staff on night duty
- Clinical teaching staff on night duty
- Work schedules
- Ward records including patient-care programmes
- Kit-book, valuables book
- Dependence-producing substances and control
- Report writing, handing over of reports
- Taking, recording and carrying out doctors' prescriptions
- Medicine and poison control
- Standard of *patient care*
- The amount of clinical teaching done in the ward and by whom; methods used; records kept
- Supervision of patient care
- Are students recognised as such and given the opportunity to learn to

  - plan patient care
  - do peer-group teaching
  - organise and manage the ward so that they will be able to function as trained nurses
  - discuss patient problems and receive instruction and guidance
  - discuss observations made in the light of learning more of patient care

- System used for the continuous assessment of student progress.

The following aspects of *teaching facilities* will be inspected:

- Class-rooms
- Library and learning resource centres: Are books up to date, used regularly, and are the centres properly controlled?
- Equipment and availability (not locked away and thus almost unobtainable)
- Charts, models, etc
- Toilets
- Refreshment facilities
- Study facilities
- Hygiene
- Noise and its control
- Heating, ventilation, lighting
- Ordering of films, etc.

Regarding *teaching personnel,* the following aspects will be inspected:

- Qualifications
- Experience
- Up-to-date in-service education programmes – provision for this as well as special efforts on the part of the staff
- Method of implementation of South African Nursing Council requirements
- Ratio of time devoted to formal lecturing and to other teaching methods
- Examination results
- Remedial teaching, if any
- Method of internal testing, examining and general assessment
- Feedback to principal and thus to matron
- Availability of journals
- Subject teaching, team teaching or other teaching strategies
- Method of dealing with students' problems, both personal and learning
- Community practica and arrangements – are students involved, or are they observers only?
- Use of workbooks, etc
- Assessment of teaching personnel capabilities
- General philosophy underlying the activities of the department
- Involvement of tutors in professional activities
- Research carried out to improve teaching methods, selection, results, etc
- Student selection
- Integration of guide and statement of the purpose of the course into all teaching programmes
- Clerical assistance with record-keeping, etc
- Availability of typing facilities, photostat facilities and other technical aids.

14.4.3 Local inspection

This is done by the principal or person in charge of a school, or as delegated by her. It can be done on a frequent basis, a formal basis or a spot-check, informal basis. A school or college is there to teach the practice of nursing. The principal or her deputy must be accountable for the college in general and the clinical matron, or the matron in charge of students for the clinical teaching. The two should co-ordinate their activities and plans.

In a properly run training school it should be possible for an inspection to be carried out on any day and at any time, without causing consternation.

When outside inspectors arrive, the normal courtesy of first going to the medical superintendent and the matron in charge of the hospital, as well as the principal of the college, must of course always be adhered to.

15 Evaluation in nursing education

15.1 DEFINITION OF EVALUATION

Chambers Twentieth Century Dictionary defines evaluation as 'determination of the value of', and value as, among others, 'worth, a fair equivalent, intrinsic worth or goodness' and 'that which renders anything useful or estimable'.

The Concise Oxford Dictionary says to evaluate is 'to ascertain the amount of' and *Websters Encyclopaedic Dictionary of the English Language* states that it is derived from the Latin *valere* = be worth, and means 'exhaustive appraisement' 'careful appraisal' or 'judgement as to worth or amount' as that 'quality of a thing which renders it valuable, merit, excellence', and appraisal 'to estimate the value of under the direction of a competent authority'.

This somewhat lengthy search for the meaning of evaluation is necessary, as it is so often seen as merely 'attaching a numerical value to', in other words, nothing more than giving a 'mark' to something. True, the end result of evaluation may take the form of a mark or a symbol, but the process must include looking for the *worth,* the *intrinsic worth* or *goodness,* whether the work or action being evaluated has anything that renders it *useful or estimable* and whether the material being evaluated has anything which renders it valuable, *meritorius, of excellence,* and includes *exhaustive and careful* appraisal, estimation of the value of under the direction of a *competent* authority.

Competent is defined by the *Chambers Twentieth Century Dictionary* as 'sufficient, legally qualified', and as 'properly qualified to' by *The Concise Oxford Dictionary*.

This latter concept, *competent* authority, has two aspects, one of which is someone duly appointed by the legal authority, be it the South African Nursing Council as is the case in most written examinations, by universities or other duly authorised bodies, or someone in the clinical field appointed by the employing or other authority to do the evaluation.

The other aspect of a competent, *properly qualified* person, implies a knowledge and expertise which enables him to make proper evaluations. This is a factor that is often overlooked in nursing evaluation for competence to undertake evaluation is seldom tested, and the workload attached to marking endless tests as well as examinations, not to mention making value judgements in clinical work, where nurse-patient relationships, emotional support, and other variables are as important as carrying out a technical skill. Competency implies more than giving a mere opinion.

Evaluation in nursing education must then be founded on the following:

- Careful gathering of information
- Knowledge of the subject, upon which to base a judgement
- Knowledge of the objectives to be achieved
- Objectivity
- The ability to form judgements on the basis of the information gathered
- Weighing the information according to the knowledge of the evaluator, expected knowledge of the person being evaluated and the set objectives.

It can thus be defined as a systematic process whereby a valid appraisal can be made of desired behaviour, skills and attitudes regarding a described level of proficiency in the art and science of nursing. This systematic process of valid appraisal must take place under the direction of a competent person or authority.

15.2 WHAT IS TO BE EVALUATED?

At a superficial glance this may seem to be a simple question: Nursing education, or the product of such education, is to be evaluated. If, however, one pauses for a moment to consider what nursing is, as discussed in chapter 1, and what the product of nursing education should be, then the question becomes far more complex.

Nursing education, as part of tertiary education, is post-Standard 10 education, and it is concerned not only with the acquisition of measurable knowledge, such as for example that acquired in the study of anatomy, but also with the application of that knowledge to the health care of *many human beings,* all of whom are unique. All humans react in different ways, physically, physiologically and psychologically to illness or its threats, to treatments and medications, and their very lives may depend on the educated judgement of the nurse who is the person to be evaluated.

Because she is continuously dealing with human beings in many different situations where contact and communication are essential, her interpersonal relationship skills must be well developed. This is another factor to consider in overall evaluation.

In the past the aim of nursing education was simply to teach a person to carry out the instructions of a doctor, which were in any case limited by his own limited knowledge, and to give physical care of a toilet type to those who could not do this for themselves. Today nursing education's aims are much wider.

15.2.1 Prescriptions

The doctor's prescriptions, because of the iatrogenic aspects of many drugs which today make up his armentarium because of the scientific advancement of medicine, require far more knowledge from the nurse. But it is *the nurse* who detects the first signs of untoward reactions, not the doctor who, in the nature of medical practice, usually sees his patient at the most for a few minutes per day.

15.2.2 Skills

The technical skills required from the nurse have changed and are everchanging. These include stitching wounds, setting up and monitoring intravenous therapy, performing vacuum extractions, performing and stitching episiotomies, giving skilled care to patients on respirators, cardiac monitors, haemodialysis, various oncological procedures, patients having had extensive surgery, including neurosurgery, and having to nurse efficiently those subjected to the marvels of modern medical science and technology.

Instant, often lifesaving reaction to emergencies such as cardiac arrest by applying defibrillation, is also expected.

Disaster planning and responsible action in such circumstances is another facet of nursing education.

15.2.3 The care of both healthy and sick people of all ages

This occurs in the community as well as in the clinic or hospital, and requires extensive background knowledge as well as community skills, the ability to plan and implement health education programmes and research programmes in the community, to say nothing of school health services, occupational health services, massive immunisation programmes, and many more.

The registered nurse today also has to practise her independent functions in an atmosphere of co-operation with the doctors and other health-care professionals.

John Sheahan (1979: 48 – 49) in his modification and application to nursing of the Technician Educational Council Aim, makes the following statement in expressing the need for education in the new era:

Every programme should aim to develop the learner's ability to think, to grasp ideas and to communicate effectively. Adaptability, curiosity, self-confidence, independence of thought and the power to make critical judgements are personal qualities that should be given every encouragement to grow. In this way the learner will learn to make decisions, to exercise initiative, to respond to change, to act as an effective member of a group and to supervise the work of others where this is required.

Thus the nurse has to be evaluated on the cognitive, psychomotor and affective levels discussed earlier.

The South African Nursing Council, in its evaluation of both basic and post-basic students, is well aware of the need for judging the abstract as well as the more concrete skills.

This is borne out by the clause now included in the latest regulations concerning several of the post-basic courses. This clause states that, among the requirements for admission of a candidate to the examination, is a certificate issued by the person in charge of the school that the candidate 'on the basis of a system of continual assessment, has been found competent and suitable in respect of attitudes, approach, insight, knowledge and skills'.

Thus, a system of continual assessment needs to be developed in order to be able to certify that the student has been found competent in abstract qualities as well as in technical skills.

15.3 THE PURPOSE OF EVALUATION

If evaluation is to be done, it must be done with a purpose in mind in order to give it direction. The *purpose of evaluation in nursing education* can be summarised as follows:

(a) To determine whether the *end product,* that is the person being evaluated, is a competent, knowledgeable, humane nursing practitioner, capable of performing her independent as well as dependent functions with educated judgement. This aspect entails the protection of society, which is the main concern of the South African Nursing Council.

(b) To *assess what progress* the student is making towards achieving the goals of the nursing education programme. This assessment can of course be repeated at stages during the course to determine the results achieved at each stage. Has the student mastered the skills required before being promoted to a further stage?

(c) To be in a position to supply the *individual student* with an idea of *his progress,* so as to enable him to maintain and improve areas of strength while at the same time, eliminating weaknesses. Knowledge of results and achievement is a motivating factor in learning.

(d) To enable nurse-educators to assess the *results* of their teaching and improve, review or renew their methodology as necessary. In class-room teaching particularly, when a large number of students appear to have the same difficulty in grasping a subject, or show the same lack of knowledge, teaching strategies need careful study so that the necessary changes in attitudes and learning will occur.

(e) To *clarify and re-define* educational objectives.

(f) To provide *certification* of satisfactory completion of a course in order to meet registration or enrolment requirements and which entitle the successful candidate to practise his profession.

(g) To determine whether a candidate is suitable or ready for *promotion*.

(h) To determine whether an applicant for a *post-basic course is a suitable candidate* for such a course.

(i) To train, by assisting and teaching and giving the opportunity for practice, *those who have not yet acquired evaluation skills*.

(j) To have *on record reliable information* about all students, pupils, or other staff members so that confidential reports can be issued when required.

(k) *To keep personnel on their toes* by a system of continual evaluation, the results of which should be made known to trained as well as untrained staff. Regular six to 12-monthly evaluations of all registered staff in terms of their patient care, teaching and administrative and interpersonal performances should be routine.

(l) To assist persons towards realistic *self-evaluation* of their abilities, strengths and shortcomings.

(m) To *develop* and continually review *evaluation procedures* and techniques so that the person(s) being evaluated is assured that the best available and tested method is being used and that the same criteria apply to all.

(n) To decide whether the programme as a *whole,* and not just the individual product, is succeeding and if not why not. Where are the weak points? Is it necessary at all? Do staff need refresher courses, assistance, a change of subject–matter to teach? Are students of the same calibre as previous years? Are the health needs of the employing authority as well as the community, and the requirements of the registering body, being met?

(o) *Student evaluation* of their courses and of teaching personnel can be a valuable exercise.

15.4 PRINCIPLES OF EVALUATION

Before discussing some of the methods of evaluation, the basic principles on which all evaluation should be based should be clearly stated:

(a) *Objectivity* should, as far as is humanly possible, be an inherent part of evaluation.

(b) *Criteria* must be defined and be possible to observe. These should be defined in terms of the following:
- *Expected student knowledge* at level of training
- *Interpersonal skills*
- *Habitual performance* as opposed to performance under examination-type conditions
- Valid *skill* performance at level of training

- *Safety of patients*
- *Relevance* to behaviour, etc, being tested
- The *ability to express,* in examinations or in ward report writing, meaning clearly and concisely without danger of incorrect interpretation
- *Normative behaviour* in terms of nursing professionalism
- *Self-control* in crisis or difficult situations.

(c) *Continuity:* Evaluation should be a continuous process, and must be seen as an integral part of the learning/teaching situation with which no nurse, however senior, is ever finished.

(d) *Feedback to students:* Discussions of weak points, the reason for a poor mark, helpful comments on returned assignments, while time consuming, are essential.

(e) Evaluation should be *carried out according to the educational programme and its stated objectives.*

(f) Valid *measuring instruments* should be used, that is they must measure accurately what they are intended to measure. They must therefore be *tested; reliable* in that the same results are likely to be obtained by different evaluators (consistency); *specific,* precise and clear so that the average intelligent student can understand and deal with the question or work assignment; designed to fit in with the *time* allocated; *realistic* and *practical;* and *directly related* to what is being tested.

(g) *As many persons as possible,* who are concerned with the education of the student, must be included in evaluation, so that prejudice on the part of one person, especially in the clinical situation, can be avoided. It would be feasible if as wide a variety of persons as possible were to assess the student independently over a long period of time, as a composite picture would then emerge.

(h) There should be *regular analysis of and research* into evaluation results, techniques, and student potential related to actual performance.

15.5 WHEN TO EVALUATE

The examining and/or registering body lays down some stipulations as to the formal examination system to be followed, while interim testing or 'college' examinations are laid down by authorities in charge of the colleges. Some decisions about testing and when it is to be done, are left to the tutor and to leaders in the clinical situation.

In the lecture-room situation testing may be done daily in the form of a short quiz or five-minute written question dealing with work covered the previous day. It can then almost be regarded as part of the teaching process. It may be more formal and occur on a weekly basis, or be divided into study-day, modular, daily release or concurrent theory and practica systems; it may be done fortnightly, monthly, when a particular portion of the work is completed, quarterly, or even once a semester.

The method chosen will depend on the tutor, the college, the students and the course.

A few pointers in this respect might assist the aspirant tutor-evaluator.

- Short, five-minute tests which are marked and discussed immediately serve to reinforce teaching, and are therefore almost a part of teaching.
- Frequent testing of a small section of the work will inevitably lead to high marks, because of the small quantity of work tested. This may lead to false ideas of capabilities, and a slackening off in study which can often be ill afforded.
- Tests must be marked and returned with as little delay as possible or the value to students is lost as is the opportunity for remedial teaching.
- Very infrequent testing does not stimulate study or attention in class.
- Short fortnightly to monthly tests, which cover a reasonable amount of the work, and can be marked and discussed, are probably best.
- Students *must know* well in advance when testing is to be done.

15.6 METHODS OF EVALUATION

There are a number of methods which may be selected, singly or in combination to evaluate nursing education. Some are of greater value in certain sections than others, but the expertise of the person setting and marking the tests is the crux of the matter.

In nursing education we do not only deal with written examinations, although these play a vital part, but we are concerned with testing technical as well as interpersonal skills, and often an interaction or combination of such skills.

Various methods of examining will now be reviewed and explained, and their applicability to nursing evaluation will be discussed in some detail.

15.6.1 Written tests

These tests can take a variety of forms, but only the best known and most frequently used ones will be discussed.

15.6.1.1 Essay-type tests

These may be of either the long-answer or short-answer type, and are familiar to most students. There are several variations of this type:

15.6.1.1.1 The long-answer type

Long-answer questions must test factual knowledge, comprehension, creativity and ability to explain, discuss and describe, as well as to select, organise and summarise relevant material. They must allow the student to show that she can think about a subject, put it into perspective, consider the patient as a person, and draw up and where necessary amend a relevant, realistic nursing care plan that will meet the needs of the given situation.

15.6.1.1.2 The problem-solving type

Here the student is presented with a particular nursing situation, given the relevant information about the patient and his health problems, and asked to discuss the subsequent nursing care or draw up a nursing care plan. As both would expect the student to discuss aspects, such as complications and their prevention and/or management, they could have great value as testing instruments. The answer would require thought and not just a regurgitation of learned facts. Problem-solving questions should be posed so that it is clear to candidates what is required.

15.6.1.1.3 The straight discussion type

The following is an example of a more straightforward approach: 'Discuss the symptoms, treatment and nursing care of a one-year-old infant admitted to a ward with acute gastro-enteritis. What precautions should be taken to prevent the spread of this infection in a paediatric unit consisting of two four-bedded, two two-bedded and six single cubicles?'

15.6.1.1.4 The factual or structured type

An example of this type is as follows: 'A patient is admitted with acute abdominal pain, nausea and vomiting.
(a) What could be the causes of this condition?
(b) Give the specific signs and symptoms of each cause mentioned.
(c) Discuss the nursing observations and care given while awaiting the arrival of the doctor, including preparation for emergency medical treatment.
(d) Which tests might be ordered?
(e) Describe the essential aspects of preparing such a patient for surgery.'

Long-answer questions may appear easy to draw up, but good ones require a great deal of thought, so that they can be answered in the time allocated, and yet are a reasonable test for the student at her level of training. They should be drawn up so that they call for careful consideration, but can be answered briefly. The marking of long-answer, essay-type questions takes considerable time.

A memorandum must be drawn up for each question against which the answer will be marked. Depending on the question, this memorandum may include essential factual knowledge required, possible nursing care plans and complications and treatment. Marks must be allocated for answers to each specific point.

Memoranda must also make it possible for the 'average' student to obtain about 50%. They must also allow for about two additional marks per question, which are allocated for additional *relevant* information, with the proviso that the extra marks thus provided do not make up more than 10% of the total marks allotted for the paper as a whole

These memoranda, in the case of nursing subjects at least, will help to eliminate subjectivity to a large extent. They would be less prone to varied interpretations. The student with a neat handwriting, and good style and language ability, will always tend to be favoured, except in the case of simple card marking for computer analysis. In any written test, legibility, spelling and grammar are always likely to influence a marker.

Usually tests requiring longer written answers can only cover a limited portion of a syllabus; and therefore the tests may not truly reflect the student's knowledge, but rather his ability to 'spot' a few questions and prepare 'model' answers for these.

If students are given a wide choice of questions the danger also exists that they are actually answering *completely different* question papers, and therefore their results are not at all comparable. It has been suggested that *no choice* be allowed in setting examination papers. The results would then, at least, be comparable.

Another reason against allowing students a choice is that it is extremely difficult to compile questions of equal complexity which will again penalise some and favour other candidates. Students are also often not good judges of their own knowledge, and may therefore choose the wrong question.

Problems such as 'spotting', will not be eliminated but can to some extent be avoided by seldom testing the same subject-matter in essay-type questions, and by compiling the whole examination paper by the use of various types of questions. This would provide more adequate sampling of student knowledge.

Another disadvantage of long essay-type answers is learner fatigue. Writing continuously for three hours at a time on long essay-type questions allows little time for thought, and as weariness seb01ts in, so errors creep in, or sheer tiredness makes the student careless and liable to leave out often essential facts, which in fact are known.

General guide-lines for essay tests include the following:

(a) Set questions clearly and unambiguously.

(b) State precisely time limits concerned, for example for the first two hours post-operative, or age, for example a child of three, adult of 24, adult of 86; also exact phase of illness and precise phase of disease. These will materially affect answers.

(c) Word questions carefully to cover a specific subject and limit the scope. For example, 'Discuss the treatment of myocardial infarction' is too wide and could take a whole book, not a 30 to 40-minute examination question to provide a satisfactory reply.

(d) Plan your tests and examinations well in advance. Setting tests or examinations at the last minute invites trouble.

(e) Be clear about the verb used in the question and make sure that it is what you mean. Describe, discuss, compare and explain have very different meanings, and therefore the verb should be the one which will produce the required answer.

(f) Percentage weighting for sections of essay-type questions, especially of the 'factual' type discussed above, should be indicated.

15.6.1.1.5 Short-answer type

Short-answer questions call for definitions, brief notes on various topics, or short explanations.

Ideally the short-answer type question should have only one acceptable answer, therefore 'write short notes on' is not a good way of phrasing a question, as many 'short notes' could be written about a subject, while phrases such as 'what do you know about' should be avoided altogether; in fact, if a student wrote in answer to such a question 'nothing', she should be awarded full marks!

In setting short-answer questions great precision is needed and students must know *precisely* what is required. Questions such as:

- Define culture
- Describe the stools of a patient with obstructive jaundice
- Name the complications of diabetes mellitus
- Give the advantages of breast-feeding

are reasonable types of questions requiring short answers, and the amount of detail required can be indicated by the marks allocated next to each short question. The answers are easy to mark, and the scope of testing can be very much wider than in the long-answer type, provided that the person setting the test is sensitive to the need for good sampling. Short-answer questions must require less information than do long-answer questions. The statement of the question itself may be longer because of the need for precision and better explanations so that a paper comprised of many short answers may have a rather formidable appearance because of its length, but students soon adapt to this format.

Because of the more factual nature of the information required, the marking can be more objective and facts are not lost, as they might be when markers have to wade through the long-answer type.

Short-answer questions have a definite place in the testing of students of nursing. With practice the tutor can draw up excellent examples of such testing, which can be used to advantage in practice.

15.6.1.1.6 The open-book test

This is a method which can be used in written examinations. In this type of testing the student may take into the examination room and use any book, document, or personal notes (as specified by the examiner). The questions are then designed to test the student's ability to find, assess and use information, rather than simply to recall what has been learnt. The student is not expected simply to quote or rephrase the content, but to assess the information and use it judiciously. An approximation of a real-life situation might be simulated in that the student would be required to demonstrate that she knows what information was needed in the particular situation, *where* to find it, and how to use it once it has been found.

15.6.1.1.7 The marking of essay-type questions

The following points are of importance, and are summarised below:

(a) A memorandum of the required answer, and the allocation of marks should be drawn up.

It is preferable to mark all the students' essay answers to the same question in order to try to obtain some uniformity. When hundreds of question papers have to be marked boredom might occur, and then it would perhaps be better to mark them in batches of say 25 to 30 of one question, then 25 to 30 of another question. In other words, a group of 250 papers could be subdivided into sets of eight to ten.

(b) Mark papers anonymously when possible.

(c) If possible, two markers should grade the same papers independently, and then award an average mark. Ideal but, with increasing tutor shortages at present, unrealistic.

(d) Marking should not take place at one sitting, unless the numbers of papers to mark is fewer than ten. Weariness on the part of the marker can adversely affect grading, and a break of even 15 minutes at regular intervals should be mandatory.

(e) Do not assume that a student knows what he has not explicitly written down. Vague answers usually indicate little knowledge, and should be

306

dealt with as such.

(f) A wrong statement would receive no mark, but if the wrong statement or omission were such that it showed that the candidate had no understanding of the subject, or was indeed unfit to practise, then marks should be deducted accordingly. A student who states categorically that one of the reasons for performing a tracheostomy is to feed the patient artificially, deserves to fail outright.

(g) If test papers are to be returned to the student, copious notes and corrections should be made as they are being marked, if it is at all possible, as this can play an important part in the learning/teaching event. Omissions and inaccuracies should not only be crossed out or marked wrong, but the correct answer or reason supplied. Discussion of the paper with each individual student can also be helpful.

15.6.1.2 Objective testing

Because of the degree of subjectivity inherent in essay-type testing and the sheer mass of work required in marking papers of large groups, the so-called 'objective testing' system has been developed.

It is possible to set objective tests which assess knowledge, understanding, educated judgement, reasoning, the application of principles, as well as abstract thinking.

One word of warning should one think that this type of testing is the answer to all our problems: Good, objective-type tests take hours to compile, to test and retest for validity and reliability, and require a great deal of skill to construct.

In the construction of objective tests certain criteria must be kept in mind:

- The test must not be so easy that it could be answered correctly by all candidates, or it would be invalid.
- It must not be too difficult, so that the candidates who answer correctly because they understand, would be so few that their number would be equal to those who obtained the correct answer by guesswork. This would again invalidate the test.
- Adjustments must be made for positive scores which could be obtained by simple guesswork.
- The test must include items which will require the student to show the ability to reason, apply principles or make deductions, and not simply to supply factual answers.
- Examinations based on objective testing should include more than one type of 'objective' question.
- Very clear instructions must be given to students, so that mistakes in completing forms (or whatever method is used) would not be due to inade-

quate directions, but to lack of knowledge.
- Language usage must be correct, simple, and incapable of being misinterpreted by anyone with a reasonable knowledge of the language. Sentences should be short.
- Clues in the alternative responses must be avoided.
- Alternatives which are completely contradictory should not be used (as in the multiple-choice type, as students can then eliminate all other answers which contain either of them).
- If written responses to questions are required, no more than two words should be required.
- In multiple-choice phrasing, responses should be kept short.

15.6.1.2.1 Advantages of the objective type-test

- A large quantity of material can be covered in a short time.
- Marking is quick.
- Students do not become fatigued by writing continuously.
- Marking can be done by anyone using a score or cover sheet, or even by a machine.
- Once a 'pool' of about 5 000 suitable, valid, reliable questions have been built up, it may be drawn on repeatedly in setting examination papers. This can even be done by a properly programmed computer.

15.6.1.2.2 Disadvantages of the use of the objective-type test

These include:

- Amount of time, expertise and man hours required to prepare valid reliable tests.
- Guessing is more possible.
- The amount of space, and thus paper required, to present the questions is considerable, and therefore costly.

15.6.1.2.3 Types of objective tests

There are many types of objective tests in use, and no doubt more will be invented. Some of the better known, and more frequently used are the following:

(a) *Short or one-word answer type* (simple recall, free response or completion)

The question should be phrased so that only one answer is possible.

A simple statement is made which has a missing word, phrase or symbol and this missing item must be supplied by the student.

This is useful for testing factual knowledge only. Examples include:

- The *causative organism* of typhoid fever is . . .
- The *name* of the bone in the thigh is the . . .
- The islets of Langerhans, in the pancreas secrete . . .
- The valve found between the left atrium and left ventricle is the . . . valve
- Inflammation of the liver is known as . . .

(b) *Sentence completion type*

Here more than one word may be left out and the student must complete the whole sentence. Care must be taken not to use direct phrases from a textbook, as the student may have learned the whole section parrot-fashion.

A few examples of this type of question are:

- Lipase acts on fats to produce . . . and . . .
- Sucrose is hydrolised into . . . and . . .
- The causative organism of urinary bilharzia is the . . ., the vector of which is the snail named . . .
- Permanently hard water is caused by the sulphates or chlorides of . . . and . . .
- Angina pectoris is a syndrome which is characterised by paroxysms of pain in the . . which are the result of insufficient . . . to the . . .

(c) *True-false type*

In this form a short statement is made and the student must decide whether it is *true* or *false*. The statement made must contain only one idea, and must be *definitely* true or *definitely* false. Answers such as 'sometimes' or 'not always' should not be possible. Never use words such as 'many', 'few', 'large', 'small', 'sometimes' or 'never', as they may all lead to confusion. Negative statements should also be avoided and the sentences should be clear and short.

It is advisable in a true-false type of test to have about an equal number of true and false items, but they should be irregularly distributed. The possibility of guessing in this type of question is fairly high and an uneven distribution helps to avoid this type of guessing:

First √   Second ×   Third √   Fourth √
and so on.

Examples of true-false questions are:

- The tenth cranial nerve is the glasso-pharyngeal nerve.
- Urinary bilharzia is caused by the *Scistosoma haematobium*.

- The pericardium is a single layer of fibrous tissue covering the heart.
- Florence Nightingale founded the St Mark's Hospital Training School in London.
- An incised wound has lacerated, jagged edges.
- The normal erythrocyte count in a male is 4 600 000 to 6 200 000 per mm^3.

The method of indicating the answer must be clear to the student:

T = True   F = False

- Ring whichever response is correct.
- Place the symbol (or write the word True (T) or False (F)) next to each statement.
- Place two columns or blocks next to the statements indicating clearly that one is *True* and the other *False* and ask them to put a cross in the appropriate block or column:

	T	F
Statement 1		
Statement 2		
Statement 3		

	T	F
or		
Statement 1		
Statement 2		
Statement 3		
Statement 4		

15.6.1.2.4 Listing tests

This type of test is related to the completion type, but there are some differences. The student is required to supply a list of items, terms or other information in answer to specific instructions. An example would be:

List four causes of mass loss

1 ....

2 ....

3 ....

4 ....

The answers may not correspond and therefore would have to be marked by a nurse-educator, but they are useful in testing recall of specific facts, while at the same time reducing the possibility of guessing from 'supplied' answers.

They test factual knowledge only, and not ability to interpret.

310

In this type a diagram with numbered parts is supplied. The student is then required to supply the correct name of the different numbered sections. An example could be a diagram of the heart. Below the numbered diagram a list of numbers with blank spaces next to them is given, so that the student can fill in the name of the particular parts, as follows:

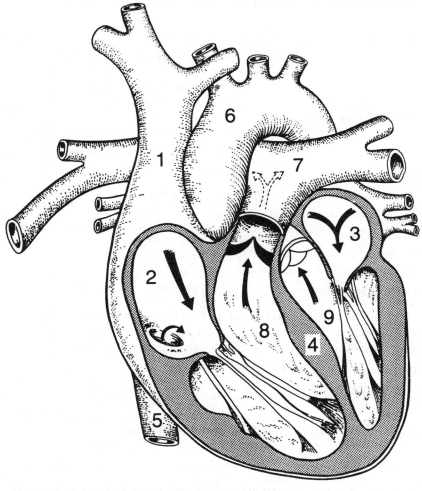

1 ....   5 ....
2 ....   6 ....
3 ....   7 ....
4 ....   8 ....

15.6.1.2.6 Matching-pair type

In this type the student is asked to select the item from column 1 which matches that in column 2, and write the number in the space provided. The number of answers should be more than the number of questions asked, to avoid obtaining the correct answer by a process of elimination.

Examples of the matching-pairs type could be:

Diseases			*Causative organisms*
Syphilis	☐	1	*Echinococcus granulosus*
Hydatidosis	☐	2	*Rickettsia prowazekii*
Epidemic typhus	☐	3	*Treponema pallidum*
Intestinal bilharzia	☐	4	*Schistosoma mansoni*
Malaria	☐	5	*Plasmodium vivax*
		6	*Schistosoma haematobium*

or

Symptom			*Name*
Pain on micturition	☐	1	Dyspnoea
Difficulty in swallowing	☐	2	Dysuria
Difficulty in breathing	☐	3	Dysphagia
Indigestion	☐	4	Dyspepsia
Diarrhoeal disease	☐	5	Dystrophy
		6	Dysarthria
		7	Dysentery

or

Names			*Reasons for fame*
Banting	☐	1	Discovery of penicillin
Barnard	☐	2	Renal dialysis
Fleming	☐	3	Discovery of insulin
Lister	☐	4	Discovery of radium
Roentgen	☐	5	Pioneer of antiseptic techniques
		6	Discovery of X-rays
		7	Heart transplantation

Various combinations could be used such as:

- Terms with definitions
- Symbols with the names of the chemicals they represent
- Causes with effects
- Drugs with side-effects

- Diseases with specific complications
- Names of specific tests with normal levels
- Instruments with their uses.

The matching-pair type of test is especially valuable in assessing student ability to recognise relationships, make associations and place items in categories. It does not test interpretations and understanding and, if badly constructed, tends to 'give away' some answers.

In constructing matching-pair tests the following should receive attention:

- There should be at least five, but no more than 12 responses per group.
- There should be more answers than questions.
- Possible answers must not be so ridiculous that they are eliminated without thought.
- The column with the single words or shorter phrases, should be on the left-hand side of the page.
- Directions for students must be explicit.
- All items constituting one section of the test should be on one page.

(a) *Advantages of matching-pair questions*
- Little time is required for reading.
- A wide variety of subject-matter can be tested quickly.
- If carefully constructed, chances of guessing are limited.
- They can be marked quickly and objectively.

(b) *Disadvantages*
- They are time-consuming to construct.
- If poorly constructed, they can 'give away' the answers.
- It is often difficult to collect sufficient related material to make up homogeneous lists, thus unimportant and irrelevant material may be included simply to construct a 'test'.

15.6.1.2.7 Multiple-choice questions

These are among the most popular of the objective-type questions.

Each question has three components. The first part or *stem* is an incomplete statement, a leading phrase, a question or a problem.

The second part is the *key* or correct answer, while the rest of the test consists of incorrect responses or *distractors*.

Various forms of multiple-choice questions exist, for example:

(a) *The single- or best-response type*
The *stem* is constructed and set out. Then the *key* and *distractors* are stated, and

the student has to make a choice of the *correct*, that is the *best* response.

Stem: How many vertebrae are there in the human vertebral column:

Distractor	a	118
Distractor	b	14
Key	c	26
Distractor	d	28
Distractor	e	24
Answer	c	

or

Stem: The term alimentation means:

Key	a	nourishment
Distractor	b	disease of bowel
Distractor	c	disease
Distractor	d	joining together
Answer	a	

(b)   *The multiple-response item*

This consists of the stem followed by several statements, where one or more may be the *key* or correct answer, and where there are also several distractors. An example of this type would be:

Stem: An adult suffering from acute leukaemia may have the following symptoms:

(a) Abscess of the mouth
(b) Haemorrhages into the skin
(c) Increased cholesterol level
(d) Lowered resistance to infection
(e) Increased uric acid blood level

Answer
1 all of above
2 (a), (b), (e)
3 (a), (b), (d)
4 none of above
5 (a), (b), (d), (e).
Answer = 5

Stem: Clinical picture of malaria includes:

(a) Rigor
(b) Splenomegaly

314

(c) Headache
(d) Myalgia
(e) Myxoedema
(f) Hypopyrexia

Answer
1 all of above
2 (a) and (b) only
3 (a), (e) and (f)
4 (a), (b), (c), (d).
Answer = 4

Setting multiple-choice questions is extremely difficult. The following points must be borne in mind:

(a) The *instructions* for the student must be very clear, for example: For each of the incomplete statements below *one or more* of the completions is correct.
Indicate on the answer sheet if
1 all are correct
2 (a), (b) and (c) are correct
3 (a) and (d) are correct
4 (a) only is correct.
(b) There should be sufficient questions for the time allowed, but not too many.
(c) Ensure that the *stem* is clearly stated.
(d) Do not use negatives in the stem or in the item. Make positive statements where at all possible. If it is absolutely necessary to use a negative then the negative word, for example *NOT*, must be *capitalised* and *underlined*.
(e) Each item should be completely independent of answers to other items.
(f) Use *plausible* distractors. It should at least appear to have something to do with the subject.
(g) Avoid clues that suggest the correct answer.
(h) Arrange the correct answers to various items in such a way that, for the test as a whole, no one letter or figure which indicates a correct answer appears much more frequently than the others.
(i) Ask only one question in one item.

All objective testing should have some form of negative marking included in the scoring to obviate guessing. Not giving an answer will not be penalised – a wrong answer will receive no mark, but if some system, such as subtracting half a mark for every wrong answer is used, and the students are aware of this, they will be less tempted to guess.

315

15.6.1.3 Programmed examination

This type of testing is between the essay and the objective-type. It can also be called a problem-solving approach.

A case history of a patient admitted to hospital, is written out in detail. The student then has to complete a form, which will take a certain format. The choice of answers is not suggested, and the student is free to complete it according to her judgement.

Observations on admission	Nursing action required	Possible outcome

A second phase can be added, which details a progress report as on the second day (or after a week). The student then completes another form:

Progress report items	Nursing action now required	Possible outcome

Several such progress insets could be made, ending up with describing the nursing action and psycho-social care required in the community.

These tests also demand a great deal of preparation, but can be very good tests of nursing competence, insight into problems and possible problems, and applications of principles. The question is put explicitly and therefore the student is more likely to stick to the point.

15.6.1.4 Oral examinations

This is where the student is directly confronted with the examiner or even a panel of examiners, and required to answer the questions put to him verbally.

The art of oral examining consists of putting the student at ease, of getting him to talk and to show what he knows. They have the advantage that the student has the opportunity to ask for clarification of ambiguous questions, while the examiner can really probe an area where the student appears hazy.

A little time thus spent may reveal whether the student really has a good knowledge of the subject.

A great deal of material can be covered in a short space of time.

Oral examinations should last a minimum of 20 minutes, and should be properly structured so that the examiner has a worked-out scheme of questions to be asked. The examiner mustalways remember that it is his task to find out *what the student knows,* and not to reduce him to a petrified figure unable to answer at all.

It is a very useful form of testing and can be used to advantage where students are 'borderline' cases – either for gaining distinction or for passing.

It is also useful where illness has prevented the student from writing an examination. Two evaluators should always be present to limit subjectivity.

15.6.2 Evaluation of clinical competence in the practice of nursing

Because nursing combines clinical skills with theoretical knowlege, it is necessary to assess the clinical competence of students as part of the total evaluation procedure. Yet, assessing clinical competence is a difficult task which is nevertheless absolutely vital. It is also imperative that nurses are taught self-evaluation of their own competence, and which should be part of their daily lives in the practice of nursing.

In order to evaluate clinical competence in the art and science of nursing, it is essential to establish exactly of what clinical competence consists.

It is generally agreed that nursing is far more than the performance of technical skills, important though these are. Before deciding on the method of evaluating clinical skills very careful thought must be given to this matter, and the criteria against which the student is to be judged, are decided upon (WHAT). Also, a decision must be taken as to WHO is the best person to assess clinical competence, WHEN this assessment is to be undertaken, WHERE the assessment is to take place, and then the method, the HOW of the assessment.

It is suggested that criteria be drawn up by a group of people most concerned with the technique, and that these are reviewed from time to time, and revised as necessary. The following criteria could be included:

15.6.2.1 *What* is to be measured?

The criteria for clinical competence are the following:

- Checking any necessary orders
- Preparing the patient and equipment
- Dexterity
- Gentleness in carrying out the procedure

- Technical skill
- Patient–nurse relationship
- Avoiding embarrassment and ensuring privacy for the patient
- Knowledge of the theory upon which the technique is based
- Knowledge of the dangers/medico–legal hazards involved in the technique, and how to avoid these
- Powers of observation
- Achievement of the objective with minimal discomfort to the patient
- Recording
- Reporting
- Ability to deal with untoward happenings during the procedure
- Professionalism.

15.6.2.2 *Who* should do the assessment?

Any registered nurse should be capable of assessing clinical competence, though some will be better at it than others.

Students in their final year *should* be taught assessment *and* given the opportunity to practise it.

Assessment of clinical competence is *not* the prerogative of clinical teaching professional nurses only, but should be part of the everyday work of every unit professional nurse. Continuous assessment means just that; it is not a once only event. The unit professional nurse who is responsible for nursing care *must* assess the clinical competence of those to whom she assigns or delegates tasks – there is no other way for her to accept her role and be accountable for the clinical care given in her unit.

15.6.2.3 *When* is the assessment done?

Although it may be necessary to do specific assessments to test clinical competence in a special area or for a specific purpose, assessment of clinical competence should be an ongoing part of clinical care.

It may be part of a training programme to formally test specific skills at certain stages to be sure that all students are at least competent in what are considered basic techniques, but this must not be seen as the most important form of assessment to be done.

The answer to WHEN therefore, is 'all the time'.

15.6.2.4 *Where* is the evaluation done?

Practical assessment of the student nurse/pupil nurse should be in the clinical situation, that is in the ward, unit or patient/client care area.

This move has made the evaluation of clinical competence less artificial, as the nurse can be observed and assessed while working in the real-life situation, but there are also administrative difficulties such as lack of 'procedures' upon which to test the nurses' technical skills, the lack of co-operation on the part of the patient, who is entitled to refuse being the subject of an evaluation procedure, and to want to preserve his privacy and dignity.

It may be difficult to carry on with ward procedures, because practical testing or 'examinations' tend to upset the routine of unit work. Real-life situations are difficult to repeat for a group of students.

The student too, may have difficulty reacting normally in an 'examination'-type situation, whereas if this evaluation was simply part of the routine work of the unit professional nurse, she would be relaxed and perform normally.

The more 'real' the situation, obviously, the better, but the value of simulation techniques outside the actual ward situation must not be forgotten. Simulation is a process of representing a real-life situation as close as possible to the actual situation. The simulation of clinical reality can be less stressful to a student, there is little or no risk to the patient or student involved, and it is possible to set up the same set of circumstances for groups of students.

Nevertheless, the use of simulation techniques must *not* replace real-life assessment in the actual clinical situation. It may be *considered*, however, when the following conditions occur:

- When real-life situations are unavailable and the testing of student competency in certain techniques is essential
- When there is real danger to a very sick patient, who should only be in the hands of skilled practitioners, and yet students need an opportunity to gain at least technical skill with apparatus, etc
- When the time to assess the care of a patient by a particular student may, because the nature of the patient's illness requires long-term care, be spread over too long a period
- When a technique can only be assessed in an actual situation such as a cardiac arrest. This cannot be arranged to order, nor could such vital care be done to assess the inexperienced. Simulation, using models can, however, assess the student's degree of competency with cardio-pulmonary resuscitation.

15.6.2.5 How can clinical competence be assessed (method)?

15.6.2.5.1 Evaluation ward round

The student, accompanied by the evaluator, makes a round of the unit (ward) in which she is working. The procedure is for the student, then, to do the following:

319

- To introduce the patient to the evaluator by name
- To give the name of the patient's doctor
- To supply the date of admission.

The following should be discussed *out of hearing of the patient:*

- Diagnosis
- Specific observations
- Medical treatment
- Nursing care plan
- Response to treatment, etc.

The depth of knowledge, powers of observation and ability to plan and comment upon nursing care, and the response to treatment would, of course, depend on the level of training of the student being assessed.

The discussion may vary from a simple explanation of the diagnosis and consideration of basic nursing care, to an in-depth examination of:

- The causes of the condition
- Signs and symptoms/nursing history
- Tests done, including reasons for them, preparation involved and interpretation
- Medical treatment, including the drugs used with their effects and possible side-effects
- Diagnosis for nursing care
- Nursing care plan
- The progress of the patient
- Prognosis
- Possible complications and their management
- Rehabilitative aspects, where applicable.

The nursing component is stressed throughout.

The evaluator may also initiate discussion of anything noticed in the ward during the course of the evaluation session, such as:

- Admission of a patient
- Ordering of diets
- Cleaning of suction apparatus and use of the machine
- Care of an indwelling urinary catheter
- Blood transfusion management and regulations
- Aseptic procedures
- Medico-legal hazards
- Ward and patient hygiene and many more, the number being limited only by her initiative, observation powers, and the time available.

320

Much can be gained from such a ward round. Not only can the evaluator assess the student's knowledge, but she can also test her ability to correlate theory and practice, her nurse/patient relationships, communication skills, ability to observe intelligently and other such abilities.

15.6.2.5.2 Observation of individual performance

This is one of the oldest means of evaluation. It is useful for assessing all manner of things, from technical skills in the clinical area, to the ability to carry out such tasks as explaining to a mother the care of her newly diagnosed diabetic child.

This method involves observation of the student at work, and should not be limited to technical skills, but include observation of the nurse/patient relationship, and whether all a patient's needs, physical as well as psychological, have been met.

Ideally a student being assessed for competency should be observed in her everyday work rather than at specially arranged opportunities. It is also important that she knows that she will be so assessed and the criteria against which she is to be assessed are made known.

Disadvantages of individual observation are the fact that a student's behaviour often changes when she is aware that she is being watched, and the possibility of subjectivity on the part of the evaluator. To help prevent this, a student should be observed on a number of occasions when performing the same type of task, and preferably by different people.

15.6.2.5.3 Rating scales used with checklists

This method is suitable for assessing competence and characteristics in a fairly formal situation:

Provided that the students are frequently subjected to such 'proficiency' testing, and are judged by more than one person for different assessments, they can give a very accurate picture of the student's competency and other characteristics. Students must be aware of the criteria against which they are being assessed, and the results discussed with them after completion of the evaluation (except, of course, in cases where a 'confidential' mark is required).

It is also a useful technique for training students and newly qualified professional nurses in evaluation techniques.

The checklist must contain the criteria and the rating scale must give different degrees of competence ranging from poor to excellent, from below average to superior, or simply use figures.

The person doing the assessment is then required to supply the appropriate degree or grade for the student's performance against each criterion.

A simple rating scale could be something like the following:

Student's name: .... Year: ....

Course:...

EVALUATION FORM

	Very poor 1	Poor 2	Aver- age 3	Good 4	Very good 5	Total
General preparation						
1 Checking of orders						
2 Becoming acquainted with patient						
3 Inspection of and decision regarding work area						
4 Inspection of apparatus need/pack						
5 Preparation of trolley/tray						
Preparation of patient						
6 Psychological						
7 Physical						
Procedure						
8 Maintenance of hygienic standard/sterility						
9 Dexterity						
10 Handling of equipment/solutions, etc						
11 Ensuring of privacy/avoidance of embarrassment						
12 Achievement of objective						
Completion						
13 Psychological support of patient						
14 Physical comfort of patient						
15 Recording/reporting						
16 Disposal of materials and equipment						
Discussion						
17 Knowledge of patient and condition						
18 Reasons for procedure						
19 Dangers						
20 Observation						

The danger with the above rating scale is that there is a temptation to simply fill in a cross (X) or something similar without giving too much thought to the characteristic being marked.

An assessment form which re-arranges the ratings for each characteristic requires more thought, and is thus more likely to give a considered assessment of a student's ability. However, it is more difficult to arrive at the final mark.

An example of this type of checklist assessment or rating would be the following:

QUALITY					
1 Interest in work	Enthusi-astic, full of interest	Interest variable	Shows little interest	Usually interested	Appears dis-interested
2 Punctu-ality	Always late	Always punctual	Some-times late	Often late	Punctual
3 Care given to patients	Good standard	Poor standard	Excellent standard	Average standard	Variable
4 Attitude to patients	Insensi-tive to needs	Very good	Variable	Brusque, off-hand	Good
5 Appear-ance	Very neat and well-groomed	Often untidy	Variable	Usually neat and tidy	Very untidy
6 Powers of observation	Usually observant	Obser-vant at all times	Unob-servant	Not yet sufficiently observant	Very un-observant

This example is given simply to demonstrate a technique, and is very incomplete. A full assessment form would be much longer. The various characteristics being observed should be grouped together. Forms could be designed to meet different assessment needs.

As with all other forms of assessment, they require careful planning with consultation, testing, reviewing from time to time and altering according to changing needs.

15.6.2.5.4 Anecdotal records, diaries and notebooks

Anecdotal records are simply brief records of actual events (they should not relate to staged events), usually regarding a student's personal or professional development and social interactions. The method should not only be used to record incidents of misbehaviour or misjudgement which put the student in a bad light, but they should include reports of good performance by the student. They should contain

(a) a factual description of the setting in sufficient detail to give meaning to the event or incident; and

(b) a factual description of what the student did and said.

The record must be objective. Any opinion or interpretation of the incident made by the recorder must be separated from the factual description and clearly noted as such, so that anyone reading the record may form his or her own opinion, which might not coincide with that of the recorder.

One anecdotal record is of little value by itself, but a series of these may be useful in assessing the behaviour, attitudes and values of a student, as they may indicate trends of behaviour over a period of time.

Anecdotal records may be completed by either an evaluator or by a student. These, together with notebooks and diaries kept by students, may form a valuable means of self-assessment. All of these should be discussed individually with the student concerned.

A comparison of the anecdotal records kept by the unit professional nurse about a student, and by the student herself could prove very interesting.

15.6.2.5.5 Confidential reports and progress reports

Tutors, unit professional nurses and sometimes clinical instructors are usually asked to write such reports. The report may be in the form of rating scales or check lists. In other cases the registered nurse is required to comment on the development of the student in a fairly structured form, with regard to reliability, leadership, initiative and other such qualities or progress in such areas as application of theory to practice. Report forms may also be unstructured, which allows for free comment, but gives little guidance.

Unfortunately, reports are often completed in a hurry at the end of a month. In addition, the person asked to give an opinion, particularly about personal qualities, may not be really qualified to do so. A tutor with a class of 50 to 60 students, for instance, cannot really know individual students sufficiently to report on various qualities beyond test marks after they have been one or possibly two months in block.

A unit professional nurse in charge is also not always present when a student exhibits certain characteristics, such as intolerance and poor nurse-patient relationships, initiative, the ability to cope with an emergency, and even technical skills. This difficulty can be overcome to some extent if she confers, in private, with the other professional nurses in the ward – although what she eventually writes will, of course, be confidential. Here, time is one of the limiting factors. One of the greatest drawbacks is that these reports tend to be influenced by the personal values and biases of the registered nurse, and will therefore be subjective. While opinions are not scientific evaluation, they nevertheless give an estimate of the effectiveness of student performance and of the nursing education programme. Again a single report is of little use and must be seen in conjunction with other such reports. It is important that confidential and progress reports be discussed in private with the student and that she be given an opportunity to discuss what has been said about her and to put her own point of view.

It is often amazing to see how consistent the reports on one student are, even though they come from a wide variety of evaluators.

Anyone who has to do any form of evaluation, and who is studying to become a teacher of the practice of nursing, would do well to study the mass of literature which is available on the various forms of evaluation. See also Mellish and Johnston (1986).

16 *Communication in teaching the practice of nursing*

16.1 DEFINITION

The word 'communicate' according to *Chambers Twentieth Century Dictionary* means to 'give a share of, to impart, to reveal', while Dance (1970) having examined 95 published definitions, came to the conclusion that the most acceptable was that of Anderson (1959):

> Communication is the process by which we understand others and in turn endeavour to be understood by them. It is dynamic, constantly changing and shifting in response to the total situation.

Norman Munn (1961) defines communication as 'A form of interaction in which the behaviour of one organism acts as the stimulus, for the behaviour of another'. Yearwood-Grazette (1978) states that:

> Communication is a social process concerned with the flow of information, the circulation of knowledge and ideas in human society and the propagation and internalisation of thoughts.

Fisher (1977: 392) says that 'Communication may be defined as the transmission of meanings to others by the use of symbols'. Highet (1950: 86) says: 'Communication is the transmission of thought from one mind to another.'

Quite a number of definitions exist. It seems to the writer that human communication is, in essence, the transference of a message by some or other means from one person or persons to another person or persons. This requires human interaction.

It is possible for two normal people to be put together in a room and, although they may not say a word to each other, they would communicate in some way. They would be aware of one another, might smile or frown, or show signs of anxiety.

16.2 PROCESS OF COMMUNICATION

For communication to take place, the following are required:

A sender or communicator; a message; a medium or means for sending that message; a recipient; a response.

Translated into the world of nursing education:

- the *sender* can be the tutor, unit professional nurse, patient, other members

326

of the health-care team, other lecturers, relatives and friends of the patient, or the student/s.

- The *message* could be in the form of theoretical knowledge, practical skills, correlation of theoretical knowledge and practical skills, or patient reaction.
- The *medium* is the written or spoken language, or non-verbal means such as gestures.
- The *recipient/s* could be the student/s, patients, relatives or friends.

16.2.1 The sender

In nursing education the *sender* of a message, which can become the means of learning something about the practice of nursing as has been indicated above, need not necessarily be the tutor. This would be to deny the great deal of information which is passed from members of the peer group, that is the students themselves, to one another. It would also leave out the patients or clients for whom the nurse is learning to care, and who are the central figures in the practice of nursing, as well as the relatives and friends who voluntarily or involuntarily supply information (ie send or communicate) which becomes part of the student's knowledge. As this work is concerned chiefly with teaching the practice of nursing in the more formal sense, we will consider the tutor, teaching professional nurse, unit professional nurse or clinical teacher as the main senders of messages. They initiate the process by which communication in nursing education occurs.

16.2.2 The message

This is the knowledge that the student is expected to acquire in order to function properly as a competent practitioner of nursing. It will vary from the natural, biological and human sciences to the technical skills that have to be mastered, and the skills in interpersonal interaction.

It will vary in complexity from simple, almost rote-type learning material to the understanding and applications of complex skills, and the ability to discern differences and how to practise educated judgement and plan expert nursing care.

The 'message' may be short or long. It may be simple or complex. It may also be a reverse message received from the recipient in the form of a test, a question or a bewildered expression which clearly says 'I do not understand!'

16.2.3 The means of communication

When communicating, human beings interact with one another in several ways:

(a) *By the use of language:* Here we have subdivisions of language which may be used between senders and recipients in more than one way:

- *Verbal communication* where the spoken word is actually used.
- *Written communication* where the language used is expressed in writing. This writing may take the form of written texts, notes, chalkboard or transparency summaries, or labelled charts.
- *Sign language:* This does not refer to 'body language' as such, which will be discussed in the next paragraph, but to specially devised sign language, which is used by the deaf to communicate words to one another, or by the use of 'braille' through which the blind can 'read' words which make up the symbols of language.
- *Body language:* This is the language which conveys a message from one person to another by facial expressions, physical withdrawal, touch, or a combination of all three. It is very easy to convey the message, 'That is the wrong thing to do!' without saying a word.

(b) By drawing, making use of symbols such as arrows →, # for a fracture, and charts. Though in some ways these convey meaning which is translated by the recipient into language, there is a subtle difference.

The message can be conveyed by many media, amongst which are:

- The tutor or registered nurse, or another member of the health team
- Films, film strips, film slides
- Tape recorders
- Synchronised slides and tapes
- Textbooks and other forms of written material
- Video cassettes
- Television (open, or in special cases closed-circuit television)
- Charts, posters, pictures
- Models
- The patient's reactions
- The observations made by the student or pupil
- Examples set by good role models
- Laboratory experiments.

The list is endless. The message, that is information required to learn the practice of nursing, offers so much scope for different and varied presentation, for formal and informal teaching, for situational teaching and observation. The whole of chapter 9 is devoted to teaching strategies which can be used to convey the message or subject-matter, and related techniques in nursing education. Therefore, further discussion is unnecessary here.

16.2.4 The recipient

In nursing education, the recipient of information is the student or the pupil.

Chapter 6 was devoted to the student of nursing, and the characteristics of the individuals who are the recipients of nursing education were discussed in some detail.

All that will be emphasised here is that students and pupils

- are individual *human beings;*
- come from different social and cultural backgrounds;
- speak different languages at home;
- learn at different rates;
- have different school backgrounds. Although they must all have Standard 10 to be able to be admitted as students, the subjects that they have studied, and the methods used to teach those subjects also differ considerably;
- need recognition, satisfaction in the work (and thus the learning) situation, encouragement and support;
- need to be able to achieve.

If these aspects are remembered by those who are the deliberate communicators or the senders of planned messages in nursing education, the recipients will have the best possible chance to learn the practice of nursing.

16.2.5 The response

The full cycle of the communication process is completed by the response of the recipient. The ultimate response it is desired to achieve, is the production of the competent nursing practitioner who is capable of independent action based on educated judgement.

Obviously responses will vary in complexity all through the period of nursing education.

The response to a question, the interaction in a class, the interaction between students, between registered nurses and students, between students and patients and between students and other members of the health team, are all part of the process of communication in learning the practice of nursing.

Formal response in the form of replies to testing of various kinds was discussed at length in chapter 15.

The response that comes from the recipient of nursing education in the form of behaviour, attitudes, exhibition of sympathy and empathy, and professionalism, is the product of the communication process.

If there is *no* response, then there is *no* communication. If there is poor response, then the message has not been properly received, and the tutor should seek the reason. It may be due to the student's abilities, her motivation, her attitudes, her state of health, or it may be due to the teaching strategy which is not meeting the needs of the class as a whole or the individual student.

16.3 THE SPOKEN WORD

Because so much teaching in nursing education is done by means of the spoken word, a short section will now be devoted to communication with groups of people by use of the spoken word or public speaking.

It is felt that many students who are studying teaching the practice of nursing could benefit from some insight into the presentation of the spoken word. This section covers far more than actually *speaking* or even the *choice of language* but points out some extremely important aspects which could make all the difference between success and failure in using the spoken word in communicating with large groups.

16.3.1 Appearance of speakers

It still appears to be common practice for tutors (and also for students sitting in class-rooms for hours on end, day after day) to wear 'uniform'.

Beyond the fact that they are the same colour, and that epaulettes with all their appendages, are worn, there is usually nothing 'uniform' about them. (What nurses wear in the wards is not a 'uniform' either, but is protective clothing, but that is another issue.)

Nevertheless, whether wearing 'uniform' or not, the appearance of the tutor before the class is important, for she is a role model for young students. Therefore her dress should be neat, tidy and appropriate at all times. When working with students and patients or clients in the practical situation in the units, proper protective clothing should of course be worn.

With this type of clothing (or so-called uniform) jewellery is inappropriate and rings and watches worn on the arm can actually injure patients when some forms of nursing care are given.

Equally inappropriate when standing in front of a class and dressed in mufti or ordinary clothes are items of apparel or adornment, such as long necklaces, charms with large pendants, dangling earrings and jangling bracelets. They distract the attention of the student from the work in hand, and can be displayed and admired outside the lecture-room setting.

The lecturer, tutor, nurse-educator, call her what you will, should always pay attention to grooming. She should have a neat hairstyle, apply make-up with discretion and varnish fingernails only with a natural colour if in 'uniform'. If one denies students the right to grow long fingernails when working with patients, then one must follow the same rules.

Tutors come in all shapes, sizes and ages. The first time one has to deliver a lecture to a class is a nerve-racking experience. Knowing that one is appropriately dressed, and avoiding fiddling with items of clothing such as scarves, ties or items of jewellery or fidgeting with a belt, a watch, a lock of hair, buttons, keys, pens or even notes, would contribute to a successful lecture.

330

16.3.2 Posture

The impression a lecturer makes before a class can be enhanced or spoiled completely by careless posture.

The class is there to hear what you have to say, to look at appropriate visual aids and to learn. You are there with a purpose – that of the communication of knowledge or ideas. The tutor is paid for her work. She has a responsibility to her class. She does not treat them as though they were of no account by adopting a slouching 'don't care' posture.

Stand tall, with the weight distributed evenly on both feet, which can be spaced slightly apart. One foot can also be slightly in front of the other, but good balance must be maintained.

Stand straight: Do not lean against the wall, the lectern, a chair or any other piece of furniture. The purpose of the furniture or the wall is not to act as a prop for the lecturer. By placing both hands firmly on the lectern, one attains balance and confidence.

If you have enough self-confidence, let your arms hang loosely at your side, use them to handle notes or visual aids. Do not fidget with them.

Stand still: There is nothing more distracting to an audience, in this case your class, than a lecturer pacing up and down like a caged lion. If it is necessary to move to use a piece of apparatus or to gain attention for a point – move purposefully and then stop. No one is going to be rooted to one spot throughout a lecture period, but nor should she hop about like a bird seeking seed. If it is necessary to move forward to emphasis a point, to bring you closer to your class, then do so, but do not move just for the sake of moving. Avoid the two extremes of being glued to one spot, and of pacing backwards and forwards.

Another important factor is that when talking to a class one should make a point of making eye contact with the audience (the students). The eyes should not concentrate on one person or group, but should move around from person to person, from group to group, backwards and forwards, from one side to the other as you are talking. In this way the class gets the feeling that they are all important, that you are interested in them all and not only a few, or in what is going on outside a window or against the ceiling. Eye contact need not be kept up constantly. It will be necessary to consult notes to point to models, charts, etc, but it is vital that rapport be established with your class by this means.

16.3.3 Gestures

A gesture is a significant movement of the hands, body or face. Therefore, when you want to illustrate a point, clarify something, count off the points of what you are saying on the fingers of your hand, point to a specific object, express approval or extreme disapproval of something, make sure that your movements are not wild gesticulations, but that they serve a purpose. Sometimes not only the hand, but the whole arm, or even the whole body can be used. Illustrating to a student what could happen to a paralysed arm and hand, and the subsequent functioning if only shoulder movement were returned, had the patient been allowed to develop a dropped wrist, the fingers had been allowed to stiffen in an open position, and the elbow to stiffen straight, by using appropriate movements can make a point about the care of a patient with hemiplegia very clear. Stiffen the elbow, leave the fingers splayed and try to hold a spoon, using shoulder movements only. Then show the same type of occurrence if the hand had been correctly positioned with the wrist cocked up, the fingertips together and the elbow bent. The gestures you make, the meaningful movements, will illustrate more readily than words how, in the first case, with 'wrong' care, and in the second case, with 'correct' care, the second patient would be able by using shoulder movement only to learn for example to feed himself.

A gesture is not just there for show, it can be a wonderful aid to lecturing. In the course leading up to qualification as a nurse-educator and in the early days of teaching, you must not only work at your lectures carefully and correctly, and select good media aids, but you must also practise delivery and the use of gestures.

16.3.4 Delivery

16.3.4.1 The voice

Some people are blessed (or cursed, depending on your point of view) with loud voices. Nevertheless it is possible to develop your voice through practice.

Modern technology comes to the aid of those who are softly spoken with microphones which can even be worn on the lapel. If the microphone should break down, however, those with weak voices are lost.

A voice has four characteristics:

(a) *Pitch:* It could be high and squeaking or low and husky. Practice can do wonders here. A tape recorder, used in the privacy of one's own room is a great help.

(b) Volume: When softly spoken, try the following:
Practise deep breathing, and use plenty of breath with each sentence. Do not raise the shoulders when breathing in. Aspirate when speaking. It is possible for a whisper to be heard at a distance if there is enough breath behind it. Yawn widely, with an open throat, and then try saying *ah, oh, oo,* starting softly and allowing the volume to increase with each sound.

(c) *Quality* is the identifying characteristic of a sound. The quality of sounds differ, for example when the sounds EEE and OH are produced.

(d) *Duration* is the length of time of a sound. With breath training and practice a sound can be held for a considerable time.

To avoid strain when using your voice, practise breaking up what you have to say into small sections, sentences or phrases, and *pause* for breath in between.

Therefore, the lecturer must concentrate on the following:

(a) *Practise concentrating on the meaning of what you are saying.* Practise talking as though you were talking to a friend on the campus three metres away. Practise frequently so that tension is gradually relaxed. Avoid tight clothing or jewellery constrictions around the neck and relax the neck muscles. It is possible to practise tensing, and then relaxing, the neck muscles at the same time gritting the teeth and then relaxing.

(b) *Stand erect,* chest well out, avoiding stiffening the shoulders or overarching the back. It must feel as though you are stretching upwards, as though your head was being pulled up by a string.

Practise sharp words of command or exclamations and say *no! no! no!* while banging on a desk.

(c) Always enunciate your consonants, and do not rush your delivery.

The above and many more, will help considerably towards improving voice projection.

Shouting is a strain and must be avoided; practising relaxation and controlled breathing exercises, and the gradual development of volume will be beneficial.

16.3.4.2 Pronunciation

There is actually no such thing as 'correct' or 'incorrect' pronunciation in any language; as too many variations occur. The following however, are characteristics of *acceptable* pronunciation:

(a) It should be what is commonly used by educated people. Not a fancy, hoity-toity 'plum in the mouth' delivery, but that which is in common use by people who have had a reasonable level of education.

(b) It should be in current use.

(c) Articulation should be clear so that words do not run into one another or are clipped. Vowels should be accorded their full value, and the consonants should be audible. Where two vowels occur in combination in a word, each should get its value, that is 'cruel' is pronounced 'kroo-el' and 'ruin' 'roo-in'.

(d) When in doubt, either avoid the word and find out from someone who knows, or make use of a good dictionary.

(e) Avoid accenting the wrong syllable, for example

contribute	= konn-TRIBB-yoot
not	= KONN-tri-byoot
demonstrate	= DEMM-on-strayt
not	= de-MONN-strayte
robust	= roh-BUST
not	= ROH-bust.

Examples are endless.

(f) *Affectations* should be avoided. This is when people go out of their way to find a different way of pronouncing words and thus drawing unwarranted attention to the *word*, rather than to *what they are saying*.

16.3.4.3 Common errors to be avoided

(a) The *er, and-er*, or *-um habit:* It is fairly common to employ the odd '-er – um', and 'and-er' in speech but used frequently it is boring and one should avoid more than one such 'error' in 45 seconds. Practise again helps to break down this habit.

(b) *Use of meaningless words and phrases:* A delivery interspersed with 'all that sort of thing', 'you know', 'something or other', 'and so forth' is poor. They make no sense and the lack of specificity spoils delivery.

(c) *Panic action:* If you drop your notes, laugh, pick them up, re-arrange them and continue as though nothing had happened. If the microphone breaks down and you cannot be heard without it, wait for it to be fixed. If a loud noise occurs, such as a jet plane passing overhead, shrug your shoulders, perhaps point upwards and wait until the noise has subsided.

 For those having difficulty with voice projection, a course on the subject with a trained teacher will do wonders. It is important that the *sender* – the tutor, transmits the *message* – the information, to the *recipient* – the student, in such a way that the *response* is learning.

This chapter on communication is only meant as a guide to persons preparing to teach the practice of nursing. A great deal has been written on the subject as a whole, to which readers are referred.

17 *International approaches to nursing education*

This chapter does not pretend to be a definitive or detailed presentation of all nursing education systems in the world. What it will try to do is to explain briefly the systems used in the countries where nursing education has progressed to a reasonable level. It must be pointed out that the developing countries can only provide the type of nursing education which it and its citizens can afford, and that the level of general education is often a deciding factor in the type of nursing education that can be provided.

In most countries of the world there are various levels of training or educating nurses. There are also variations in the way in which nurses are prepared in each category.

17.1 CATEGORIES OF NURSES

The various categories are:

(a) Those being prepared for practice as professional nurses, with some form of licensure or registration
(b) Those being prepared for a semi-professional function, usually for licensing (the licensed practical nurse in America) or for enrolment
(c) Those being prepared to assist the first two categories. These are the nursing assistants, nurses' aides and licensed auxiliary nurses.

The above categories obviously have overlapping areas of practice where the functions carried out by one group are similar to those carried out by another, but basically the pyramid is the same.

Professional nurse

Practical nurse

Assistant to the above categories
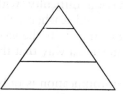

Preparations for registration, that is for the first category, take place in various countries by means of baccalaureate degrees conferred by universities which are associated with hospitals in some way or other for provision of practica; by means of associate degrees conferred by community colleges; by diplomas or certificates achieved through universities; and hospital training schools with or without attached colleges.

The system used depends on the country concerned.

Preparation for enrolment or licensure of the second category, such as the enrolled nurse and the licensed practical nurse, takes place at hospital nursing schools, sometimes in association with the nursing colleges. In some countries it may also form part of the general secondary education system of the country, at special vocational schools, or within the community college system.

The third category is a very large category where the preparation is perhaps the least satisfactory, and where less control is exercised. These nurses may be trained at hospital schools, or at hospitals themselves, at geriatric units and in the psychiatric hospitals. Many of them, as has been shown by recent research, are functioning at levels far beyond their training, and thus beyond levels for safe practice.

Despite the move towards educating more and more nurses at degree level, the vast majority of professional nurses are prepared at hospital nursing schools.

17.2 COURSES OFFERED IN VARIOUS COUNTRIES

A brief discussion of the types of courses offered and their duration, as well as other details of selected countries follows:

17.2.1 Republic of South Africa

17.2.1.1 Courses offered

17.2.1.1.1 For registration

(a) Degrees are offered by universities, the name and the type of course depending on the faculty in which it is offered.

All must meet basic South African Nursing Council regulations, but subjects may be added or increased in depth. Thus we have BSc(Nursing), BA(Nursing), BCur and BSocSc(Nursing) degrees.

- *Duration of course:* Varies from 4 to 4½ years
- *Registration obtained:* General nursing, psychiatric nursing, midwifery and community nursing
- *Minimum lecture periods:*
  - Fundamental nursing science, ethos and professional practice – at least one (1) academic year
  - General nursing science – at least three (3) academic years
  - Psychiatric nursing science – at least two (2) academic years

336

- Midwifery – at least two (2) academic years
- Community nursing science – at least two (2) academic years
- Biological and natural sciences – at least two and a half (2½) academic years
- Pharmacology – at least half (½) an academic year
- Social sciences – at least two (2) academic years

- *Minimum practica hours:* 700 general; 800 midwifery; and 800 psychiatric nursing, and 320 community nursing with periods specified for various units and/or specified practica, as required
- *Entry requirements:* Matriculation or matriculation exemption, that is 12 years of schooling with proper subject choice and level of passing
- *Examination:* To be set by the university concerned
- *Designation on completion:* Registered nurse (professional nurse)
- *Registration body:* South African Nursing Council
- *Finance:* Students at university pay fees. They receive a training allowance from the authorities offering the training.

(b)   Diploma offered at Nursing colleges in association with universities:

- *Duration of course:* four years
- *Registration obtained:* General nursing, midwifery and psychiatric nursing community nursing
- *Minimum lecture periods:* As for degree
- *Minimum practica hours:* As for degree
- *Entry requirements:* A Standard 10 certificate (12 years of schooling)
- *Examination:* Nursing colleges in association with universities
- *Designation on completion:* Registered nurse (professional nurse)
- *Registration body:* South African Nursing Council
- *Finance:* Students pay fees. They receive a training allowance from the authorities offering the training.

(c)   Diploma offered at hospital nursing schools (being phased out):

- *Duration of course:* Three years
- *Registration obtained:* General nurse
- *Minimum lecture periods:* 960
- *Minimum practica hours:* 3 000
- *Entry requirements:* Standard 10 (12 years of schooling) or registration as a midwife or as a psychiatric nurse
- *Examination:* South African Nursing Council
- *Designation on completion:* Registered nurse (professional nurse)
- *Registering body:* South African Nursing Council
- *Finance:* At present students pay no fees and receive a training allowance throughout the course.

17.2.1.1.2 For enrolment

(a)   Certificate for enrolment as a nurse:

- *Duration of course:* Two years
- *Enrolment:* As an enrolled nurse
- *Minimum lecture periods:* 270
- *Minimum practica hours:* Not laid down. Have to be done over a two-year period
- *Entry requirements:* Standard 8 (ten years of schooling)
- *Examination:* Conducted by the South African Nursing Council
- *Designation on completion:* Enrolled nurse (staff nurse)
- *Enrolling body:* South African Nursing Council
- *Finance:* Pupil receives a training allowance throughout the course.

(b)   Certificate of enrolment as a nursing assistant:

- *Duration of course:* 100 days
- *Enrolment:* As enrolled nursing assistant
- *Minimum lecture periods:* 50
- *Minimum practica hours:* 100 days
- *Entry requirements:* Not laid down
- *Designation on completion:* Enrolled nursing assistant
- *Enrolling body:* South African Nursing Council
- *Finance:* Pupil receives a training allowance and pays no fees.

(c)   Diploma for registration as a psychiatric nurse:

- *Duration of course:* In South Africa psychiatric nursing is usually offered as part of a comprehensive course or as a one-year course following on general nursing
- *Registration obtained:* Psychiatric nurse
- *Minimum lecture periods:* 360
- *Minimum practica hours:* 960 (integrated course), with specified times in various areas of psychiatric nursing
- *Entry requirements:* Standard 10 certificate or registration as a nurse or midwife
- *Examination* (except in the case of integrated courses at universities who conduct their own examination): South African Nursing Council
- *Designation on completion:* Registered psychiatric nurse (professional nurse)
- *Registering body:* South African Nursing Council
- *Finance:* At present students pay no fees and receive a training allowance throughout the course.

(d)   Diploma for registration as a midwife:

- *Duration of course:* Except in comprehensive courses, one year for registered nurses, and two years for enrolled nurses
- *Registration:* Registered midwife/accoucheur
- *Minimum lecture periods:* 300
- *Minimum practica hours:* 960 hours (one-year course), with specified times in various areas of midwifery and/or specified practica, as required
- *Entry requirements:* Registration as a general nurse; registration as a psychiatric nurse; or enrolment as a nurse
- *Examination:* South African Nursing Council
- *Designation on completion:* Registered midwife (professional nurse/accoucher)
- *Registering body:* South African Nursing Council
- *Finance:* Students pay no fees and receive a training allowance throughout their course. This course will remain until all professional nurses in practice are prepared by the comprehensive course.

(e)   Post-basic courses: Post-basic degrees for registered nurses, conferring additional qualifications.

Honours, masters and doctoral post-graduate study are available at various universities, and at present courses leading to the following post-basic qualifications are offered by various bodies:

- Community nursing science
- Oncological nursing science
- Paediatric nursing science
- Advanced paediatric nursing science
- Advanced midwifery and neonatal nursing science
- Operating theatre technique
- Intensive nursing science
- Orthopaedic nursing science
- Ophthalmic nursing science
- Geriatric nursing science
- Nursing administration
- Nursing education (nurse–educators or tutors), usually at university level – others are offered at technikons and hospital schools.

Short post-basic courses are also offered leading to a certificate in:

- The nursing of spinal injuries
- Occupational health nursing

The regulations in the RSA are given above in some detail. Like all regulations they are subject to amendment. Any student would therefore be well advised to consult the most recently published regulations.

A short sketch will subsequently be given of the nursing education in several other countries so that the reader can see how they vary. Again, these regulations and systems will alter from time to time, and the reader should always seek up-to-date information.

17.2.2 Great Britain

The majority of schools are hospital nursing schools which offer general, midwifery and psychiatric nursing courses.

Degree courses in nursing are also offered at three universities, Edinburgh, Manchester and Cardiff, while a number of universities offer nursing science and art as an optional course for other degrees. These are not proper nursing degrees as we understand them. The whole nursing curriculum is recognised by these universities as only one subject.

The diploma courses extend over three years.

Nursing education in Great Britain is controlled by the Central Council for Nursing, Midwifery and Health Visiting for the United Kingdom, whose function it is to make provision for the education, training, regulation and discipline of nurses, midwives and health visitors, and to maintain a single professional register. Under this Central Board are four National Boards, one each for England, Scotland, Northern Ireland and Wales, whose functions within the statutory rules of the Council are to provide, at institutions approved by them, for courses of training which meet the requirements of the Central Council regarding content and standard, to hold such examinations as are necessary, to enable persons to satisfy requirements for qualification, and to carry out investigations into alleged misconduct.

Entrance requirements for *enrolment* courses, is simply good general education. No special school certificate is required. Duration of this course is two years.

Registration course
Minimum hours   960 – theory
                 4 760 – clinical

On completion, the student is registered as: State Registered Nurse (SRN) or Registered General Nurse (RGN)
If training is in mental nursing: Registered Mental Nurse (RMN)
If training is in the nursing of the mentally subnormal: Registered Nurse for the Mentally Subnormal (RNMS)

Enrolled nurse
Minimum hours: 350 theory
               + 80 clinical teaching
                 3 330 clinical practica

Training for nurse-tutors and health visitors is provided at the level of universities and polytechnics or institutes for advanced education.

Other post-basic courses which include Registered Sick Children's Nursing (RSCN), Clinical Teaching, District Nursing, Ophthalmic Nursing and Orthopaedic Nursing, are offered at staff college or hospital school level.

The Joint Board of Clinical Nursing Studies which was concerned mainly with training in post-basic courses, now falls under the Central Council.

Students receive a salary during training.

At the moment proposals are being made for a change. A three-year course with two years common to all and a third elective specialist year is being suggested.

17.2.3 New Zealand

The general pattern is very similar to that in Great Britain, with training done at hospital nursing schools, although polytechnics now offer nursing courses and the policy is to move all nursing education into such institutions in time. University education for nurses is limited to post-registration courses.

The *registering body* is the New Zealand Nursing Council.

Admission requirements: Full secondary education is not required for training in New Zealand, except of course for university courses.

General, midwifery and psychiatric and psychopaedic training courses are offered. The basic general nursing course is three years. Enrolled nursing courses exist, varying in duration from 12 to 18 months. Nurses in training receive a salary at hospital schools but not at polytechnics.

17.2.4 Australia

There are eight nurses' registration boards in Australia, each state having its own, as do the Australian Capital Territory and the Northern Territory.

In all these states the pattern of nursing education is still similar to that in Great Britain, the nursing schools are all hospital based and students receive a salary while training. Entrance requirements do not stipulate full secondary school education.

Colleges for advanced education now also offer courses in basic nursing education. Admission to these courses does require full secondary education. Students in these courses receive the allowances that are paid to all students at higher education institutions in Australia. These colleges have to make arrangements with the hospitals for practica.

There is no basic degree course in nursing in Australia. Courses offered are in general nursing, midwifery and psychiatric nursing. Enrolled nurses are also trained and post-basic courses include midwifery, intensive care nursing and geriatric and rehabilitation nursing. Degrees in Applied Science are offered for registered nurses at Institutes of Health Science (Institutes of Technology).

17.2.5 Canada

Basic registration in Canada may be obtained by following a baccalaureate degree or a diploma course.

There are 11 registration areas and diploma graduates have to write the registration examination set by one of these registration bodies. University courses vary from four to five years' duration and lead to a baccalaureate degree in nursing. Post-basic degrees exist for registered nurses and post-graduate education facilities are excellent.

Before 1964 all diploma courses were offered in hospital schools. Diploma programmes varying in length from two to three years are increasingly being offered at post-secondary level at schools within the general provincial educational system. These courses appear to be phasing out the hospital school system. This is in keeping with the trend towards placing *all* post-secondary education under the auspices of educational authorities, and the higher status accorded to education in 'junior' colleges and universities.

Educational programmes of ten to 18 months for nursing assistants (practical nurses or nurses' aides) are provided at hospital nursing schools and are approved either by the provincial nurses' association, the Department of Health, or a Board of Registration of nursing assistants.

In all except two provinces this category of worker is licensed. No educational admission requirement is stated.

Psychiatric nurses are trained in the four western provinces (British Columbia, Alberta, Saskatchewan and Manitoba only).

17.2.6 The United States of America

In the United States a separate registration body exists for each state, all of which set their own State board examinations.

Diploma courses are offered at hospital nursing schools, although the policy is to phase these out, and to train all professional nurses at degree level. The diploma courses still accept three years as the norm although some are shorter. The clinical component varies considerably, the average being 3 200 hours.

Registered professional nurse students must have full secondary education. The degree courses vary in length from four to five years.

The practical component of nursing education is supplied by hospital and health institutions, several of which are affiliated to the larger universities.

It appears as though the controlled practical experience varies between 1 000 and 2 000 hours. Theoretically the students are supernumerary and are under constant supervision by faculty members, the ratio varying from five to 12 students to one instructor. Night duty experience is very limited.

Associate degree programmes: These are two-year programmes offered at community colleges, and are financed by municipalities or city councils of the various states. The fees are low.

The practical component is very low indeed, being limited to 84 'activities', which vary from carrying out specific procedures to being assigned to full care of one patient for a period of time.

Nursing graduates from four- to five-year university degree programmes, from two-year community colleges, and from three-year hospital school diploma courses, all have to write the State board examinations and are all called *registered nurses*.

All nursing students pay for their education. Some of the hospital schools make a small allowance to students, but only in the third year of study.

Practical training for *licensing as practical nurses* is offered in junior colleges or vocational colleges. This is a one-year course to which the educational entrance requirement is equivalent to ten years of schooling (Standard 8).

Nurses' aides, orderlies and nursing assistants are also trained to meet the needs of the service. These courses are of a short, intensive pre-service or a form of in-service, on-the-job training.

Post-basic education facilities are excellent, most of them at post-graduate level. Midwifery is not generally offered.

17.2.7 Belgium

Basic nursing education is of two types, the three-year course which requires an education entrance level of 12 years' general education, and a two-year course.

The nursing schools are independently organised and financed and are linked to hospitals.

Some courses in the technical education system are also linked to hospitals. Undergraduate, post-graduate and post-basic nursing education are well developed.

Post-basic specialisation can be done in paediatric nursing (one year); midwifery (one year); psychiatric nursing (one year); nursing education (two years) and social work (nursing) (two years).

Post-graduate degrees are offered in nursing education and administration, and nursing education in these disciplines is also offered at diploma level.

The Ministry of Health supervises the examination and registration of nurses.

The theory and practica component of courses is more or less as follows:

For the three-year programme:	1 800 hours theory
	2 500 hours practica
For the two-year programme:	960 hours theory
	2 400 hours practica

17.2.8 The Netherlands

Basic training is offered in general nursing or psychiatric nursing (course I) for which the entrance requirement is ten years of schooling, or for the *higher vocational* training for nurses programme, which is of 11 or 12 years' duration (course II).

Secondary vocational training for nurses also has a ten-year general education admission requirement (course III).

The Ministry of Health is the supervisory, certification and licensing authority.

The theoretical and practical requirements are as follows:

Course I:	1 060 hours theory
	3 540 hours practica
Course II:	2 220 hours theory
	2 600 hours practica
Course III:	2 150 hours theory
	1 556 hours practica

Post-basic courses exist in sick children's nursing, public health nursing, social psychiatric nursing, nurse-tutor training, clinical teaching, middle management and administration. Maternity nursing and midwifery courses are also available.

17.2.9 Switzerland

Nursing education in Switzerland offers preparation for *registered general nurses, registered maternal and child-care nurses, and registered psychiatric nurses.*

In the first two categories the supervisory function is exercised by the Swiss Red Cross Society. They also certify competence by examination. The third category is supervised by the Swiss Association for Psychiatry. Nursing schools are run by religious organisations. Both Catholic (nuns) and Protestant (deaconesses) schools are private foundations, which enter into contract with certain hospitals to supply clinical experience to their students. There are now also many public hospitals which set up their own nursing schools.

17.2.10 The Scandanavian countries

In Norway, Sweden and Denmark, nursing schools have been set up. They are administered and financed separately from hospitals. Some of the schools are privately owned and some are municipal hospitals financed by municipal or state funds.

General and midwifery training is provided, and the Ministries of Health in each country supervise the training and examinations and register those who qualify.

Denmark offers post-basic nursing education for tutors and nurse-administrators at university level.

In Finland the pattern is similar, but the schools are established and supervised by the Ministry of Education, thus giving nursing education tertiary education status, which is not the case in the other countries.

In Denmark the training period is three and a half years, the theory component being 1 500 hours and the practica 4 500 hours.

17.2.11 Nursing schools in France, Spain, Italy, Portugal and Greece

Most provide two to three-year courses of training in general nursing. The schools are organised in the same way as are the Swiss schools and supervision is exercised by the Ministries of Health, which are also the registering or licensing bodies.

Clinical experience is obtained on contract with hospitals and students pay for their courses, although a few hospitals pay the students a small allowance when they are doing clinical practica there. In France (Royal College of Nursing 1977), theory occupies 1 328 hours and practica 2 152 hours. Admission to nursing schools in these countries is ten years of schooling (Standard 8).

So far none have developed a university system for educating nurses at either a basic or post-basic level.

A few schools offer some form of post-basic specialisation.

17.2.12 The Far East

17.2.12.1 Hong Kong

The programmes of nursing education follow the British pattern and registered general nurses and midwives and enrolled nurses are trained. Public health nursing courses for registered nurses are of nine months' duration, and in-service courses in various specialities such as orthopaedic nursing, paediatric nursing, psychiatric nursing and the nursing management of medical and

345

surgical nursing, are given. The pattern of general nursing education and midwifery is also based on the British pattern, that is general nursing takes three years, midwifery one year, enrolled nursing two years. All training is hospital- and nursing school based. Community health courses are the only post-basic ones available, and they are not registrable as post-basic qualifications.

Basic or post-basic education at university level does not exist. In order to qualify as nurse-tutors or to specialise in any other field of nursing, nurses have to leave Hong Kong. Australia and the USA are usually selected for post-basic study mainly because of the geographical proximity, which makes fares less expensive than travelling to the United Kingdom.

17.2.12.2 Japan

Nursing education is controlled by the Public Health Nurse, Midwife and Nurse Law.

The basic course consists of a three-year programme, which includes 3 375 theory hours and a minimum of 1 770 hours of clinical practica. The students are required to pass a national examination after the minimum three-year training. Admission to these courses is completion of high school education (12 years of schooling). Hospital schools, some of which are national hospitals, and some of which are private institutions offer the course.

There is also a four-year degree course available for the training of professional nurses at university level.

Junior colleges of nursing also offer professional nurse training, which is of three years' duration.

Before licensure by the Ministry of Health and Welfare all nurses, whether trained at universities, junior colleges or hospital schools, have to pass a national examination.

A two-year course leading to licensure as a nurse also exists. The total theoretical instruction required is 2 250 hours with 915 hours of clinical practica. The syllabus is the same as that of the three-year course. Admission to this course is nine years of ordinary schooling, plus a three-year high school nursing course. The same national examination must be passed.

A two-year assistant nurse course is also offered. An examination conducted by the prefectures leads to licence as an assistant nurse.

Three years' experience as a licensed assistant nurse can lead to admission to the three-year course for full national licensure.

Midwifery and public health are studied at post-basic level, and courses also exist for registered nurses to qualify as tutors. All require the passing of a national examination before licensing.

Student nurses in Japan enjoy supernumerary status. There are as yet no post-graduate nursing courses.

17.2.12.3 Taiwan

There are three ministries concerned with health and education.

- *The Ministry of Health (Health Yuan)* is concerned with all aspects of community health and the licensing of all medical and nursing personnel. The Commissioner of Health makes the final decision in cases of disciplinary action, which are usually dealt with by the institutions concerned or the courts in the case of a serious offence.
- *The Ministry of Education* controls the educational standards of the medical and nursing courses.
- *The Ministry of Examinations* is concerned with the standards of all professional examinations.

There are Health Boards within the framework of these authorities, and one or two nurse representatives serve on these boards.

- *Public health nurses:* The one-year post-basic training was stopped in 1975. Public health is integrated into the general nursing curriculum. Each nurse has between 8 000 and 8 500 members of the population under her care.
- *Teaching and training* of medical students and senior nursing students is done at the National Taiwan University. Each student is placed under supervision of a public health nurse after one week's orientation period, and she is assigned to take care of ten families. Health workers and foreign health workers are given orientation and refresher courses at the Centre.

17.2.12.3.1 Nursing education

All nursing education is offered by universities or colleges. There are no hospital-based diploma schools for professional nurses in Taiwan.

The system of general education entails six years' primary schooling, three years' junior high, and three years' senior high school, after which the person is eligible for entry to university.

There are, however, two categories of nurses, vocational and professional, and both have to write licensing examinations.

The vocational nurse completes nine years of basic schooling and a three-year nursing course at a technical school. She is then qualified to give direct nursing care, and may take an additional one-year course in midwifery in preparation for a rural practice.

The integration of general nursing and midwifery is not favoured. Nurse leaders believe that nurses should follow only one of the two and that to follow both entails a 'waste of education'. However, the professional course includes a substantial component of maternity nursing, psychiatric nursing and community health, together with general nursing.

Provision is made for professional education at technical schools on the basis of nine years' schooling, plus a five-year nursing course, or 12 years' schooling and a two-year nursing course, on the pattern of the USA Associate Degree courses.

University education is highly valued and admission to a nursing course requires strict selection. The university takes only top school graduates, and an entrance examination is required of all applicants.

Nursing rates approximately 25th on the list of career choices. Chemistry and physics are often the most desired courses; however, there is stiff competition for the 40 places offered annually at the National Taiwan University.

17.2.12.3.2 The National Taiwan University

The university consists of a number of colleges, the School of Nursing being part of the College of Medicine. There are five other schools within the College including a School of Public Health, which has a graduate nurse-lecturer on the staff.

The Dean of each school sits on the Board of the College of Medicine, and the rotating chairman is a member of the senate of the university.

The bachelor of science degree in nursing was offered for the first time in 1956. It is a four-year course requiring 156 credits, which are acquired on a semester basis.

The credit system is calculated as follows:

Theory: 14 to 16 hours = one credit

Practica: Three to four hours per week for 16 weeks = one credit.

The total requirement for practical work would appear to be in the region of 1 200 hours.

The baccalaureate programme aims to prepare nurse-teachers and administrators.

Practical training is undertaken at the National Taiwan University Hospital which accepts only university students, except perhaps in the vacation when students from the Technical College may be admitted. Apart from one vacation in their third year, the students are not required to work during their vacation.

All faculty members hold joint appointments. They are university lecturers, as well as hospital supervisors in the area of their speciality. The students are regarded as supernumerary. At present there is one supervisor to every eight students (one to four is regarded as ideal).

(a) *Examinations:* The final licensing examination is of the multiple-choice type. Eight or nine papers are written in two days. Each paper usually consists of 100 questions to be answered in 100 minutes. On graduation, the student is equipped to function as a general nurse and tutor.

(b) *Fees:* The students pay for their education and training; scholarships are available from the government or city authorities.

(c) *Midwifery courses:* There are one-year courses for students of vocational schools, and schools for midwives provide a two-year course. However, information on midwifery training is scarce. Deliveries are done by the doctors, who approximately equal the nurses in number, hence the need is for maternity nurses, not independent midwives. Only the rural areas require midwives.

(d) *Psychiatric nursing:* There is no separate licensure, and no community psychiatric service. Patients attend the day hospital and clinic. Although the family is very much involved in their care, the nurse has the first and lasting contact with the patient, and a psychiatric social worker is not needed. Short in-service psychiatric courses are offered to registered nurses by the nurse-instructor/supervisor.

(e) *Public health nurses:* Nurses may read for a master's degree at the School of Public Health, but the majority undertake graduate studies in the USA. In-service training is undertaken, the registered nurse then being employed in the field and drawing a full salary.

(f) *Other post-basic courses:* The university offers short in-service courses (of two months' duration) in either medical or surgical intensive nursing care.

Although there is said to be no discrimination between the sexes, male nursing students are not encouraged.

(g) *Nurse aides:* Apparently there are currently few people in this category. They apparently receive little training.

17.2.13 The Soviet Union

Nursing is part of an integrated medical service, and not a separate profession. All teaching personnel at nursing schools are doctors, with the exception that senior nurses may supervise students during their practical experience. Evening school programmes are available in basic nursing education but they take a year longer than the full-time course.

About five per cent of the best students are selected for medical school at the end of the nursing course. Other nurses, if suitable, may continue to higher medical school after the obligatory three years' service, following completion of their nursing course (Quinn 1968: 80, 82).

Nurses are in the middle medical category along with feldshers and midwives. The latter two categories are prepared to work much more independently than the nurse.

The education of nurses, as of other middle medical workers, is the responsibility of the Ministry of Health of the USSR, which plans and approves the educational programme. This programme is uniform throughout the Soviet Union, being financed by the State.

Nursing students with eight years of schooling can be admitted to the course which is then of two years and ten months' duration. If the student has full secondary education, the programme is one year shorter.

Feldsher courses are four years in length for those with eight years of general education and three years for those with full secondary education.

17.2.14 Africa

The nursing education that has developed in the African States has followed the pattern of the colonising powers, and the level of general education that the populace has achieved under colonial rule. This pattern also applies throughout the world.

All this will have shown the considerable variation in the nursing education of the various countries.

Nursing education is dynamic and as educated students become available so the nursing education pattern will develop until the most sophisticated needs are met. This takes time and vision on the part not only of those responsible for health services, but also on the part of those providing basic education.

18 *Special aspects of training nurse-tutors*

18.1 MICRO-TEACHING

This is a useful teaching strategy for the training of nurse-educators.

Micro-teaching aims at reducing the many aspects of teacher training into its various components.

In order to carry out micro-teaching, a special laboratory is necessary. This consists of a small basic class-room with all the necessary technical facilities available such as desks and seats, a chalkboard, an overhead projector with its special, fixed slanted screen, a slide and a film projector, the facilities for hanging charts, and for using other teaching aids. The seating facilities should accommodate about eight to ten students. A video-tape machine must be available, which then records the whole process for review, for students to recognise and correct their own faults, as well as for the instructor to be able to point these out.

Small groups work together. Students are required to prepare a short teaching session, with a clear statement of objectives, a planned methodology and the planned use of learning aids.

To commence the exercise the student should be given five minutes to become familiar with facing a camera. This time can be used in various ways, for example by telling a short story, introducing herself and her background, and relating an actual experience.

After this exercise, the student presents the prepared lesson for the period of time decided upon, usually eight to ten minutes. Fellow members of the group act as students. Throughout the entire teaching session, that is the student's presentation and the reaction of those being 'taught', is filmed.

The video-tape of this lesson is then played back, which enables the presenter to criticise her own performance.

Aspects to be considered, are the following:

- Posture
- Any irritating mannerisms or habits of speech
- The use of the voice (audibility, flexibility and whether understood), and of language (suitability – explanation of 'strange' terms, etc)
- The manner of presentation
- The content
- The handling of teaching aids
- The reaction of the 'class' (fellow students) to her teaching.

351

The student group and the instructor also view the tape and render appropriate *constructive* criticism and suggestions.

The student presenter can play the video-tape back herself to reassess her strengths and weaknesses, and she can also use the video-tape apparatus for recording practice sessions on her own. It is quite frightening to see and hear oneself for the first time, but groups working together learn from the mistakes and good points of others, and it is invaluable for self-evaluation.

After review the student should repeat the lesson, aiming at improvement of methodology and presentation as a whole.

The instructor must ensure that student confidence is built up and not broken down. Micro-teaching is excellent preparation for the further stage of teaching in the real-life situation. It is an *aid* to teaching would-be teachers how to teach, and not the whole of it. Actual practice in the live situation cannot be replaced by micro-teaching.

18.2 CREATIVITY IN THE TRAINING OF NURSE-TUTORS*

The Concise Oxford Dictionary defines creativity as the 'state of originating', while Chambers explains it as 'the act of bringing into being, making, producing or designing'.

Listening to the radio I heard someone describing creativity as man's inherent denial of the inevitable – death: his way of seeking immortality by producing something new, be it in art form, in building, in the laboratory or in the written word, or in any other sense. He likened man's creativity to the four slaves or captives depicted by Michaelangelo, slaves striving to escape from the bonds that hold them fast in stone. An interesting thought: Is the motivation of those training nurse-tutors to try to achieve a form of immortality by producing those who will carry on where they leave off? The Reader's Digest book *Use the right word – a guide to modern synonyms* (1968) supplied the following – 'Creative suggests the entire process whereby things that did not exist before are conceived, given form and brought into being'. It further suggests that to be creative 'originality', 'imagination', 'inventiveness', 'resourcefulness' and 'ingenuity' are necessary. From all this I have deduced that creativity is the state of producing something which did not previously exist – and that originality, imagination, inventiveness, resourcefulness, and ingenuity are all part of creativity.

These thoughts on creativity could now be related to the training of nurse-tutors, and a creative approach to this task suggested.

Nurse-tutors, or nurse-educators are at present in very short supply. Many people who are nurses, but not necessarily trained nurse-tutors, are

*Freely adapted from a paper presented by Mellish at a symposium to celebrate 25 years of degree training at the University of Pretoria, July 1981.

engaged in teaching the practice of nursing.

In many professions, the practitioner teaches the neophytes. Thus the practice of medicine is taught by medical men, the practice of law by legal persons, the practice of dentistry by dentists, the practice of physiotherapy by physiotherapists, and so on. It is therefore to be expected that the practice of nursing should be taught by nurses. What is perhaps unique is that the nursing profession actually trains some of its practitioners in the art and science of teaching. This may stem from the fact that every nurse has a teaching responsibility of some sort and therefore the realisation that better teaching will be done by trained teachers is more readily perceived. Another profession that regularly makes use of trained teachers to educate its neophytes is that of teaching itself.

It is not suggested that all the teaching of student and pupil nurses should be done by trained tutors. This would be to deny the extremely important role of the unit professional nurse in educating the young nurse.

However, to say that the unit professional nurse is without any form of training in teaching is also wrong, for General Nursing Art and Science III of the South African Nursing Council requires, according to the regulations, three papers of three hours' duration each; an oral examination in clinical practica (including ward administration, *clinical instruction* and professional practice), and the directive on Nursing Art and Science III states that ward administration, *clinical instruction,* and professional practice must be examined in paper 3.

What we are concerned with here is the training of nurse-educators or tutors who for the most part at present, function in our nursing colleges and universities, and who follow a university course leading to a diploma in nursing education.

There are some tutors trained thus, who have been appointed nursing service managers in charge of large training schools, where their background or nursing education is invaluable, and a few, sadly only a handful, who are in the field of clinical teaching, where they can supply a dimension to nursing education which is of inestimable benefit to the education of a nurse as a whole. Perhaps, when present shortages have been eliminated, there will be more trained nurse-educators functioning outside nursing colleges. Furthermore an exchange system could be organised, which would bring the college tutor back into the clinical field for short periods of time to clearly keep in mind the teaching of the *practice* of nursing.

Creative teaching, according to Schweer (1972: 40, 41) is 'providing unlimited opportunities for individuals and groups to assume their own responsibility for furthering their learning experiences', it is 'approaching each teaching experience as a new and unique assignment, which demands understanding and concern for the individual students, and the utmost skill

353

in working with the subject matter'.

How then can we go about using and fostering creativity in the training of this elite corps of nurses, the nurse-tutors, so that they in turn will produce that which did not previously exist, that is the registered nurse or enrolled nurse, from the student or pupil?

The tutor herself should be capable of creative thinking, should display originality, imagination, inventiveness, resourcefulness and ingenuity, characteristics which should have been fostered in her own training or education.

18.2.1 Search for suitable candidates

In order to train nurse-tutors, with or without creativity, one has to have the would-be tutor to train. Finding and selecting suitable candidates for this important task is not easy, and in many instances the approach is haphazard, to say the least.

Producing future registered and enrolled nurses is the responsibility of all and I mean *all* those who are concerned with nursing as a profession. Perhaps a creative approach to the *search for suitable candidates* is where we should begin.

It is suggested that every nursing service managers in charge of a hospital should have some means of seeking potential tutors from amongst her registered personnel. These would be registered nurses who, in their activity in the unit, use their imagination, resourcefulness and ingenuity in creating learning situations for students and pupils. The future registered or enrolled nurse is, for a large part of her training programme, entrusted to the care and guidance of the unit professional nurse to learn the practice of nursing. Many registered nurses demonstrate teaching potential in this way. The means for identifying them should not only be there, but the responsibility clearly stated, and accepted by all nursing service managers (nurse-administrators).

It should also be policy for regular reports to be made on particularly gifted students who have shown promise during their course or training. These reports should not only give an idea of how the ex-student is faring as a registered nurse, but should specifically state any teaching potential observed. Unfortunately there are those nurse-administrators who actively discourage applicants for post-basic courses which are not clinical, because they fear they will lose good unit professional nurses. Such nurse-administrators lack the imagination and resourcefulness that should be displayed in seeking those who could benefit the profession as a whole, by training to teach the future generations of registered nurses. They are also likely to lose the professional nurse in any case for if she is interested in furthering her studies, she will seek an employer who will make it possible for her to do so.

It is also suggested that nursing colleges could play a part in identifying possible future tutors amongst their students. The progress of such persons could then be watched carefully as they gain the necessary experience in carrying out the duties of registered nurses, to see whether teaching potential is also displayed.

It should also be the clearly defined policy of the head offices of the nursing service departments to actively and systematically recruit student tutors amongst the entire personnel. Only in this way could sufficient suitable applicants for nurse-tutor courses be found. Here creativity could again be brought into play. Originality in notices calling for applications, resourcefulness in visiting hospitals, speaking at 'sisters' meetings, and ingenuity in ensuring that all potential tutors are aware of the availability of study facilities should all be displayed.

Potential candidates must then be encouraged to apply in good time and given every reasonable opportunity to make use of such facilities. It is not suggested that nothing of this sort is done – only that the approach could be more creative in order to produce better results. All programmes for training nurse-tutors are at present under-subscribed. This is a cause for concern.

In a country that in 1980 had about 21 000 student nurses, as well as many pupil nurses in training, only 40 extra tutors were added to the register. On the registers of the South African Nursing Council there were only 1 223 tutors, many of whom, as we are all well aware, are not actively engaged in teaching. Some are retired, some are not practising and some are working as nursing service managers in areas where little or no training falls within their ambit.

Shortages of tutors are likely to be perpetuated if this aspect of *seeking and finding* does not receive immediate attention.

18.2.2 Creativity in the training programme

Once the suitable applicants have been found, it is the duty of all those concerned with their education to produce something *that did not previously exist,* the nurse-tutors who in their turn will display creativity in their teaching role. But first we all need to take a long hard look at our present programmes and the methods which are used to achieve tutor registration.

The student tutor enters the course with a background of at least a diploma in general nursing, usually in midwifery as well, and often with some further post-registration diploma in one or other clinical field. She will probably also have at least two years of clinical practice as a registered nurse behind her.

This means that she has a certain amount of knowledge and experience. How then are we to provide as Schweer said, those 'unlimited opportunities for her to assume responsibility for furthering her learning experiences, which is creative teaching'?

Those teaching in the course must now approach the education of the student or group of students as a unique assignment, with understanding and concern for the individual students, and the utmost skill in working with the subject-matter. Many students will come to the course with preconceived ideas and with expectations of having the subject-matter presented to them in much the same manner as it was done in their basic, or even post-basic courses. While it is known that colleges of nursing do attempt to present subject-matter by means of projects, modules, assignments, mini-courses and learning programmes, the tutor standing before the class, delivering a formal lecture is still the method most commonly employed. This is due to the system, the time factor and the shoab01tage of tutors, all of which allow little opportunity for individual work.

The product of such programmes will not be able to adjust easily to the creative approach in the presentation of subject-matter in the tutor course.

Concern for the difficulties of individual students and assistance so that they can assume responsibility for their own learning experiences, must be shown. Students may never have had to decide for themselves how much time they need on each subject, or how to go about drawing up a study timetable. They may not know how to actually tackle study itself, especially when this does not simply entail what has been presented, but entails self-activity in the form of assigned reading, among other things.

Beyond the sheer mass of work which has to be covered, the new student will also be unfamiliar with the new surroundings, with the library, even with the town in which she finds herself. All these need understanding and sometimes ingenuity to prevent frustration.

Having overcome initial difficulties the student now settles down to study.

18.2.3 Are tutors' courses too short?

This is a moot point. Potential tutors are already products of an education programme which is in fact a programme of tertiary education. Three years of nursing education, post-Standard 10, should be sufficient background for student tutors. That it is not always the case is not the fault of the student, but of the way in which the course has been presented to her. It also depends on whether she has really mastered the subject-matter, or only been able to reproduce it for an examination, and thus forgets it immediately afterwards. Another factor is whether post-course study is encouraged and made possible by continuous in-service education programmes.

The object of the tutor course should be to build on existing knowledge of the student tutor, to develop creative thinking and the ability to establish priorities, to encourage and facilitate learning in the student nurses of the future and to develop her own potential to the full.

Many courses are overloaded and the student is chased from pillar to post, constantly struggling to keep up with the assignments, and to pass the tests and examination which will enable her to register as a nurse-tutor. There is little time for her to do much self-directed study or to develop critical judgement and the ability to think independently.

On the other hand, one is also aware of the effect that degree courses which last for a minimum of three years have on students. It is true that most of our post-registration degrees offer triple registration, and are therefore also very heavy. However, the extra time taken for a degree does give students something that they miss in many of the diploma courses. Is it not time that all tutors be prepared at degree level? Degrees that are planned for tutor registration only, and are not marathon survival courses, providing multi-disciplinary registration.

In fostering creativity in the training of nurse-tutors, it is suggested that the following be considered:

- Careful statement of general and specific objectives
- Co-ordinated planning by all departments offering the course
- Consideration of the need for a degree course in nursing education to prepare the student tutor more effectively for her future role
- Devising and applying proper recruitment techniques in order to find the maximum number of potential candidates for nurse-tutor courses to meet future needs
- Re-designing courses to allow for more guided independent study
- Incorporation of pre-testing so that students with good background knowledge can proceed more rapidly to the more difficult sections by independent study
- Constant reviewing of existing programmes to ensure that they meet not only present, but also future needs
- Re-orientation of those concerned with the training of nurse-tutors so that they understand the creative approach to teaching and that in *bringing into being, originating or designing* nurse-tutor programmes, *to produce that which did not previously exist* – the trained nurse-tutor – they must be allowed to escape from the bonds that bind them to the conventional approach.

A creative approach means that *originality* is used, *imagination* is given free rein, *inventiveness* is displayed, *resourcefulness* is practised, and *ingenuity* is employed.

The need of the profession for many, well-prepared nurse-tutors is well known. Let us *find* the potential tutors, and then use *a creative approach* in their training, so that they in turn may help to produce many, well-equipped, well-educated, creative nurses, for the ultimate benefit of all our patients and clients, whom it is our privilege to serve.

Whether, in so doing, those preparing nurse-tutors would achieve immortality, is difficult to decide. But they would be able to pass on to the future generations of tutors the ability to continue to help produce the quality of registered nurses of whom we can be justly proud.

18.2.4 Presentation of subject-matter

In most university programmes, different subjects are presented by those with special knowledge in the field.

The natural and biological sciences often present the greatest stumbling blocks. Here the department responsible for the overall co-ordination of the course can do much to point out to the departments concerned just what the objectives of the course are and the level of knowledge students need. This can present many difficulties, as anyone who has ever tried to explain to a lecturer studying towards a doctorate in physics, what background knowledge is needed by the student tutor for a course in anatomy and physiology, will know.

Student tutors have to be prepared to lecture to student nurses in the elementary aspects of physics and chemistry, and in anatomy and physiology, microbiology, parasitology, pathological anatomy and pharmacology. But they do not have to become physicists or chemists in 120 easy lectures. Nor do they have to become anatomists, physiologists, microbiologists, pharmacologists or pathologists.

Perhaps this is one of the areas where creativity could be employed. A clear statement of objectives, inventiveness in drawing up a programme, which may involve many periods of guided self-study, and resourcefulness in its use might be the answer. Inventiveness is a practical kind of creativity, combining the qualities of an analytical mind with a common-sense approach to the needs of students. Resourcefulness, that is solving the problem despite its limitations, finding the available means and adapting them to the end in view, could perhaps resolve many of the difficulties which confront student tutors.

Despite the fact that lecturers are extremely busy people, and that they change from time to time, a positive move to sort out the needs and difficulties could be attempted. Round-table discussions and a clear delineation of objectives, both general and specific, for all the aspects of the course where doubt might exist, would be a creative move and facilitate the work in the long run.

The teaching of teaching skills is usually left to an education department which is surely fully aware of the need to use creative teaching and to instil creativity into student tutors.

It is, however, often the responsibility of the nursing science department to translate what is taught by the educationalists into subject didactics, and

358

to apply this to teaching the practice of nursing. Here creativity can be brought into play, provided it is approached not only with enthusiasm, but with realism.

We are all aware of the various teaching strategies that are available to us, for example the lecture, the demonstration, assignments, projects, group discussions, case studies, workbooks, field trips, tutorials, programmed learning, seminars, role play and other simulation techniques, to name a few, and in the clinical field, use of the teachable moment (situational teaching), ward rounds, nursing rounds and clinics, patient-centred discussions, problem solving in the unit, nursing care plans and the application of the process of nursing (nursing methodology to patient care), writing and giving of reports, peer-group teaching, and many more.

Although all of these are usually taught theoretically to student tutors, they are often required to give formal lectures and are examined in this technique. One could ask, however, how much practice is possible or required in our present courses when mastering many of the other techniques? Opportunities for practice appear to be very limited. True, the student tutor will be given assignments, but working out your own study is quite different from allocating and assessing those of others.

18.2.5 The use of teaching aids

All courses which train nurse-tutors contain a section devoted to the use of technical teaching aids or media. This aspect of tutor training is surely one area where creativity can be allowed full play. Just how much this contributes towards making the student tutor proficient in the preparation of material such as transparencies, models, charts, even slides and films or videotape presentations, varies considerably. Student tutors are introduced to the use of technical software and hardware as teaching aids, they are encouraged to produce suitable material to use in formal lectures.

Some go so far as to arrange exhibitions of teaching aids produced by students. The student tutor must have the time and opportunity to develop skills in the preparation of teaching aids. Many students, when first required to produce teaching aids, are absolutely horrified at the idea, and yet when given an outline of simple techniques, the opportunity to practise under expert guidance, as well as the materials with which to do so, are amazed at what they can do. Perhaps time is again the limiting factor.

Ingenuity, resourcefulness and imagination come into play in the creation of something which did not exist before.

Skill at handling slide and film projectors and the effective use of overhead projectors, the proper use of commercially prepared charts and models are only some of the skills that creative teaching can develop.

18.2.6 Evaluation techniques

Tutors, when they are qualified, will be expected to set and mark tests and examinations. In order to develop their skills in this direction, they need more than a course of lectures on the subject. They need to be given the opportunity to draw up various types of tests or examinations. They need to be able to try out proposed tests and to gain experience in assessing the validity of the testing instruments that have been drawn up. They need to be able to draw up memoranda against which various test questions will be marked. They need to be able to mark test papers independently and compare results.

Surely creativity in the training of nurse-tutors can be used to good effect in this section of the course. The pure educationalists need assistance from the nurse-educationalists in the assessment of what is relevant (an overworked word), what is important in subject-matter for the student tutor to include in the proposed test, and what value should be allocated to each point in a factual answer. Again a plea is made for greater co-ordination between the lecturers in different sections of the course, so that objectives are spelt out clearly and are for the benefit of all.

18.3 IN-SERVICE EDUCATION AND NURSE-TUTORS*

Mellish (1978) defined in-service education as meeting the following requirements:

- It is given to people while they are employed.
- It is deliberately planned.
- It is designed to meet specific needs, to fill gaps in learning or to remedy deficiencies in the knowledge and skills of employees.
- It aims at more efficient functioning on the part of the employee.
- It aims at better functioning of the organisation.
- It usually follows on a period of pre-service education.
- It is only a part of continuing education.

She identified the nurse-educators as one of the groups that required in-service education. It may be asked why this group of nurses, who undergo a very stiff university training in order to qualify for tutor registration, should at all require continuing or in-service education?

Besides the fact that it is mandatory, according to the South African Nursing Council, for registered nurses (let alone tutors) to keep abreast of developments in nursing, and within the profession after registration (Directive, South African Nursing Council, 1979) the tutor has an added responsibility. To her is entrusted the education of the young neophyte in the

*Freely adapted from a paper read by Mellish at a symposium presented at the University of the Witwatersrand's Department of Continuing Medical Education.

profession, and it is her bounden duty to ensure that the student is guided in her learning, so that she is able to function as a competent practitioner of nursing. The newly registered nurse must be capable of exercising educated judgement, of planning and implementing nursing care, of teaching and guiding young students in her unit. She must also ensure that the best quality of nursing care that it is possible to give according to today's and even tomorrow's knowledge, and not according to what was thought to be correct only last year, is given.

There are some subjects in medical and in nursing education that alter very little. After all, the femur is the femur is the femur. It may change its name, but that is about all. To all other subjects upon which modern medical and nursing practice are based, new knowledge is added daily, even hourly. This knowledge can drastically alter the treatment given to a patient, which adds to the technological management skills required of nurses and which increases the psychological stresses on the patient. The registered nurse thus also needs psychological skills.

Many forms of treatment which I was taught in my training, which was of course some time ago, would be ridiculed today. Can you imagine treating a badly shocked patient, with already disturbed electrolyte balance because of fluid loss, by putting him under a huge metal cradle, filled with electric light bulbs, in order to raise his body temperature? After all, a cold clammy skin was and still is a symptom of shock, so it seemed logical to warm him up! What one did to his physiological processes by almost 'cooking' him and thus increasing his fluid loss is unthinkable today, and yet 35 years ago this was standard practice for the treatment of all forms of shock! This may be a somewhat drastic example to use, but it illustrates the point.

Before expanding further on the methods which can be used for and the role of the authorities in providing in-service education opportunities for tutors, it would be as well to make one or two general points.

It is known that we live in an era of tutor shortages, and that the number of candidates for tutor training is alarmingly small. Perhaps it would be as well to examine some of the frustrations of tutors, and also to consider how much of it is due to their own practices.

18.3.1 The functions of the nurse-tutor

These functions are the following:
(a) To guide the learning of students
(b) To help produce competent, knowledgeable, independent, thinking practitioners of nursing, who are capable of:
- exercising educated judgement in the care of patients

- planning, implementing and evaluating that care
- carrying out their independent functions as befits a professional person
- forming an important part of the multidisciplinary team that makes up the modern practice of nursing
- giving psychological as well as physical support to their patients
- guiding the students and enrolled personnel under the jurisdiction towards the giving of that care

(c) To maintain her own professional competence in the clinical as well as the theoretical field

(d) To act as a role model for the student, who may one day also consider joining the tutor ranks

(e) To promote the professional image of the nurse among students and public alike

(f) To continue self-development in her chosen profession.

You will notice that nowhere is mentioned the aspect of *getting students through examinations*. Passing of examinations, before licensure to practise is a characteristic of professionalism, in nursing no less that in other professions, but teaching *only* for students to pass examinations is a sterile exercise which, to quote Shakespeare, is *not* 'a consummation devoutly to be wished', (Hamlet, act 3, scene 1) but rather one *devoutly* to be *deplored*.

It is possible to teach people, of not even very high intelligence, to quote, parrot-fashion, subject-matter they have learnt by heart. Teaching by using old examination papers and working out model answers which students copy or learn by heart, may produce passes at examinations, but it does not produce *good registered nurses*.

In 16 years as an examiner with the South African Nursing Council, I saw many examples of such teaching, where large numbers of students would reproduce stereotyped answers almost word for word! They also sometimes landed in difficulties because the question was phrased differently from that for which the answer had been worked out, and therefore their answer was not valid.

It is hoped that such sterile, futile so-called 'teaching' no longer exists. Tutors do tend to be measured against the results their students obtain in examinations, while little thought is given to the quality of material with which they have to work. There is also often complete disregard for the end product of nursing education and the quality of care which the patient will receive from people taught in this way. The whole purpose of nursing education is negated by such methods and attitudes.

Many tutors become frustrated when they are forced to work under such a system, unable to be individual and creative in their teaching, and in some cases actually rigidly regulated to the exact number of periods which must be devoted to a small segment of the syllabus, without regard for student abilities and needs. In their university courses student tutors are taught various teaching methods, are enthusiastic and interested, and are ready to try out new ideas, only to be obstructed by the system. Many of them ultimately seek other posts, and are therefore lost to teaching and will continue their in-service education in more rewarding areas. Potential student tutors are also discouraged because they learn of this and the reasons why their friends give up teaching. This contributes to the continuing shortage of tutors.

Having looked at functions of the tutor, the reasons for the need for in-service education are almost self-evident, but they should be pointed out again.

(a) *To guide the learning of students:* If her own learning is rusty and out of date, then the tutor cannot fulfil this function.

(b) *To maintain her own professional competence in the clinical as well as the theoretical field:* This means moving out of the class-room and into the units to see for herself what is new and to gain proficiency in new skills as well as maintaining those already gained.

(c) *To help produce the competent, knowledgeable, independent, thinking practitioner of nursing* who is capable of exercising educated judgement in the care of patients, and planning, implementing and evaluating that care: If the tutor is out of date, or out of touch with current practice, she also cannot do this.

(d) *Continuing self-development in her chosen profession:* Florence Nightingale said that to stand still was to go backwards. Therefore, the tutor who imagines that when she receives her diploma, she knows it all, is like a motor car which is put into reverse at the top of a hill and careers backwards out of control until it lands as a wreck at the bottom of the hill.

Lancaster (1972: 72) says:

> It would seem that opportunities to continue and to extend their professional education is as important for nurse teachers as for other grades of nursing staff. Subject content, teaching methods and curriculum development are areas in which all teachers require periodic refreshment . . .
>
> Unless educational standards are maintained at a high level it would seem that there must inevitably be a decline in the standard of nursing practice. Trained nurse teachers should be better equipped than many other nurses to keep themselves updated, in fact they owe it to their students to do so.
>
> Nevertheless, the sheer pressure of coping with frequently changing classes in a 'block' system, may leave them little time for personal reading and research. They need encouragement in the form of arranged 'inservice' courses, and other 'inservice' activities to stimulate their self-

learning activities. It is unfortunately true that there are 'sister-tutors' to be found, and that far too frequently, who have used the same methods and presented the same material for the past 10 – 15 years. These old 'sister-tutors' often stifle the enthusiasm and readiness for change that teaching courses attempt to engender in their products.

Recently qualified nurse teachers become disheartened, and, in their turn stagnate.

Nurse teachers are not the only category of teacher that fall prey to this type of teaching practice, or rather lack of activity. Teachers, who need to be initiators of change, are so often the brake on others who are trying to prepare the up and coming neophytes to deal with and to prevent *Future shock*.

Let me hasten to assure you that I know that there is a shortage of tutors, that classes are too large, that marking of tests and the like leaves little time for preparation, that many tutors are grossly overworked and that, with constantly changing blocks, there is little time for professional refreshment.

This is something which we have to live with at the moment, but there are nevertheless many tutors who still find time, despite their heavy loads to take part-time post-basic courses at residential universities, or to study for degrees and diplomas through Unisa.

WHERE THERE IS A WILL THERE IS A WAY – BUT WHAT WAY?

Let us now examine some of the opportunities available for in-service education.

18.3.2 Strategies for in-service education for tutors

A great deal of in-service education is or can be done on a relatively informal basis such as:

- Informal discussions with colleagues over a cup of coffee or a meal, which are often valuable contributions to individual in-service education, even if they do no more than make one of the group realise that she was unsure of what was being discussed, and either make her ask a question or look up the facts in a reference book
- By regular reading of professional literature
- By the formation of journal clubs in colleges where tutors read up on specific topics in professional journals, and then meet regularly to inform one another in summarised form of anything new they have read on the specific subject
- By visiting wards and units with or without students to keep in touch with the reality of a hospital unit as well as to learn the latest techniques used in the practical situation

- By organising regular film shows on modern methods or new techniques
- By arranging for *experts* to lecture to tutors on a monthly basis on interesting aspects of their work or new developments in medicine and in nursing. Remember that there are *nurse experts* as well as medical ones and that paramedical experts are also available. Patient care is a multidisciplinary exercise and the contribution of knowledge by anyone who is part of a patient care team should be encouraged.

More formal and perhaps less easily arranged in-service strategies include attending symposia, workshops, short courses and conferences; use of self-learning modules prepared with the continuing in-service education of nurse-tutors in mind; and membership of special interest professional societies, either in the education field or in the clinical field. Tutors, after all, are teaching the theory of clinical nursing and their interest in these societies should be actively encouraged.

It is also important that part-time study be undertaken either at residential universities or by means of teletuition. Tutors within reach of residential universities could attend courses in subjects where they feel rusty.

18.3.3 The role of the authorities responsible for the provision of nursing education

Although the tutor has an individual, professional responsibility to keep up to date, the authorities for whom she works and whose students she teaches, also have responsibilities with regard to tutor in-service education.

They should provide learning resources such as all the professional journals, the most up-to-date library material, photocopying facilities and programmed, up-to-date instruction material prepared especially for tutors' needs.

Suitable reference material, which is readily available when needed, aids the informal or unstructured, even unplanned in-service education, which is as important as formal, structured, planned programmes and courses.

By readily available, I mean just that – of course there has to be some control, but access must be so simple and for such long periods of each day that tutors will really make use of such resources.

Where special technological apparatus is needed this should also be readily available.

A programme needing a tape-recorder and facilities for showing slides is of no use if they cannot be obtained easily, between classes or in the evenings if desired.

It should be made possible for all tutors to attend at least one short course or symposium every year. It would be quite impossible for all tutors to attend everything, as too many could not be released at the same time, but it should be obligatory for tutors attending special courses or symposia to report both verbally and in writing, to the other tutors in the college, on their return.

Special symposia or short courses should be arranged in various parts of the country so that as many people as possible can attend.

Tutors should be allowed sufficient time for study when following part-time courses.

We have thus seen that tutors need in-service education, that there are various methods by which it can be obtained, and that those that are responsible for nursing education also have a role to play in ensuring that tutors have the opportunities to keep up to date, to grow and develop professionally. However, the ultimate responsibility for maintaining professional competence and knowledge remains that of the tutor.

As a tutor myself of many years' standing, I still find it exciting to read new material, to try out new teaching methods, and to attempt to stimulate the young to life-long learning.

A few apt quotations to stimulate thought:

'By their fruits ye shall know them' (St Matthew VII:15)

Let the products of your teaching be the fruits by which you will be proud to be known.

'Nature that fram'd us of four elements . . .
Does teach us to have aspiring minds' (Marlowe)

May your minds be constantly aspiring towards new knowledge.

'Let knowledge grow from more to more' (Tennyson)

This can be achieved by in-service education.

Let no one say of you, because you have not kept up to date by in-service education of some form or other: 'Who is this that darkeneth counsel without knowledge?' (Job XXXVIII:2)

Let me also ask the question posed by Paracelsus:

'I am he that aspired to knowledge, and thou?'

It is hoped that the present shortage of student tutors will soon be resolved.

It is also hoped that despite present difficulties, tutors will continue to find teaching satisfying and fulfilling, and that no matter how difficult, they will not only make use of what in-service opportunities already exist, but will actually create new ones.

We dare not fail our students, for in so doing we are failing our patients, whose need for trained care is the reason for our existence.

Let us say to ourselves, and to others who doubt the future:

But screw your courage
To the sticking-place
And we'll not fail (Shakespeare: Macbeth, act 1, scene 7).

19 Research and the nurse-educator

Whenever the word 'research' is mentioned to most nurses, a shutter seems to come down in their minds which either prevents them from getting on with much-needed research, or from realising that they are actually engaged in some form of research.

It is essential that those who are to be engaged in nursing education are clear on what research is all about, are able to teach students the fundamentals of research techniques, and are able to help and guide students in research projects, as well as becoming involved in their own research into nursing education.

19.1 WHAT IS RESEARCH?

The word 'research' is derived from the Latin *circare* (= to go about) via the French *chercher* (= to try to find, to seek) and *re* (= again).

It thus means a careful search for, or systematic examination of knowledge, finding reasons for occurrences, giving answers to problems.

Research, therefore, requires a scientific approach, an enquiring mind, and a subject to investigate.

Francis Bacon very aptly stated that 'Crafty men condemn studies and principles thereof. Simple men admire them, and wise men use them.'

In the scientific approach, the scientific method of investigation is used. This method consists of several steps:

19.1.1 Definition of the problem

This requires clear definition of concepts and terms, delineations of the area or boundaries of the subject to be researched, and its limitations in *clear, unambiguous terms,* so that anyone who reads it cannot misunderstand what is being investigated, the extent of the investigation, and its purpose.

19.1.2 Statement of hypothesis

A hypothesis is a tentative answer to the problem. The researcher considers the problem from all angles, studies the question posed by the problem, and forms an idea of what he thinks might be the answer to the problem. This is then clearly stated, and the research process of finding out whether or not his hypothesis is correct, is under way.

The hypothesis, or tentative solution, provides a definite starting or focal point, helps the researcher to decide on the way he will go about seeking an answer, states the facts which are applicable, and upon which he must concentrate, and cuts out those which are not relevant to the enquiry.

A researcher must keep an open mind and be as ready to accept a negative finding, which shows his hypothesis to be incorrect, as he is to accept a positive finding.

19.1.3 Orientation

No proper investigation of a problem can occur unless those concerned with the study have a wide background knowledge of the subject. One cannot expect an expert in music to be able to investigate intelligently the occurrence and causes of cross-infection in a hospital ward, about which he knows absolutely nothing. The researcher must of necessity have studied his subject thoroughly. This is why a nurse should do nursing research, and a nurse–educator research in nursing education. Despite his original background, it is necessary for every researcher to read widely and selectively on the subject to be researched, so that the problem can be studied objectively, and can be seen in broad context.

It is also of no use to study background material which reflects only one school of thought. It is essential to seek various viewpoints so that the actual research is conducted without bias.

19.1.4 Collection of data

In order to investigate a problem, to answer a question or to test any hypothesis, facts must be collected. This is done in many ways. *Observations,* both visual and auditory, may be made by the researcher or properly briefed field workers, and recorded in a planned format. In the field of natural sciences especially, *controlled experiments* may be conducted, and the results noted down.

Interviews, both structured and unstructured, may be undertaken and the findings written down. Many of the recorded findings will be coloured by subjective observations, and subjective answers will always influence recording. An interviewer should note down whether an interviewee exhibits marked bias in answering questions. Interviews are very valuable in research, but they must be undertaken with care and insight.

Case studies can be undertaken with specific observations being made and recorded.

Carefully compiled *questionnaires,* or other research instruments, can be devised and presented to the target population.

The method to be used for the accumulation of data, must be carefully considered, and must be relevant to the problem being researched. The method/s selected must be tested in pilot studies, and adjusted as needed. It must be the medium judged most likely to render the information best suited to helping to test the hypothesis, and thus contribute towards a solution of the problem.

Several techniques may be used to investigate one problem, and to collect data relating to it. Some aspects may be investigated more thoroughly by one method, and some by another. What is important is the collection of reliable, accurate, objective data.

19.1.5 Classification and analysis of collected data

This is a vital aspect of the whole research process, as a mass of unclassified information, which cannot be systematically analysed is of no value to anybody.

The data *must* be organised in a systematic, meaningful manner so that it can be studied carefully, the important facts be distinguished and used to determine whether or not the hypothesis was correct. The method to be used for analysing findings must be carefully considered when the research instrument is decided upon and tested.

19.1.6 Interpretation of the data

Once the data has been classified, systematised, and analysed, it must be carefully studied and interpreted, so that valid conclusions are arrived at, which either reject or confirm the hypothesis.

As this chapter is not intended to do more than introduce the subject of research to the nurse-educator student, and to stimulate her interest in the subject, further details are not given. There are many excellent reference books available to those who seriously wish to tackle research.

Nurses are constantly involved in making observations, drawing inferences from these, and coming to conclusions upon which they act. It is part of the life-world of nursing to make judgements and act upon them.

In both scientific experiments and day-to-day occurrences, observations are made and conclusions drawn. The differences between the observations of a scientist, and those of a layman, is that in scientific activity, the onus is on the scientist to draw his conclusions so that the logic of his reasoning is clear for all to see. 'Common sense' conclusions have no place in the scientific method, for they are based on value judgements and unsubstantiated beliefs, and not on carefully analysed observations of patients and their symptoms, of changes in condition, of response to treatment and of the behaviour patterns of those who receive nursing care.

It should not be difficult for the nurse to take part in *organised* research, or to initiate it, for it is almost a way of life, a part of her normal working life.

19.2 TYPES OF RESEARCH

By the very nature of things any form of systematic enquiry will have different forms of approach, with often more than one method being used in investigating a problem. The most common forms of research being used are the following:

19.2.1 Historical research

This involves looking into the past, finding and studying documents, reports, archive material, Acts of Parliament, Hansard reports, letters, and other primary material, as well as a study of secondary material such as comments upon, and summaries and evidence of effects which legislation, for example, has made on the population. The researcher collects all her information, analyses it, and relates it to the study which she is undertaking. An example of historical research is to be found in the doctoral thesis of Professor C Searle (1965).

19.2.2 Empirical research

This is the collection of material relevant to the problem being investigated, from the 'real' world. In other words research is undertaken into for example nursing problems or phenomena, the manner in which nursing care can be improved, the effectiveness of new forms of wound care, the reasons for student wastage, criteria for student selection, etc. The facts are to be found in the actual work situation or the life-world of the nurse. Empirical research relies on what *is,* in the here and now.

19.2.3 Descriptive research

This is simply the description of a situation by means of the scientific method. The terms used must be precisely defined, accurate documentation is essential, and it may be necessary to draw up special forms for this, to ensure collection of all the data for complete description. Precise measurements must be made where these are appropriate for the description to be complete.

The data collected by various descriptions of the course of treatment and progress of several patients suffering from similar conditions, could then be compared. The effect of prematurity on maternal bonding could be a subject for descriptive research. It is a type of research that requires time, great care and patience. Results cannot be obtained quickly, but worthwhile findings can be obtained. A five-year study of the career patterns of registered nurses after qualification is another type of descriptive research that might be undertaken.

19.2.4 Experimental research

This form of research is the most difficult to apply in nursing as one is dealing with people, and their health needs come before any research plan. Experimental research is based on the principle that there is a control group and an experimental group, and that the groups are as similar as possible in all respects, such as age, sex, health status, and socio-economic status.

The experimental group then receives some form of input, such as a different form of treatment, a new type of bed, wound protection, or any other variable, which the control group does not receive.

It is an extremely difficult form of research to undertake. To find comparable groups and maintain them as such, that is holding the variables constant, can be almost impossible. While it is possible to undertake it, it can only be done with the greatest care by the most experienced researchers, and with due consideration for the specific patients involved. One could also hardly jeopardise student qualification by experimenting too drastically with teaching methods. Nevertheless, it is a field for experimental research within reasonable limits.

19.2.5 Action research

This is similar to experimental research, with the researcher investigating a local problem, and evaluating the effect of specific changes in treatment on people who are being cared for in a unit. It is also related to descriptive research. Investigating skin care of paraplegic patients is an example of action research. It differs from experimental research in that the researcher does not try to keep anything constant, but allows changes according to the needs or reactions of patients. A scientifically organised description of the results of actions taken are prepared, which could conceivably give pointers towards handling this type of nursing care problem.

19.2.6 Philosophical research

This type of research studies logic and reason attaching to words and their meaning as they are used in nursing practice. It endeavours to study concepts, ideas, values and norms through the application of the academic discipline of philosophy, and in so doing to bring about greater understanding of the art and science of nursing.

A topic for this type of research could be, 'What is meant by "quality nursing care", and how can it be assessed?'

Many of the terms and concepts used glibly in the teaching of the ethos of nursing could bear scientific research and clarification by means of philosophical research. (According to *The Concise Oxford Dictionary*, philosophy is 'Love of wisdom or knowledge, especially that which deals with the ultimate reality, or with the most general cause and principles of things'.)

19.3 SOME FUNDAMENTALS REGARDING RESEARCH IN NURSING

In any form of research there are fundamental considerations which must be borne in mind. They apply even more stringently in nursing than in some other fields, because the main consideration must be the welfare of the patient or client, whose health needs are the nurse's responsibility, and for whose nursing care she is individually accountable.

In nursing education the nurse-educator is accountable for the education of the student, and thus research planned in this field, although less difficult, must always adhere to the ethical standards required from all researchers.

These standards may be summarised as follows:

19.3.1 Valid aim and purpose

Research in nursing aims at adding to available knowledge, and at contributing to the common good. The search for methods to improve patient care, and to avoid student wastage could contribute to knowledge and thus to the common good, and are therefore *valid* research projects.

19.3.2 Consideration of patients and personnel

While undertaking research, care should be taken that unnecessary discomfort, hazards and disturbances or difficulties to patients be avoided, and consideration duly given to problems of personnel and difficulties which research might entail. Apart from paying special attention to the welfare of the patient, no research project which entails extra efforts from the staff will succeed unless their full co-operation is obtained, and as many inconveniences as possible are eliminated.

19.3.3 Confidentiality and anonymity

Unless patients and staff alike can be assured that they will not be identified in their responses, and authorities are assured that all matters will be handled in the strictest confidence and that anonymity will be preserved, they can quite legitimately refuse to be part of research. Research is not done to find fault or to point out a specific person's weaknesses, but to add knowledge for the common good. No one should be used for any form of research without his consent, and authorities responsible for services must always be approached before research is done in that field. A research report may not include names of participants or any other label by which it may be possible to identify them, unless their permission for such identification is obtained beforehand. This is rarely necessary.

19.3.4 The researcher's capabilities, attitudes and qualifications

By reason of their temperament, lack of insight, and lack of skill in research techniques, some people are not sufficiently competent to do research. Therefore the person to do research, should be selected with care.

19.3.5 Use of research findings

No research should be allowed unless the aim and purpose thereof have been clearly defined, and unless the use to which the findings are to be put, is reasonable and ethical. Of course much research is carried out on behalf of, or by authorities themselves. Research findings should be formulated carefully, and therefore expert guidance is necessary. Findings should be put together in an organised whole and be made available, even if only on a limited scale, to anyone interested. Research for the sake of research and not for practical use by nurses, has little place in nursing.

19.4 RESEARCH TECHNIQUES

Some of these have already been mentioned. Those commonly in use are the following (for further information the nurse-educator should consult the appropriate literature): interviews – structured, semi-structured and unstructured; questionnaires and schedules; analysis of reports, statistics, Acts, etc; literature study; use of resource persons; case-study data; and observations.

Such matters as pilot studies, random and other forms of sampling, variables, probabilities, research instruments and statistical significance should all be studied and understood before research projects are undertaken.

19.5 AREAS OF RESEARCH IN NURSING

These are legion – especially in this country, where little has as yet been done. Such areas include:

- Absenteeism among students, registered nurses, enrolled nurses
- Student wastage

374

- Registered nurse wastage
- Selection criteria
- Nursing establishment needs in hospitals
- Job descriptions
- Various forms of improvement in patient care
- Nursing care in specialist areas
- Nurse-patient interaction
- Student nurse-registered nurse interaction
- Recording methods
- Patient fears and anxieties in a variety of situations
- Methods of preparation of various categories of nurses
- Image of the nurse
- Needs of specific groups of nurses
- Care of terminally ill patients
- Manpower utilisation in hospitals
- Cost control studies
- Career patterns in nursing
- Effects of technology on the nurse and patient
- Centralisation of services
- Danger of depersonalisation of the patient
- Teaching methods and technology
- Clinical teaching
- Registered nurses – are they nursing or supervising?

The role of the nurse-educator in this field is to read more about research, understand the methodology, be able to read research reports with understanding, and to encourage her students to meaningful participation in research projects, and to eventual initiation into such activities by developing in the student an active enquiring mind which will stimulate her to life-long learning. Research will then get off the ground.

Bibliography

A Books

Baly, ME. 1973. *Nursing and social change*. London: Heinemann.

Byge, ML. 1964. *Learning theories for teachers*. New York: Harper & Row.

Bloom, BS. 1956. *Taxonomy of educational objectives*. New York: McKay.

Chambers. 1901. *Chambers Twentieth Century Dictionary*. London: Chambers of London.

Clark, C. 1978. *Classroom skills for nurse educators*. New York: Springer.

Consolidated Book Publishers. 1969. *Websters Encyclopaedia Dictionary*. Chicago: Consolidated Book Publishers.

Dance, FEX. 1970. *Communication in organisations*. Porter & Roberts.

Fisher, EE. 1977. *Psychology for nurses*. Cape Town: Juta.

Gagné, RM. 1970. *The conditions of learning*. London: Holt, Reinhart & Winston.

Guilbert, JJ. 1977. *Educational handbook for health personnel*. Geneva: World Health Organisation.

Gunter, CFG. 1977. *Aspects of educational theory*. Stellenbosch: University Publishers and Booksellers.

Heidgerken, L. 1965. *Teaching and learning in schools of nursing*. London: Pitman.

Highet, G. 1950. *The art of teaching*. London: Metheun.

Huckaby, LMD. 1980. *Conditions of learning and instruction in nursing*. St Louis: Mosby.

Hughs, AG & Hughes, EH. 1959. *Learning and teaching*. London: Longman & Green.

Hyman, RT. 1974. *Ways of teaching*. 2nd ed. Philadelphia, London, Toronto: Lippincott.

ICN. 1952. *The basic education of the professional nurse*. London: ICN.

James, DE. 1975. *A guide for teachers of nurses*. Oxford: Blackwell Scientific.

Kimble, GA & Garmenzy, N. 1963. *Principles of general psychology*. 2nd ed. London: Ronald.

Knowles, M. 1971. *The practice of adult education*. New York: Associated Press.

Lancaster, A. 1972. *Nurse teachers*. London: Churchill Livingstone.

Lyman, K. 1961. *Basic nursing education programmes, a guide to their planning*. Geneva: WHO.

Mellish, JM. 1978. *Theory and method of inservice education.* Pretoria: SANA.

Mellish, JM. 1980. *Unit teaching and administration.* Pretoria: Butterworths.

Mellish, JM. & Johnston, SU. 1986. *Evaluation in clinical nursing.* Durban: Butterworths.

Miller, H. 1964. *Teaching and learning in adult education.* New York: MacMillan.

Munn, NL. 1961. *Psychology, the fundamentals of human development.* London: Harrap.

Odorne, GS. 1970. *Training by objectives.* London: MacMillan.

Oxford University Press. 1951. *The Concise Oxford Dictionary.* 4th ed. Oxford: Oxford University Press.

Oxford University Press. 1966. *The Shorter Oxford Dictionary.* Oxford: Oxford University Press.

Rautenbach, C. 1981. *A definition of the role and function of various categories of nursing personnel in the Republic of South Africa and an analysis of the effectiveness of the preparation of nursing practitioners to fulfil these functions.* Unpublished doctoral thesis. University of Port Elizabeth.

Reader's Digest. 1968. *Use the right word – a guide to modern synonyms.* Reader's Digest.

Royal College of Nursing and National Council for Nurses of the United Kingdom. 1964. A Reform of Nursing Education. *Platt Report,* London: RCN & National Council for Nurses of the United Kingdom.

Royal College of Nursing. 1977. *A background to nursing in the EEC.* London: RCN.

Schweer, JE. 1972. *Creative teaching in clinical nursing.* St Louis: Mosby.

Searle, C. 1965. *The history of the development of nursing in South Africa, 1652-1960. (A socio-historical survey).* Pretoria: SANA.

Searle, C. 1975. *Some aspects of nursing education.* Pretoria: SANA.

Searle, C. 1979. *Instructa '78.* Durban: Butterworths.

Searle, C. 1980a. Credo. In *Unisa Guide NUE 003/1.* Pretoria: Unisa.

Searle, C. 1980b. *Unisa Guide NUE 001/1.* Pretoria: Unisa.

Searle, C. 1980c. *Unisa Guide NURED 1/2.* Pretoria: Unisa.

Searle, C. 1980d. Exposition of independent and dependent functions of the nurse. In *Unisa Guide NUE 003/1.* Pretoria: Unisa.

Searle, C. 1986. *Professional Practice, A South African Nursing Perspective.* Durban: Butterworths.

Tracey, WR. 1971. *Designing training and development systems.* American Management Association.

Waldren, A. 1974. Educational strategies for the health professions. In *Public Health Paper 61.* Geneva: World Health Organisation.

Yura, H. & Walsh, MB. 1973. *The nursing process.* New York: Appleton-Century-Crofts.

B Acts, Ordinances, Regulations

Cape (Province). Ordinances, etc. *Hospital Ordinance,* no 12 of 1948.

South Africa (Republic). Laws, statutes, etc. *The Health Act.* 1977 (Act 63 of 1977). Pretoria: Government Printer.

377

South African Nursing Association. *Statement of view of the Board regarding supernumerary status of student nurses.* Pretoria: The Association nd.

South African Nursing Council. 1981. Directives. *Post-registration courses,* Pretoria: The South African Nursing Council.

South African Nursing Council. 1978. *Regulations.* Pretoria: South African Nursing Council. 10 March, nos 480, 481, 482.

Transvaal (Province). 1958. Ordinances etc. *Hospital Ordinance,* no 14 of 1958.

World Health Organisation. 1956. *Statement on student status.* Geneva: WHO.
1966. *Report of the Expert Committee on Nursing.* Geneva: WHO.

C Articles

Goldsmid, B & Goldsmid, MI. 1973. Modular instruction in higher education. *Journal of Higher Education,* vol 3.

Quinn, S. 1968. Nursing in the Soviet Union. *International Nursing Review,* vol 15, no 1.

Rothenburg, A. 1978. Psychological tests in selection of students to schools of nursing in Israel. *Curationis,* September.

Sheahan, J. 1979. Measurement in Education. *Journal of Advanced Nursing Education,* no 4.

Shore, BM. 1973. Strategies for the implementation of modular instruction and their application in university education. *Journal of Higher Education,* vol 44.

Yearwood-Grazette, HS. 1978. An Anatomy of Communication. *Nursing Times,* 12 October.

Index

379